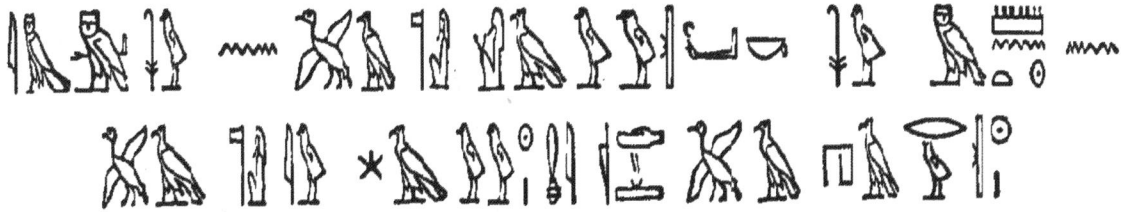

*Amma su en Pa Neter sauu - k su emment en
Pa Neter au tuanu ma qeti pa haru*

"Give thyself to God, keep thou thyself daily for God;
and let tomorrow be as today."

*A Guide for Kamitan Initiates: How to Start
Practicing Shetaut Neter (Kemetic Spirituality,
Ancient Egyptian Religion) and Smai Tawi
(Egyptian Yoga)*

INITIATION INTO EGYPTIAN YOGA
The Secrets of Sheti:

Sheti (Shedi): Spiritual discipline or program, to go deeply into the mysteries, to study the mystery teachings and literature profoundly, to penetrate the mysteries.

The Personal Daily Program of Prayers, Exercises and Meditations of Shetaut Neter

For New Initiates

Sixth Edition Expanded

Cruzian Mystic Books
Sema Yoga
P.O.Box 570459
Miami, Florida, 33257
(305) 378-6253 Fax: (305) 378-6253

First U.S. edition 1996
Second edition 1997 By Reginald Muata Ashby
Fourth edition 2001 By Reginald Muata Ashby
Fifth edition 2002 By Reginald Muata Ashby
Sixth edition 2005 By Reginald Muata Ashby

The author is available for group lectures and individual counseling. For further information contact the publisher.

Ashby, Muata
Initiation Into Egyptian Yoga. ISBN: 1-884564-02-X

Library of Congress Cataloging in Publication Data

1Yoga Philosophy, 2 Egyptian Philosophy 3 African Mythology 4 Meditation, 5 Self Help.

Edited by Karen "Dja" Clarke-Ashby and Galina Clarke

Cover painting and design by Muata

Also by the same author:

Egyptian Yoga: The Philosophy of Enlightenment
Egyptian Proverbs: TemTTchaas, Mystical Wisdom Teachings and Meditations
Initiation Into Egyptian Yoga: The Secrets of Sheti
The Egyptian Yoga Exercise Workout Book
The Egyptian Yoga Exercise Workout Video

For a complete listing
of current books and tapes
from see the back section of the book.

For a complete listing of titles send for the free
Egyptian Yoga Catalog.

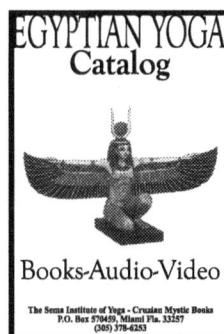

EGYPTIAN YOGA
Catalog

Books-Audio-Video

The Sema Institute of Yoga - Cruzian Mystic Books
P.O. Box 570459, Miami Fla. 33257
(305) 378-6253

DEDICATION

Dua!
(Adorations!)

I want to also express my undying appreciation to my Spiritual Preceptors, whose illuminating teaching has allowed me to peer into the depths of world myths, ancient lore, Yoga and mystical philosophy in order to bring out the beauty and glory of the Divine.

Swami Jyotirmayananda,
Dr. Joseph Campbell,
Swami Satchidananda,
Sage Ptahotep,
Sage Ani,
Sage Amenemope,
Sage Vasistha

and Lady Rekhat,
who is the embodiment of wisdom, the Supreme initiator of all Sages,

and to Vijaya, who edited this work and made it possible
through her love and devotion to the teaching.

THE SEMA INSTITUTE AND TEMPLE OF SHETAUT NETER

Sema Institute of Yoga

Sema (𓊃) is an Ancient Egyptian word and symbol meaning union. The Sema Institute is dedicated to the propagation of the universal teachings of spiritual evolution which relate to the union of humanity and the union of all things within the universe. It is an organization that recognizes the unifying principles in all spiritual and religious systems of evolution throughout the world. Our primary goals are to provide the wisdom of ancient spiritual teachings from the Neterian Culture of Ancient Africa in books, courses and other forms of communication. The Institute is open to all who believe in the principles of peace, non-violence and spiritual emancipation regardless of sex, race, or creed. The Sema Institute is recognized by the United States of America Internal Revenue Service as a Nonprofit Spiritual Organization with 501(C3) status. All donations to the Sema Institute are tax deductible.

<u>The Sema Institute and Temple of Shetaut Neter is dedicated to:</u>

✓ **The dissemination of Neterian Wisdom (Sema and Shetaut Neter) in books,**
✓ **Neterianism is the modern day reference to Shetaut Neter (Ancient Egyptian Religion),**
✓ **Promoting the practice of Shetaut Neter Religion**
✓ **Training Neterian Aspirants,**
✓ **Promoting World Peace, human dignity and equality between cultures, genders and the care of the environment.**

AUTHOR SEBAI MUATA ASHBY Ph. D., D.D., P.C., Y.U.

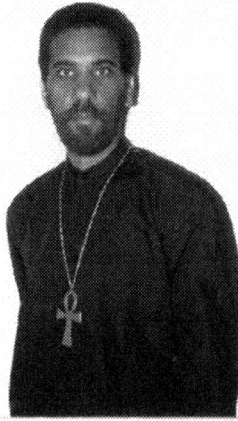

Sebai Muata Ashby was born in New York City but grew up in the Caribbean. Displaying an early interest in ancient civilizations and the Humanities, he began to study these subjects while in college but put these aside to work in the business world. After successfully running a business with his wife for several years they decided to pursue a deeper movement in life. Mr. Ashby began studies in the area of religion and philosophy and achieved doctorates in these areas while at the same time he began to collect his research into what would later become several books on the subject of the origins of Yoga Philosophy and practice in ancient Africa (Ancient Egypt) and also the origins of Christian Mysticism in Ancient Egypt. Muata Ashby discovered the vast philosophy of *Shetaut Neter* and *Sema* (Yoga mystical spirituality) practiced in ancient Africa and has written several book on this subject, detailing its history and practice for modern times. Muata Ashby also discovered the keys to understand the mystical code of the main traditions of Ancient Kamitan (Egyptian/African religion) known in ancient times as *Shetaut Neter*.

Muata Ashby holds a Doctor of Philosophy Degree in World Religion and Myth, focusing on African and Indian Religion, and a Doctor of Divinity Degree in Holistic Healing. He is also a Pastoral Counselor and Teacher of Yoga Philosophy and Discipline. Dr. Ashby received his Doctor of Divinity Degree from and is an adjunct faculty member of the American Institute of Holistic Theology and the Florida International University. Dr. Ashby is a certification as a PREP Relationship Counselor. Dr. Ashby has been an independent researcher and practitioner of Egyptian, Indian and Chinese Yoga and psychology as well as Christian Mysticism. Dr. Ashby has engaged in Post Graduate research in Yoga at the Yoga Research Foundation. He has extensively studied mystical religious traditions from around the world and is an accomplished lecturer, artist, poet, screenwriter, playwright and author of over 30 books on yoga and spiritual philosophy. He is an Ordained Minister and Spiritual Counselor and also the founder the Sema Institute, a non-profit organization dedicated to spreading the wisdom of Yoga and the Ancient Egyptian mystical traditions.

Dr. Muata Ashby has dedicated his life to educating all those interested in the mystical teachings of Yoga philosophy from Ancient Egypt. He conducts classes in Miami Florida on all aspects of Yoga wisdom and lifestyle.

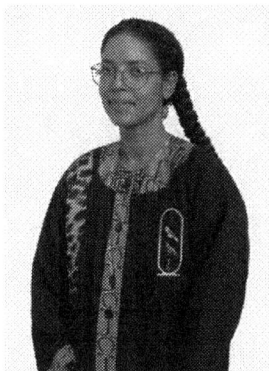

Hemit Dja Un Nefert Ashby, "Dja" is the spiritual partner of Dr. Muata Ashby. Seba Dja) was born in Guyana, South America, a heritage including African, Native American and European cultures. In 1975 her family moved to the United States. She is a Kamitan (Ancient Egyprian) priestess, initiate of the Temple Shetaut Neter-Aset (Egyptian Mysteries), Sema Tawi-Egyptian Yoga, and an independent researcher, practitioner and teacher of Sema (Smai) Tawi (Kamitan) and Indian Integral Yoga Systems, a Doctor of Veterinary Medicine, a Pastoral Spiritual Counselor, a Pastoral Health and Nutrition Counselor, and a Sema (Smai) Tawi Lifestyle Consultant." Dr. Ashby has engaged in post-graduate research in advanced Jnana, Bhakti, Karma, Raja and Kundalini Yogas at the Sema Institute of Yoga and Yoga Research Foundation, and has also worked extensively with her husband and spiritual partner, Dr. Muata Ashby, author of the Egyptian Yoga Book Series, editing many of these books, as well as studying, writing and lecturing in the area of Kamitan Yoga and Spirituality. She is a certified Tjef Neteru Sema Paut (Kamitan Yoga Exercise system) and Indian Hatha Yoga Exercise instructor, the Coordinator and Instructor for the Level 1 Teacher Certification Tjef Neteru Sema Training programs, and a teacher of health and stress management applications of the Yoga / Sema Tawi systems for modern society, based on the Kamitan and/or Indian yogic principles. Also, she is the co-author of "The Egyptian Yoga Exercise Workout Book," a contributing author for "The Kamitan Diet, Food for Body, Mind and Soul," author of the soon to be released, "Yoga Mystic Metaphors for Enlightenment."

Overture

WHAT IS SHETAUT NETER,

AND WHAT WILL YOU BE INITIATED INTO?

Long ago, before any other civilization on earth arose, the Ancient Kamitian (Egyptian) Sages developed an extensive system of mythology and psychology as a means to assist human beings to develop to their full potential. This philosophy was called *Smai Taui* or *Smai Heru Set* (Egyptian Yoga). Who am I and what is this universe? These are questions which have perplexed humanity since the beginning of civilization. However, the Sages of ancient Africa were able to discover the secrets of the universe and of the innermost nature of the human heart. This discovery allowed them to create a civilization which lasted for tens of thousands of years and it enabled the creation of the magnificent monuments (Sphinx, Great Pyramids and Temples, which stand to this day. Also, Ancient Egyptian religion influenced and continues to influence the religions of Africa and other world of today such as Christianity, Hinduism and Islam. So what does this mean for us today? Many people have visited Egypt and have studied the work of Egyptologists but how many have been transformed into higher minded, more content, more powerful human beings who can rise to the challenges of life and aspire to achieve material and spiritual success? Many people have read about and studied Ancient Egyptian mythology but how is it possible to gain a deeper understanding of the mystical principles and how is it possible to integrate them into one's life so as to transform oneself into a higher being as the texts describe? How is it possible to go beyond the limited understanding of religion and the philosophy of modern culture which have not brought peace and prosperity to the world? In order to Succeed in Shetaut Neter one must also practice the Sema Tawi (Yoga) disciplines. When one practices the disciplines of Sema Tawi in Shetaut Neter this is called *Shedy* or *"Studies and practices to penetrate the mysteries."* In order to become an effective practitioner of the mysteries one must be initiated into them, to be taught how to discover the higher Self and the path to immortality.

What is Initiation?

There are Three Major Levels of Neterian Initiation.

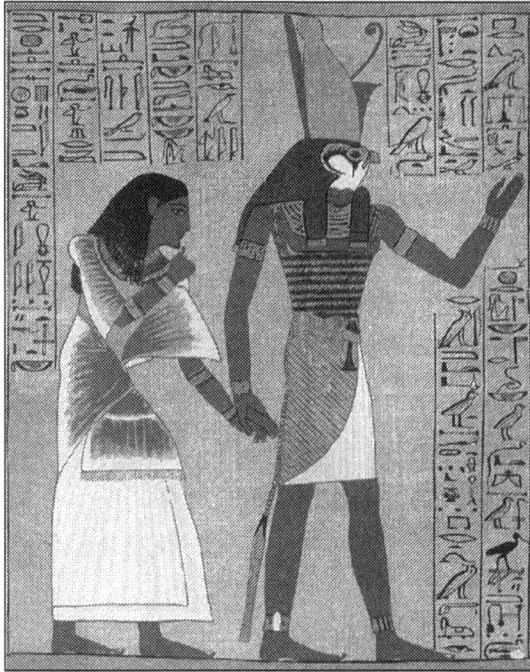

SHEMSU INITIATION

1– The first is the Shemsu Initiation. This is the neophyte level. Shemsu means follower, one who has adopted the path of Shetaut Neter and their religion, their personal spiritual path. There are varied levels of initiation into the temple. Birth is an initiation into life, which is presided over by parents. They provide a person their cultural name and general conditions for life. What a human being does with those conditions is up to them, through their actions. This is what makes human beings have the capacity to stand above nature. One of the ways of affirming your decision to move towards your chosen path is changing your cultural or ethnic name. At this level many neophytes choose a cultural name that reflects their Kamitan aspirations. Neophytes must learn the Great Truths of Shetaut Neter and the Neterian Creed.

For more on Shemsu see the EPILOG section of this book.

TEMPLE INITIATION

2-The second is the Temple Initiation– The Temple Initiation or Asar Initiation is for those who want to be temple level practitioners of the path of Shetaut Neter, engaging in intensive *Shedy* studies of the mysteries. At this level the aspirant formally receives the Temple Initiate name.

HEMU INITIATION

3-The Hemu Initiation or priesthood initiation is the level for those who want to seriously dedicate their lives to the path of Shetaut Neter and to teach it to other. The first level of priesthood is UNUT and is open to mature men and women.

Initiation is the ancient tradition of ritual and process of initiating your steps on the chosen spiritual path. It is a personal choice to enter into a spiritual tradition and relationship with a specific teaching and preceptor who will lead you to discover the nature of Self. It is a means to facilitate your ability to assimilate the teaching and it is a more powerful way to practice spirituality as opposed to studying on your own. Initiation strengthens your bonds to the teaching and the teacher and psycho-mythologically redirects your personality to become a proper vessel for the teaching.

NOTE: This book deals with the First Level of Initiation and Introduction to the Second Level.

The General Principles of Shetaut Neter Religion

(Teachings Presented in the Kamitan scriptures)

What We Believe and Uphold

1. The Purpose of Life is to Attain the Great Awakening-Enlightenment-Know thyself.
2. SHETAUT NETER enjoins the Shedy (spiritual investigation) as the highest endeavor of life.
3. SHETAUT NETER enjoins that it is the responsibility of every human being to promote order and truth, justice and non-violence.
4. SHETAUT NETER enjoins the performance of Selfless Service to family, community and humanity.
5. SHETAUT NETER enjoins the Protection of nature.
6. SHETAUT NETER enjoins the Protection of the weak and oppressed.
7. SHETAUT NETER enjoins the Caring for hungry.
8. SHETAUT NETER enjoins the Caring for homeless.
9. SHETAUT NETER enjoins the equality for all people, regardless of ethnicity, or religion.
10. SHETAUT NETER enjoins the equality between men and women.
11. SHETAUT NETER enjoins the justice for all.
12. SHETAUT NETER enjoins the sharing of resources equally.
13. SHETAUT NETER enjoins the protection and proper raising of children to be responsible adults who care for nature and other human beings.
14. SHETAUT NETER enjoins the movement towards balance and peace.

The Neterian Creed: What I Believe as a Neterian Follower

(based on the Scriptures and Traditions of Shetaut Neter)
By
Sebai Maa and Seba Dja Ashby

As a *Neterian,* I follow the Ancient African-Kamitan religious path of *Shetaut Neter*, which teaches about the mysteries of the Supreme Being, *Neberdjer*, the All Encompassing Divinity. I believe that from *Neberdjer* proceed all the *Neteru* (gods and goddesses), and all the worlds, and the entire universe. Since *Neberdjer* manifests as the *Neteru, Neberdjer* can be worshipped as a god or a goddess. I believe that there is only one Supreme Being, *Neberdjer*, and that the gods and goddesses are expressions of the One Supreme Being, *Neberdjer*. As a Neterian, I strive to come into harmony with the gods and goddesses, the *Neteru*, by developing within my personality the different virtuous and divine qualities they symbolize; this will lead me closer to *Neberdjer*. As a Neterian, I also believe that Supreme Being I call *Neberdjer* is the same Supreme Being that is worshiped by other religions under different names.

I believe that *Neberdjer* established all creation on *Maat,* righteousness, truth, and order, and that my actions, termed *Ari*, determine the quality of life I lead and experience. If I act with *Maat* (positive *Ari*) my path will be free of suffering and pain. When I forget *Maat* and act in an unrighteous manner (negative *Ari*), I invite suffering and pain into my life.

As a *Neterian* I believe when my body dies, my heart's actions will be examined against *Maat*. If it is found that I upheld *Maat* during my lifetime, I will have positive *Ari*, and my *Akhu* (spirit) will become one with *Neberdjer* for all eternity. This is called *Nehast,* the Spiritual Awakening-Enlightenment. If it is found that I acted with selfishness and greed, I will have negative *Ari,* and my *Ba* (soul) will suffer after death and then be reincarnated again to live in the world of time and space again. This is called *Uhemankh* (reincarnation).

As a *Neterian* I believe in the teaching of *Shemsu*, following the path of *Shetaut Neter,* by practicing the disciplines of *Shedy*, which include: Study of Wisdom teachings (*Rech-Ab*), Devotion to God (*Uashu*), Acting with Righteousness (*Maat*) and Meditation (*Uaa*). *Neberdjer* provided the *Shetitu,* the spiritual teaching that was written in *Medu Neter* (hieroglyphic scripture) so that the *Shemsu* (followers) might study the wisdom teaching of Shetaut Neter. Two most important *Neterian* scriptures are the *Pert M Hru* and the *Hessu Amun,* and the most important *Neterian* myth is the *Asarian* Resurrection.

By the practice of the disciplines of Shedy, I will discover the *Shetaut* (Mysteries) of life and become *Maakheru*, Pure of Heart. I will become one with God even before death, and I will discover supreme peace, abiding happiness and fulfillment of my life's purpose, and promote peace and harmony for the world.

INITIATION INTO EGYPTIAN YOGA

Table of Contents

Foreword

Amma su en Pa Neter! Give thyself to The Divine! What a fantastic notion. But what does it really mean? Many people want to give themselves to things in life. There is a universal human desire to give of oneself to something greater than oneself. This instinctive need is due to the feeling of imperfection or incompleteness within the heart. It manifests in many ways as a person evolves. Some give themselves to patriotism, others to filial relationships and others to selfish goals for personal gain, fame, fortune, power, etc. Do these things really bring happiness? How many people think about giving themselves to the Divine? Many spiritual philosophies include teachings about surrendering to the Divine and about sublimating the ego as a prominent part of their scriptures. However, do they show the benefits of giving oneself to spiritual life and the means give themselves to what is good, pure, true and beautiful in life? Why is it that most people give themselves to egoistic ways of life or to the pleasures of the life and then only think of spiritual matters when there is some adversity in life? Is there a better way of life which will allow a person to experience the joy of life and reduce the pain and sorrow?

In Ancient Egypt the leaders of society saw the need to lead life in such a way that one is able to discover the mystery of life. They called this discipline *Sheti*. Sheti is leading a spiritual life, a life that relates you to your spiritual roots and to the Supreme Being (Pa Neter). This kind of life is glorious because it allows a person to discover the true source of happiness and how to lead a rich and productive life. It leads a person to discover inner peace and spiritual enlightenment in the world as well as in the hear after. But what is this Sheti. Is it some mysterious way of life which occultist lead. Is it some long lost art spoken about by Sages of ancient times for people of ancient times? Sheti is the very essence of all spiritual traditions. It is the life of every spiritual tradition but how is Sheti to be practiced?

In modern times the word "Yoga" has become popular in society. However, most people think of Yoga as an exercise or as meditations to calm the mind. This is a very limited understanding. Yoga is a vast philosophy of spiritual life which encompasses several spiritual disciplines to aid a person in succeeding in the struggle of life and discovering their Higher Self. Therefore, Sheti is nothing more than Yoga disciplines which the Ancient Egyptians practiced many thousands of years ago. In this volume we will see how their teachings were adopted by Christians and Yogis in India and then we will begin to study the teachings of Sheti so that we may begin to spiritualize our lives. Thus we will concentrate our study on Egyptian Yoga, Indian Yoga and Christian Yoga. The relationship between these three spiritual philosophies will become evident. One important similarity is that they all used the symbol, ☥ , known as the *Ankh* of ancient Egypt.

So what is Yoga? The word "Yoga" is a Sanskrit term meaning to unite the individual with the cosmic. In Ancient Egypt the term "Smai" meant the same thing. The English terms have been used in certain parts of this book for ease of communication since the word "Yoga have received wide popularity in recent years. The disciplines of Yoga fall under five major categories. These are: *Yoga of Wisdom, Yoga of Devotional Love, Yoga of Meditation, Tantric Yoga* and *Yoga of Selfless-Righteous Action.* Within these categories there are subsidiary forms which are part of the main disciplines.

So the practice of any discipline that leads to oneness with the Supreme Consciousness can be called Yoga. If you study, rationalize and reflect upon the teachings, you are practicing *Yoga of Wisdom.* If you meditate upon the teachings and your Higher Self, you are practicing *Yoga of Meditation.* If you practice rituals which identify you with your spiritual nature, you are practicing *Yoga of Ritual Identification* (which is part of the Yoga of Wisdom and the Yoga of

Devotional Love of the Divine). If you develop your physical nature and psychic energy centers, you are practicing *Serpent Power* (*Kundalini or Uraeus*) *Yoga* (which is part of Tantric Yoga). If you practice living according to the teachings of ethical behavior and selflessness, you are practicing *Yoga of Action* (Maat) in daily life. If you practice turning your attention towards the Divine by developing love for the Divine, then it is called *Devotional Yoga* or *Yoga of Divine Love*. The practitioner of yoga is called a yogin (male practitioner) or yogini (female practitioner), and one who has attained the culmination of yoga (union with the Divine) is called a yogi. In this manner, yoga has been developed into many disciplines which may be used in an integral fashion to achieve the same goal: Enlightenment. Therefore, the aspirant should learn about all of the paths of yoga and choose those elements to concentrate on which best suit his/her personality and practice them all in an integral, balanced way.

All forms of spiritual practice are directed toward the goal of assisting every individual to discover the true essence of the universe both externally, in physical creation, and internally, within the human heart, as the very root of human consciousness. Thus, many terms are used to describe the attainment of the goal of spiritual knowledge and the eradication of spiritual ignorance. Some of these terms are: *Enlightenment, Resurrection, Salvation, The Kingdom of Heaven, Moksha or Liberation, Buddha Consciousness, One With The Tao, Self-realization, Know Thyself*, etc. Also, many names have been used to describe that transcendental essence: *God, Allah, Asar, Aset, Krishna, Buddha, The Higher Self, Supreme Being* and many others.

INTEGRAL YOGA

The personality of every human being is somewhat different from every other. However the Sages of Yoga have identified four basic factors which are common to all human personalities. These factors are: Emotion, Reason, Action and Will. This means that in order for a human being to evolve, all aspects of the personality must progress in an integral fashion. Therefore, four major forms of Yoga disciplines have evolved and each is specifically designed to promote a positive movement in one of the areas of personality. The Yoga of Devotional Love enhances and harnesses the emotional aspect in a human personality and directs it towards the Higher Self. The Yoga of Wisdom enhances and harnesses the reasoning aspect in a human personality and directs it towards the Higher Self. The Yoga of Action enhances and harnesses the movement and behavior aspect in a human personality and directs it towards the Higher Self. The Yoga of Meditation enhances and harnesses the willing aspect in a human personality and directs it towards the Higher Self.

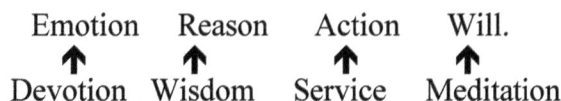

Emotion	Reason	Action	Will.
↑	↑	↑	↑
Devotion	Wisdom	Service	Meditation

Thus, Yoga is a discipline of spiritual living which transforms every aspect of personality in an integral fashion, leaving no aspect of a human being behind. This is important because an unbalanced movement will lead to frustration, more ignorance, more distraction and more illusions leading away from the Higher Self. For example, if a person develops the reasoning aspect of personality he or she may come to believe that they have discovered the Higher Self, however when it comes to dealing with some problem of life, such as the death of a loved one, they cannot control their emotions, or if they are tempted to do something unrighteous, such as smoking, they cannot control their actions and have no will power to resist. The vision of Integral Yoga is a lofty goal which every human being can achieve with the proper guidance, self-effort and repeated practice. There is a very simple philosophy behind Integral Yoga. During the course of the day you may find yourself doing various activities. Sometimes you will be quiet, at other times you will be busy at work, at other times you might be interacting with people, etc. Integral Yoga gives you the opportunity to practice yoga at all times. When you have quiet time you can practice meditation, when at work you can practice righteous action and selfless service, when you have leisure time you can study and reflect on the teachings and when you feel the sentiment of love for a person or object you like you can practice remembering the Divine Self who made it possible for you to experience the company of those personalities or the opportunity to acquire those objects. From a higher perspective you can practice reflecting on how the people and objects in creation are expressions of the Divine and this movement will lead you to a spontaneous and perpetual state of ecstasy, peace and bliss which are the hallmarks of spiritual enlightenment. The purpose of Integral Yoga is therefore to promote integration of the whole personality of a human being which will lead to complete spiritual enlightenment. Thus Integral Yoga should be understood as the most effective method to practice mystical spirituality.

The important point to remember is that all aspects of yoga can and should be used in an integral fashion to generate an efficient and harmonized spiritual movement in the practitioner. Therefore, while there may be an area of special emphasis, other elements are bound to become part of the yoga program as needed. For example, while a yogin may place emphasis on the Yoga of Wisdom, they may also practice Devotional Yoga and Meditation Yoga along with the wisdom studies. Further, it must be understood that as you practice one path of yoga, others will also develop automatically. For example, as you practice the Yoga of Wisdom your faith will increase or as you practice the Yoga of Devotion your wisdom will increase. If this movement does not occur your wisdom alone will by dry intellectualism or your faith alone will be blind faith. So when we speak of wisdom here we are referring to wisdom gained through experience or intuitional wisdom and not intellectual wisdom which is speculative. If you do not practice the teachings through the Yoga of Action, your wisdom and faith will be shallow because you have not experienced the truth of the teachings and allowed yourself the opportunity to test your knowledge and faith. If you do not have introspection and faith, your wisdom and actions you will externalized, agitated and distracted. Your spiritual realization will be insubstantial, weak and lacking stability. You will not be able to meet the challenges of life nor will you be able to discover true spiritual realization in this lifetime or even after death. Therefore, the integral path of yoga, with proper guidance, is the most secure method to achieve genuine spiritual enlightenment.

Isis is the Greek name for the Ancient Egyptian Goddess who was regarded as the very embodiment of wisdom. Her Ancient Egyptian name was Aset. The wisdom teachings in the temple of Aset were known as Shetaut Aset. We will concentrate on the wisdom teachings of the temple of Aset for our study on Sheti.

This book was created for those who, after reading *Egyptian Yoga: The Philosophy of Enlightenment*, wanted to embark on the spiritual life. This book contains the "nuts and bolts" of spiritual practice. It is written in such a way that a person may have an understanding of the essentials of spiritual life and thus be able to effectively begin the spiritual journey of life.

May you discover the Joy of Sheti!
Dr. Muata Abhaya Ashby 1997

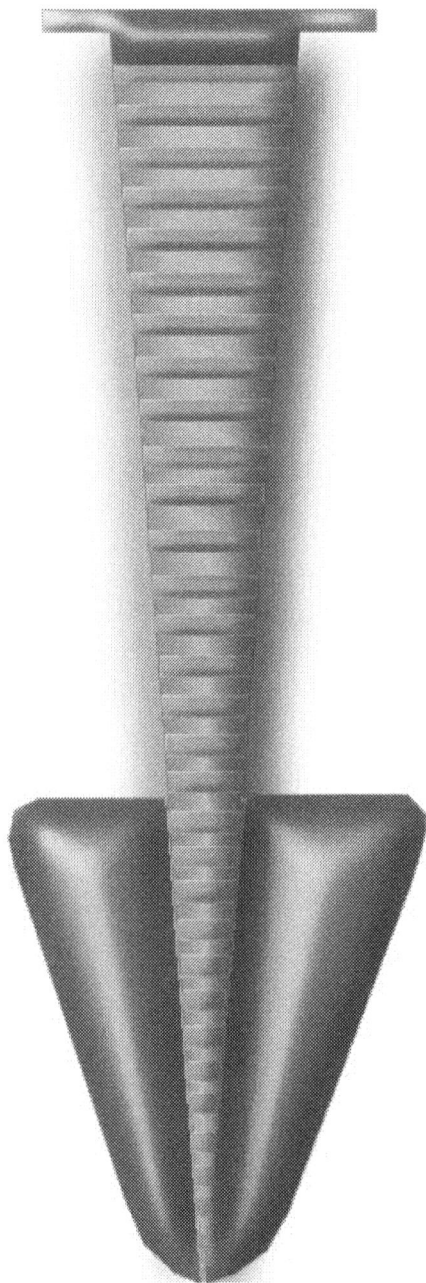

Sema

(Union)

PREFACE: A Brief History of Shetaut Neter

Early Beginnings: The First Religion

Ancient Egypt was the first and most ancient civilization to create a religious system that was complete with all three stages of religion, as well as an advanced spiritual philosophy of righteousness, called Maat Philosophy, that also had secular dimensions. Several temple systems were developed in Kamit; they were all related. The pre-Judaic/Islamic religions that the later Jewish and Muslim religions drew from in order to create their religions developed out of these, ironically enough, only to later repudiate the source from whence they originated. In any case, the Great Sphinx remains the oldest known religious monument in history that denotes high culture and civilization as well. Ancient Egypt and Nubia produced the oldest religious systems and their contact with the rest of the world led to the proliferation of advanced religion and spiritual philosophy. People who were practicing simple animism, shamanism, nature based religions and witchcraft were elevated to the level of not only understanding the nature of the Supreme Being, but also attaining salvation from the miseries of life through the effective discovery of that Transcendental being, not as an untouchable aloof Spirit, but as the very essence of all that exists.

NETERIANISM 10.000 B.C.E. – 2001 A.C.E.

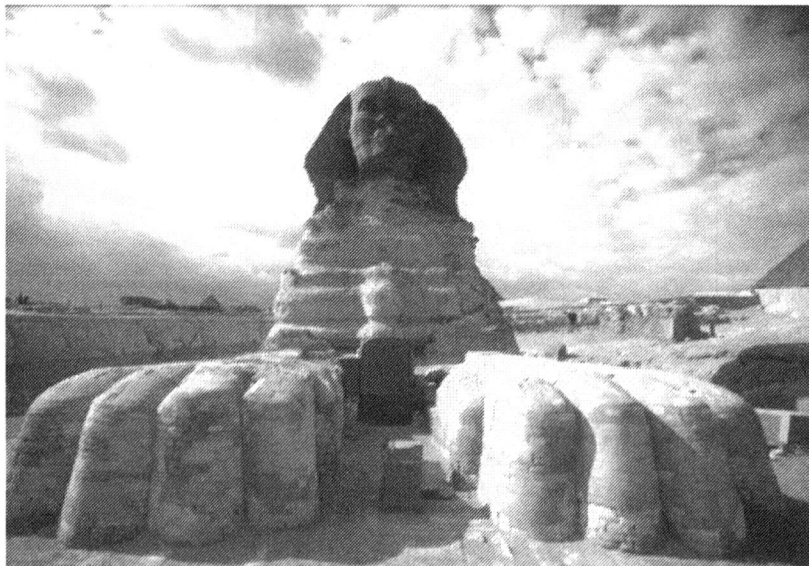

A Long History

For a period spanning over 10,000 years the Neterian religion served the society of ancient Kamit. It is hard to comprehend the vastness of time that is encompassed by Ancient Egyptian culture, religion and philosophy. Yet the evidence is there to be seen by all. It has been collected and presented in the book *African Origins of Civilization, Religion and Yoga Philosophy.* That volume will serve as the historical record for the Neterian religion and as record of its legacy to all humanity. It serves as the basis or foundation for the work contained in all the other books in this series that have been created to elucidate on the teachings and traditions as well as disciplines of the varied Neterian religious traditions.

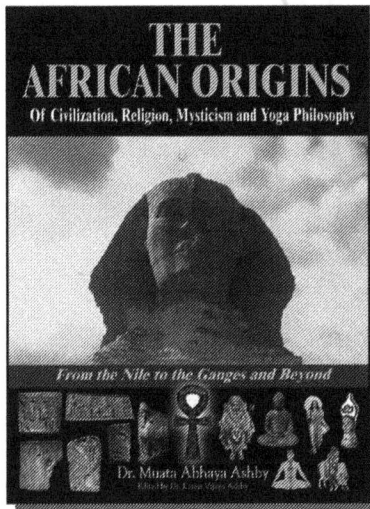

The book *African Origins of Civilization, Religion and Yoga Philosophy,* and the other volumes on the specific traditions detail the philosophies and disciplines that should be practiced by those who want to follow the path of Hm or Hmt, to be practitioners of the Shetaut Neter religion and builders of the Neterian faith worldwide.

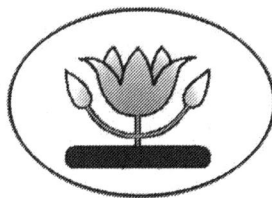

Where Was Shetaut Neter Practiced in Ancient Times?

Below left: A map of North East Africa showing the location of the land of *Ta-Meri* **or** *Kamit,* **also known as Ancient Egypt and South of it is located the land which in modern times is called Sudan.**

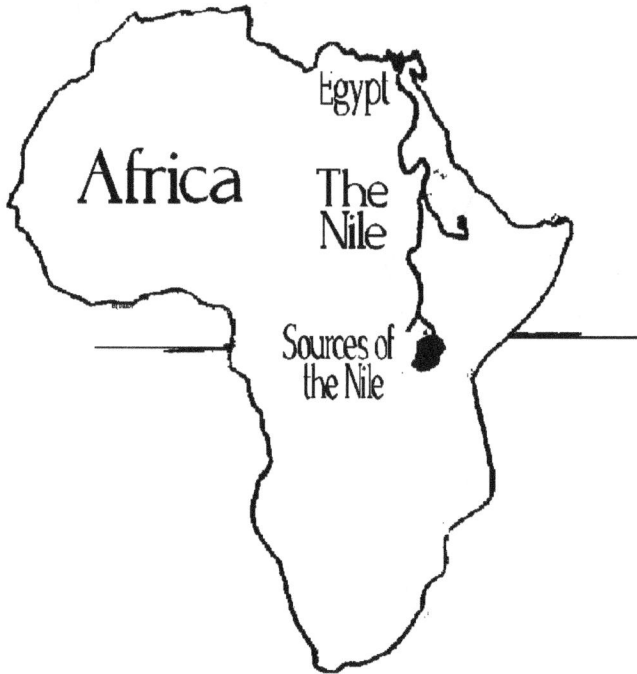

The Land of Kamit in Africa

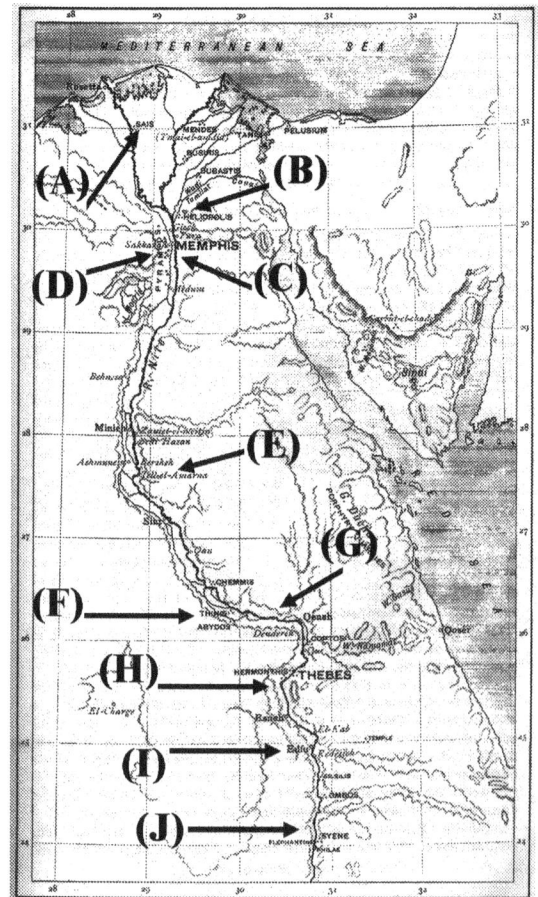

Above right- The Land of Ancient Egypt-Nile Valley

The cities wherein the major theologies of Neterianism developed were:

A-   Sais (temple of Net),
B-   Anu (Heliopolis- temple of Ra),
C-   Men-nefer or Hetkaptah (Memphis, temple of Ptah),
D-   Sakkara (Pyramid Texts),
E-   Akhet-Aton (City of Akhenaton, temple of Aton),
F-   Abdu (temple of Asar),
G-   Denderah (temple of Hetheru),
H-   Waset (Thebes, temple of Amun),
I-   Edfu (temple of Heru),
J-   Philae (temple of Aset). The cities wherein the theology of the Trinity of Asar-Aset-Heru was developed were Anu, Abydos, Philae, Edfu, Denderah and Edfu.

The Term Kamit and the Origins of the Ancient Egyptians

Ancient Origins

The Ancient Egyptians recorded that they were originally a colony of Ethiopians from the south who came to the north east part of Africa. The term "Ethiopian," "Nubian," and "Kushite" all relate to the same peoples who lived south of Egypt. In modern times, the land which was once known as Nubia ("Land of Gold"), is currently known as the Sudan, and the land even further south and east towards the coast of east Africa is referred to as Ethiopia (see map above).

Recent research has shown that the modern Nubian word *kiji* means "fertile land, dark gray mud, silt, or black land." Since the sound of this word is close to the Ancient Egyptian name Kish or Kush, referring to the land south of Egypt, it is believed that the name Kush also meant "the land of dark silt" or "the black land." Kush was the Ancient Egyptian name for Nubia. Nubia, the black land, is the Sudan of today. Sudan is an Arabic translation of *sûd* which is the plural form of *aswad*, which means "black," and *ân* which means "of the." So, Sudan means "of the blacks." In the modern Nubian language, *nugud* means "black." Also, *nuger*, *nugur*, and *nubi* mean "black" as well. All of this indicates that the words Kush, Nubia, and Sudan all mean the same thing — the "black land" and/or the "land of the blacks."[1] As we will see, the differences between the term Kush and the term Kam (Qamit - name for Ancient Egypt in the Ancient Egyptian language) relate more to the same meaning but different geographical locations.

As we have seen, the terms "Ethiopia," "Nubia," "Kush" and "Sudan" all refer to "black land" and/or the "land of the blacks." In the same manner we find that the name of Egypt which was used by the Ancient Egyptians also means "black land" and/or the "land of the blacks." The hieroglyphs below reveal the Ancient Egyptian meaning of the words related to the name of their land. It is clear that the meaning of the word Qamit is equivalent to the word Kush as far as they relate to "black land" and that they also refer to a differentiation in geographical location, i.e. Kush is the "black land of the south" and Qamit is the "black land of the north." Both terms denote the primary quality that defines Africa, "black" or "Blackness" (referring to the land and its people). The quality of blackness and the consonantal sound of K or Q as well as the reference to the land are all aspects of commonality between the Ancient Kushitic and Kamitan terms.

---

[1] "Nubia," *Microsoft® Encarta® Africana.* © 1999 Microsoft Corporation. All rights reserved.

The Hieroglyphic Text for the Name Qamit

Qamit - Ancient Egypt

Qamit - blackness – black

Qamit - literature of Ancient Egypt – scriptures

Qamiu or variant -

Ancient Egyptians-people of the black land.

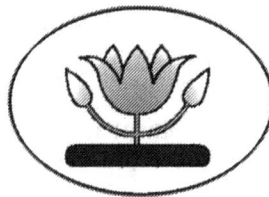

When Was Neterian Religion Practiced?

c. 65,000 B.C.E. Paleolithic – Nekhen (Hierakonpolis)
c. 10,000 B.C.E. Neolithic – period

PREDYNASTIC PERIOD

c. 10,500 B.C.E.-7,000 B.C.E. Creation of the Great Sphinx Modern archeological accepted dates – Sphinx means Hor-m-akhet or Heru (Horus) in the horizon. This means that the King is one with the Spirit, Ra as an enlightened person possessing an animal aspect (lion) and illuminated intellect. Anunian Theology – Ra - Serpent Power Spirituality
c. 10,000 B.C.E.-5,500 B.C.E. The Sky GOD- Realm of Light-Day – NETER Androgynous – All-encompassing –Absolute, Nameless Being, later identified with Ra-Herakhti (Sphinx)
>7,000 B.C.E. Kemetic Myth and Theology present in architecture

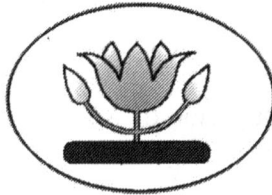

OLD KINGDOM PERIOD

5500+ B.C.E. to 600 A.C.E. Amun -Ra - Ptah (Horus) – Amenit - Rai – Sekhmet (male and female Trinity-Complementary Opposites)
5500+ B.C.E. Memphite Theology – Ptah
5500+ B.C.E. Hermopolitan Theology- Djehuti
5500+ B.C.E. The Asarian Resurrection Theology - Asar
5500+B.C.E. The Goddess Principle- Theology, Isis-Hathor-Net-Mut-Sekhmet-Buto
5500 B.C.E. (Dynasty 1) Beginning of the Dynastic Period (Unification of Upper and Lower Egypt)
5000 B.C.E. (5th Dynasty) Pyramid Texts - Egyptian Book of Coming Forth By Day - 42 Precepts of MAAT and codification of the Pre-Dynastic theologies (Pre-Dynastic period: 10,000 B.C.E.-5,500 B.C.E.) Coming Forth By Day (Book of the Dead)
4241 B.C.E. The Pharaonic (royal) calendar based on the Sothic system (star Sirius) was in use.

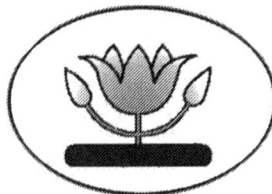

MIDDLE KINGDOM PERIOD

3000 B.C.E. WISDOM TEXTS-Precepts of Ptahotep, Instructions of Any, Instructions of
    Amenemope, Etc.
2040 B.C.E.-1786 B.C.E. *COFFIN TEXTS* Coming Forth By Day (Book of the Dead)
1800 B.C.E.-Theban Theology - Amun

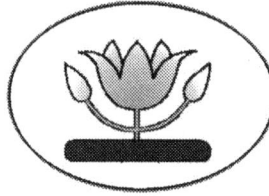

NEW KINGDOM PERIOD

1570 B.C.E.-Books of Coming Forth By Day (Book of the Dead)
1353 B.C.E. Atonism- Non-dualist Pre-Dynastic Philosophy was redefined by Akhenaton.
712-657 B.C.E. The Nubian Dynasty
657 B.C.E. - 450 A.C.E. This is the last period of Ancient Egyptian culture which saw several
invasions by foreigners from Asia Minor (Assyrians, Persians) and Europe (Greeks and Romans)
and finally the closing of the temples, murdering of priests and priestesses, the

Who Were the Ancient Egyptians and What is Yoga Philosophy?

The Ancient Egyptian religion (*Shetaut Neter*), language and symbols provide the first "historical" record of Yoga Philosophy and Religious literature. Egyptian Yoga is what has been commonly referred to by Egyptologists as Egyptian "Religion" or "Mythology", but to think of it as just another set of stories or allegories about a long lost civilization is to completely miss the greatest secret of human existence. Yoga, in all of its forms and disciplines of spiritual development, was practiced in Egypt earlier than anywhere else in history. This unique perspective from the highest philosophical system which developed in Africa over seven thousand years ago provides a new way to look at life, religion, the discipline of psychology and the way to spiritual development leading to spiritual Enlightenment. Egyptian mythology, when understood as a system of Yoga (union of the individual soul with the Universal Soul or Supreme Consciousness), gives every individual insight into their own divine nature and also a deeper insight into all religions and Yoga systems.

Diodorus Siculus (Greek Historian) writes in the time of Augustus (first century B.C.):

"Now the Ethiopians, as historians relate, were the first of all men and the proofs of this statement, they say, are manifest. For that they did not come into their land as immigrants from abroad but were the natives of it and so justly bear the name of autochthones (sprung from the soil itself), *is, they maintain, conceded by practically all men..."*

"They also say that the Egyptians are colonists sent out by the Ethiopians, Asar having been the leader of the colony. For, speaking generally, what is now Egypt, they maintain, was not land, but sea, when in the beginning the universe was being formed; afterwards, however, as the Nile during the times of its inundation carried down the mud from Ethiopia, land was gradually built up from the deposit...And the larger parts of the customs of the Egyptians are, they hold, Ethiopian, the colonists still preserving their ancient manners. For instance, the belief that their kings are Gods, the very special attention which they pay to their burials, and many other matters of a similar nature, are Ethiopian practices, while the shapes of their statues and the forms of their letters are Ethiopian; for of the two kinds of writing which the Egyptians have, that which is known as popular (demotic) *is learned by everyone, while that which is called sacred* (hieratic), *is understood only by the priests of the Egyptians, who learnt it from their Fathers as one of the things which are not divulged, but among the Ethiopians, everyone uses these forms of letters. Furthermore, the orders of the priests, they maintain, have much the same position among both peoples; for all are clean who are engaged in the service of the gods, keeping themselves shaven, like the Ethiopian priests, and having the same dress and form of staff, which is shaped like a plough and is carried by their kings who wear high felt hats which end in a knob in the top and are circled by the serpents which they call asps; and this symbol appears to carry the thought that it will be the lot who shall dare to attack the king to encounter death-carrying stings. Many other things are told by them concerning their own antiquity and the colony which they sent out that became the Egyptians, but about this there is no special need of our writing anything."*

The Ancient Egyptian texts state:

*"Our people originated at the base of the mountain of the Moon,
at the origin of the Nile river."*

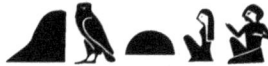

"KMT"
"Egypt", "Burnt", "Land of Blackness","Land of the Burnt People."

KMT (Ancient Egypt) is situated close to Lake Victoria in present day Africa. This is the same location where the earliest human remains have been found, in the land currently known as Ethiopia-Tanzania. Recent genetic technology as reported in the new encyclopedias and leading news publications has revealed that all peoples of the world originated in Africa and migrated to other parts of the world prior to the last Ice Age 40,000 years ago. Therefore, as of this time, genetic testing has revealed that all humans are alike. The earliest bone fossils which have been found in many parts of the world were those of the African Grimaldi type. During the Ice Age, it was not possible to communicate or to migrate. Those trapped in specific locations were subject to the regional forces of weather and climate. Less warmer climates required less body pigment, thereby producing lighter pigmented people who now differed from their dark-skinned ancestors. After the Ice Age when travel was possible, these light-skinned people who had lived in the northern, colder regions of harsh weather during the Ice Age period moved back to the warmer climates of their ancestors, and mixed with the people there who had remained dark-skinned, thereby producing the Semitic colored people. "Semite" means mixture of skin color shades.

Therefore, there is only one human race who, due to different climactic and regional exposure, changed to a point where there seemed to be different "types" of people. Differences were noted with respect to skin color, hair texture, customs, languages, and with respect to the essential nature (psychological and emotional makeup) due to the experiences each group had to face and overcome in order to survive.

From a philosophical standpoint, the question as to the origin of humanity is redundant when it is understood that *ALL* come from one origin which some choose to call the "Big Bang" and others "The Supreme Being."

"Thou makest the color of the skin of one race to be different from that of another, but however many may be the varieties of mankind, it is thou that makes them all to live."
—Ancient Egyptian Proverb from *The Hymns of Amun*

"Souls, Heru, son, are of the self-same nature, since they came from the same place where the Creator modeled them; nor male nor female are they. Sex is a thing of bodies not of Souls."
—Ancient Egyptian Proverb from *The teachings of Aset to Heru*

Historical evidence proves that Ethiopia-Nubia already had Kingdoms at least 300 years before the first Kingdom-Pharaoh of Egypt.

"Ancient Egypt was a colony of Nubia - Ethiopia. ...Asar having been the leader of the colony..."

"And upon his return to Greece, they gathered around and asked, "tell us about this great land of the Blacks called Ethiopia." And Herodotus said, "There are two great Ethiopian nations, one in Sind (India) and the other in Egypt."

Recorded by Egyptian high priest *Manetho* **(300 B.C.)**
also Recorded by *Diodorus* **(Greek historian 100 B.C.)**

The pyramids themselves however, cannot be dated, but indications are that they existed far back in antiquity. The Pyramid Texts (hieroglyphics inscribed on pyramid walls) and Coffin Texts (hieroglyphics inscribed on coffins) speak authoritatively on the constitution of the human spirit, the vital Life Force along the human spinal cord (known in India as *"Kundalini"*), the immortality of the soul, reincarnation and the law of Cause and Effect (known in India as the Law of Karma).

Color Plate 1: Below-left, Egyptian man and woman-(tomb of Payry) 18th Dynasty displaying the naturalistic style (as people really appeared in ancient times).

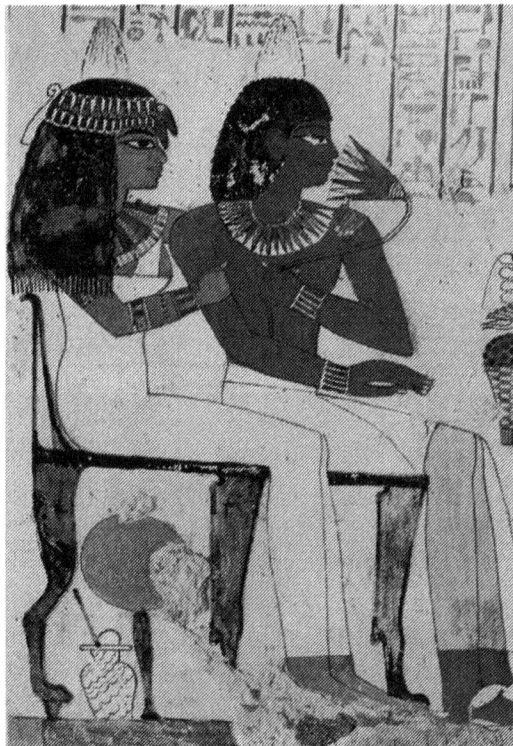

What is Yoga Philosophy and Spiritual Practice

Since a complete treatise on the theory and practice of yoga would require several volumes, only a basic outline will be given here.

When we look out upon the world, we are often baffled by the multiplicity which constitutes the human experience. What do we really know about this experience? Many scientific disciplines have developed over the last two hundred years for the purpose of discovering the mysteries of nature, but this search has only engendered new questions about the nature of existence. Yoga is a discipline or way of life designed to promote the physical, mental and spiritual development of the human being. It leads a person to discover the answers to the most important questions of life such as Who am I?, Why am I here? and Where am I going?

The literal meaning of the word YOGA is to *"YOKE"* or to *"LINK"* back. The implication is: to link back to the original source, the original essence, that which transcends all mental and intellectual attempts at comprehension, but which is the essential nature of everything in CREATION. While in the strict or dogmatic sense, Yoga philosophy and practice is a separate discipline from religion, yoga and religion have been linked at many points throughout history. In a manner of speaking, Yoga as a discipline may be seen as a non-sectarian transpersonal science or practice to promote spiritual development and harmony of mind and body thorough mental and physical disciplines including meditation, psycho-physical exercises, and performing action with the correct attitude.

The disciplines of Yoga fall under five major categories. These are: *Yoga of Wisdom, Yoga of Devotional Love, Yoga of Meditation, Tantric Yoga* and *Yoga of Selfless Action.* Within these categories there are subsidiary forms which are part of the main disciplines. The important point to remember is that all aspects of yoga can and should be used in an integral fashion to effect an efficient and harmonized spiritual movement in the practitioner. Therefore, while there may be an area of special emphasis, other elements are bound to become part of the yoga program as needed. For example, while a yogin may place emphasis on the yoga of wisdom, they may also practice devotional yoga and meditation yoga along with the wisdom studies.

While it is true that yogic practices may be found in religion, strictly speaking, yoga is neither a religion or a philosophy. It should be thought of more as a way of life or discipline for promoting greater fullness and experience of life. Yoga was developed at the dawn of history by those who wanted more out of life. These special men and women wanted to discover the true origins of creation and of themselves. Therefore, they set out to explore the vast reaches of consciousness within themselves. They are sometimes referred to as "Seers", "Sages", etc. Awareness or consciousness can only be increased when the mind is in a state of peace and harmony. Thus, the disciplines of meditation (which are part of Yoga), and wisdom (the philosophical teachings for understanding reality as it is) are the primary means to controlling the mind and allowing the individual to mature psychologically and spiritually.

The teachings which were practiced in the Ancient Egyptian temples were the same ones later intellectually defined into a literary form by the Indian Sages of Vedanta and Yoga. This was discussed in my book *Egyptian Yoga: The Philosophy of Enlightenment*. The Indian Mysteries of Yoga and Vedanta represent an unfolding and intellectual exposition of the Egyptian Mysteries. Also, the study of Gnostic Christianity or Christianity before Roman Catholicism will be useful to our

22

study since Christianity originated in Ancient Egypt and was also based on the Ancient Egyptian Mysteries. Therefore, the study of the Egyptian Mysteries, early Christianity and Indian Vedanta-Yoga will provide the most comprehensive teaching on how to practice the disciplines of yoga leading to the attainment of Enlightenment.

The question is how to accomplish these seemingly impossible tasks? How to transform yourself and realize the deepest mysteries of existence? How to discover "who am I?" This is the mission of Yoga Philosophy and the purpose of yogic practices. Yoga does not seek to convert or impose religious beliefs on any one. Ancient Egypt was the source of civilization and the source of religion and Yoga. Therefore, all systems of mystical spirituality can coexist harmoniously within these teachings when they are correctly understood.

The goal of yoga is to promote integration of the mind-body-spirit complex in order to produce optimal health of the human being. This is accomplished through mental and physical exercises which promote the free flow of spiritual energy by reducing mental complexes caused by ignorance. There are two roads which human beings can follow, one of wisdom and the other of ignorance. The path of the masses is generally the path of ignorance which leads them into negative situations, thoughts and deeds. These in turn lead to ill health and sorrow in life. The other road is based on wisdom and it leads to health, true happiness and enlightenment.

Our mission is to extol the wisdom of yoga and mystical spirituality from the Ancient Egyptian perspective and to show the practice of the teachings through our books, videos and audio productions. You may find a complete listing of other books by the author in the back of this volume.

How to study the wisdom teachings:

There is a specific technique which is prescribed by the scriptures themselves for studying the teachings, proverbs and aphorisms of mystical wisdom. The method is as follows:

The spiritual aspirant should read the desired text thoroughly, taking note of any particular teachings which resonates with him or her. The aspirant should make a habit of collecting those teachings and reading them over frequently. The scriptures should be read and re-read because the subtle levels of the teachings will be increasingly understood the more the teachings are reviewed. One useful exercise is to choose some of the most special teachings you would like to focus on and place them in large type or as posters in your living areas so as to be visible to remind you of the teaching.

The aspirant should discuss those teachings with others of like mind when possible because this will help to promote greater understanding and act as an active spiritual practice in which the teachings are kept at the forefront of the mind. In this way, the teachings can become an integral part of everyday life and not reserved for a particular time of day or of the week.

The study of the wisdom teachings should be a continuous process in which the teachings become the predominant factor of life rather than the useless and oftentimes negative and illusory thoughts of those who are ignorant of spiritual truths. This spiritual discipline should be observed until Enlightenment is attained.

May you discover supreme peace in this very lifetime!

(HETEP - Supreme Peace)

INTRODUCTION

Who Am I?

Who am I? What is this mind which perceives? What is this universe made of? Is there a God?

Throughout history, these and many other questions have followed humanity from generation to generation. The need of human nature to experience, to evolve and understand has led to the invention of philosophies which assist the human mind in grasping the realities it seems to perceive in the world as well as those which it seems to perceive with the heart but which remain intellectually unknowable. In ancient times these philosophies developed as myths, religions, yoga systems and in modern times they have taken the form of sciences called psychology, physics and non-religious philosophies such as Marxism and existentialism. Yet with all the developments of the past, humanity as a whole remains in search of the answers to happiness, health and peace. Has religion and science failed? Most importantly, throughout all the teachings embodied in religions and the discoveries of modern science, has humanity missed out on the benefits of religion and science? Is there anything useful in these endeavors for humankind? A deeper study into the history, meaning and practice of ancient teachings reveals a remarkable concordance with modern scientific discoveries. In essence, modern sciences such as Quantum Physics are leading scientists to contemplate life and our understanding of reality in terms which ancient philosophers and Sages espoused thousands of years ago. Science is a discipline which professes to shun non-rational thoughts, a common feature to both mythology and religion. So how is it possible that it would lead to the same conclusions about existence as mystical religions and Yoga philosophy?

Two of the most important areas we will look into are psychology and mythology. We will look at these from a yogic or mystical-symbolic point of view rather than a rational, literal or logical way. The reasons for doing this will become clear as we progress through the program. Mythology and spiritual symbolism were never intended to be understood as factual events which occurred in a particular place in time exclusively. Rather, they are to be understood as ever recurring principles of human life which need to be understood in their deepest sense in order for them to provide humanity with the benefit of their wisdom.

Psychology has been defined as the study of the thought processes characteristic of an individual or group (mind, psyche, ethos, mentality). In this work we will focus on religious mythology as a psychological discipline for understanding the human mind, its development and transformation. Mythology can be understood as a language, however, it is a unique kind of language. Certain languages are similar because they are part of a family of languages. For example: Italian and Spanish. This similarity makes it possible for a person whose native language is Spanish to understand the meanings of some Italian words so as to somewhat be able to follow along a conversation in Italian. Mythology is much more intelligible than an ordinary human language. Mythology is more akin to music in its universality. If the key elements of this language are well understood, it is possible to understand and relate any mythological system to another and thereby gain the understanding of the message being imparted. Setting up your own personal spiritual program will require that you develop a profound understanding of the psychological principles upon which ancient mythology is based in order to discover your special path on the spiritual journey.

In order to gain insight into the *"Psycho-Mythology"* or psychological implications of religious and spiritual mythology which promote the psycho-spiritual transformation of the individual leading to the attainment of Enlightenment, we must first define what is meant by the terms psycho and mythology. Here, the term *psycho* must be understood as far more than simply that which refers to the mind and its thoughts. We will be using *psycho* to mean everything that constitutes human consciousness in all of its stages and states. *Mythology* here refers to the codes, messages, ideas, directives and beliefs which affect the psyche through the conscious and unconscious mind of an individual, specifically those effects which result in transpersonal or transcendental changes in the personality as well as those which constitute anti-yogic, anti-transcendental movements.

While our study begins with Egyptian Mythology, Religion and Yoga Philosophy, it also necessarily relates to all mythologies, religions and philosophies around the world. Briefly, Egyptian religion is the oldest recorded religion in this historical era and in our book, *Egyptian Yoga*, we compiled the correlations between the religion which developed in Egypt and those which developed later around other parts of Africa as well as in Asia*. Through an intense study of Eastern Religions and Yoga, it becomes evident that what has been called Egyptian Mythology is in reality a highly sophisticated and advanced system of Yoga Philosophy. Yoga is a system of personal transformation by which we are able to discover our true Self wherein lies the answers to all of our questions about the purpose of our existence, who we are, how to overcome adversity and promote prosperity, and why we are in the situations of life in which we find ourselves. Most importantly, the idea is not to amass mountainous amounts of wisdom teachings but to discover their meanings and how to apply them in ordinary life to rise above it, as a lotus rises above the muddy waters without retaining a single drop of the dirty water on its petals. If this does not occur, then one is not practicing philosophy, religion or yoga but something else. Initiation is therefore the process of coming into a philosophy and way of life which allows you to become free of any restrictions or impediments to your happiness. It is also a process of discovering how to end pain and suffering in life. Thus, it is a process of becoming established in your own inner support and inner peace without depending on the world. *(Asia includes Europe)

What is Human existence?

Human life is a process in which a human being experiences various situations ranging from pain and suffering to happiness and pleasure between the time span of birth and death. From a yogic point of view, all human situations are painful because they are distractions from the true source of bliss and abiding happiness within the heart. Attachment to objects and relationships outside of oneself seems like the normal course of human life, but the masses of people adopt this mode of existence out of ignorance. Ignorance of what? Ignorance of their deeper Self. If they had knowledge of the deeper Self within, there would be no need to seek personal fulfillment through worldly achievements, worldly possessions or worldly relationships. This endless search leads every ignorant human being to engage in various situations and entanglements, which in the beginning, seem to hold the possibility of bringing about a happy circumstance, but which invariably leads to pain, suffering and frustration.

You do not have to turn on the television or read a newspaper to see the miserable condition of most people. Think about your own life. Has there been any situation where happiness was abiding? Have you experienced any relationship with someone who never disappointed you or caused you pain? Has there been any possession you acquired which did not lose its power to bring you happiness or that you did not become bored with, even though it made you happy to possess it in the beginning?

Even those people who say they are happy with life as it is, are deluding themselves into believing that the happy moments balance the painful ones. This is not true because even the happy moments are setting you up for some painful disappointment in the future because all worldly situations and relationships come to an end. Thus, your happy moment causes longing for more happy moments, and when these are not possible, there is disappointment and frustration. The longing and frustration does not end at the time of death. When the body dies, the mind continues to hold the deep rooted desires for worldly fulfillment and this causes the soul to be impelled toward countless new lifetimes of karmic entanglements in search of worldly fulfillment. All of this occurs out of ignorance of one's true Self.

However, becoming free from the clutches of ignorance is not as simple as learning about its cause. Even if you are honest and truly believe in the philosophy of yoga and mystical spirituality, all of your mental efforts to negate the ignorance will fail in the beginning because your mind has spent many hours over a period of days, months, years, lifetimes and eons, believing in the illusion of human life. Even if you were to understand that it is your worldly attachments which are causing you mental agitation and suffering, the process of attaining Enlightenment it is not as simple as saying "O.K. since my possessions are distracting me and causing me agitation and worry, I will give them up and have peace." Even if you were to find yourself without possessions, your mind would be grieving over their loss, or preoccupied with how to regain them or how to survive without them.

Even if you give everything up and go to a distant cave away from civilization, you cannot escape from the world. There will still be ants and mosquitoes to bite you, cold weather, rain, wild animals, and the restless wandering of your mind thinking of the life you left! Initiation into spiritual life is the process of learning an art of living which leads to freedom even while involved in the world. Your goal is to become as the Lotus which rises up from the muddy waters, able to exist in the world without being soiled by it, and having discovered the bliss of inner spiritual discovery, always abiding in that wondrous glory in any situation which life presents to you. Once the teachings of spirituality are understood and you have a firm conviction as to their reality, then you can begin the process of making them your reality. Spiritual realization requires sustained effort over a period of time wherein spiritual disciplines are directed toward overturning the mountainous creations which the mind has produced in the past due to ignorance. The mind is like a river. Ignorant ideas are like logs, rocks, branches and dams in the river which block, divert or distort the flow of water. With the correct equipment (correct understanding and practice of the yoga disciplines) and through sustained effort, the obstacles to spiritual realization can be removed allowing the river of the mind to flow freely toward the ocean of self-discovery.

If you have developed enough spiritual sensitivity to understand that there is no abiding peace or happiness to be found in human existence, you are qualified to study the deeper mysteries of spiritual life. This is the process of Initiation which leads from ignorance to Enlightenment and self-discovery. Where is there an inexhaustible source of bliss and happiness which does not depend on external factors? Where is it possible to find unending peace and tranquillity and a joy which is not subject to external conditions of either prosperity or adversity? The initiatic process shows the way.

In order for the teachings of mystical spirituality to come true in your life, you must make them the central force in your life. You must center your life around them and infuse them into every aspect of your life. In this way you will become transformed into the ideal of what the teachings describe: an Enlightened human being. It is not possible to gain higher spiritual understanding of the practices in any other way except to live them. Thus initiation is a way of life and not a single event. It is a continuous process which leads to greater and greater awareness and expansion culminating in the highest levels of Self-Knowledge.

What is Initiation?

What does it mean to tread the spiritual path of yoga? Being an initiate is not what most people think of when they hear of a yoga practitioner. There are many misconceptions about the teachings of yoga and there are many misconceptions about those who practice yoga. Sometimes the image of a cross-legged man with matted locks comes to mind. Sometimes wandering ascetics come to mind. Sometimes an image of an incredibly limber person in some impossible posture comes to mind. Sometimes a figure in a meditation posture transcending the world comes to mind. Also sometimes people think that yoga can drive you crazy so they picture a fanatical person uttering intelligible words. Sometimes the image of the media and from the traditional church has promoted an image of occult, mysterious and unnatural personalities as practitioners of yoga so they also picture cults and fanaticism.

What is Initiation? The great personalities of the past known to the world as Isis, Hathor, Jesus, Buddha and many other great Sages and Saints were initiated into their spiritual path but how did initiation help them and what were they specifically initiated into?

Many people think of initiation, when associated with spiritual studies, as some kind of fantastic event which will in and of itself cause a major transformation in a person's life. Initiation should be thought of less as an event and more as the process of embarking on a journey of spiritual living which will lead to spiritual enlightenment. With this broad understanding it should be clear that this entire book is initiating you, the reader, into the higher teachings of life. Every time you turn a page you are learning more and more about the world and as you do you are learning more about yourself. In this section we will discuss the process of initiation and the way in which spiritual knowledge is imparted.

From time immemorial the tradition of teacher and student has been carried on by Sages and Saints the world over. This is evident even in the world religions. Hethor of Ancient Egypt was initiated by Djehuti. Horus of Ancient Egypt was initiated into the mystical teachings by Aset (Isis). Rama (a form of Krishna from India) was initiated into the teachings by Sage Vasistha. Jesus was initiated into the teachings by John the Baptist. As in any other discipline of life spiritual studies require an authentic teacher. However, even the greatest teacher cannot teach a person who is not qualified to learn. Therefore, we will begin by enumerating the ten virtues of a spiritual aspirant. These imply the qualities that anyone desiring to practice spirituality needs to work on to develop.

The teachings of Yoga and Mystical religion are the means by which an ordinary human being can rise to the state of spiritual enlightenment, inner fulfillment, peace and abiding happiness in life. These teachings were in ancient times passed on through an exact system which involves listening to, study of and meditation upon the teachings in a proper environment and with proper guidance. This method of teaching is known as *Initiatic Way of Education.* There are many styles of Yoga, although their goals are all the same: Union with the divine. These include: Yoga of Intuitive Wisdom of the Divine, Yoga of Devotional Union with the

Divine, Yoga of Meditation and Mind Control, Yoga of Virtuous Living, Yoga of Cultivation of the Latent Life Force Energy (Serpent Power).

THE INITIATIC WAY OF EDUCATION

Yoga philosophy originated at the dawn of civilization in the present era of human history beginning with the emergence of the Ancient Egyptian civilization. The temple system provided a unique format for education and government which was able to sustain and provide for the needs of Ancient Egypt for over 5,000 years. Therefore, it is useful here to briefly describe the Temple System of education and a method in which its wisdom can be applied to modern society.

Since the teachings of yoga and mystical spirituality have been traditionally passed on through the teacher-student relationship for over two millennia, this system of education is integral to the study of transpersonal disciplines. While in modern times the local parish priest, the counselor or psychotherapist have taken the place of the Sages, they have not adopted the wisdom nor the ancient method of education employed by their forebears. Thus the *Guru-disciple relationship* and the *Initiatic way of education* are important areas of study for the aspiring Transpersonal Studies student or professional.

The need for a true teacher of spirituality cannot be overemphasized in the course of spiritual practice. This is the reason why so many "new age" teachers and even members of the traditional establishment have gone to "sit at the feet," so to speak, of Eastern teachers of yoga and mystical philosophy. This is also the reason why much of the research done by early transpersonal researchers, beginning with Carl Jung, focuses on the Initiatic relationship, as well as the wisdom which is imparted through it. An aspirant is like an athlete. He or she needs coaching and practice in order to attain mastery over the lower nature. In every area of your life where you have achieved success, it is because you studied and practiced, if not in this lifetime, in a previous one. Spiritual Enlightenment cannot be achieved through magic or through unnatural means. It is achieved through understanding and hard work, not ordinary work, but those activities which lead to purification of the heart.

It is possible to promote spiritual growth through the books written by genuine spiritual preceptors. The new forms of media such as audio and video have gone even further in conveying the message of the teachings to the entire world. However, at some point, books and tapes can only go so far in explaining the fruits of the true practice of spirituality. This is because the mind can develop many misconceptions and illusions about spirituality just as in any area of ordinary worldly life. Therefore, a guide or coach who is advanced in its practice should be sought out and approached with humility and honesty to ask questions and dispel subtle forms of ignorance. This is the process of spiritual teaching called Initiation. The aspirant is initiated into a philosophy and way of life which he or she needs to learn and practice by studying, reflecting and meditating on the teachings. Initiation is a conscious choice to adopt a teaching and to embark on the task of basing one's life on it in order to purify one's mind and body through the teaching, so that one may become a conduit of transcendental forms of experience.

One of the main problems of society is the relative lack of interest in the scriptures and secondly, the relatively small number of authentic spiritual preceptors available to teach those who are interested. Many people do not find spirituality attractive because they feel they would "lose" out on life if they became seriously involved. Others see the prospect of spirituality as being too remote for their understanding.

An authentic Spiritual Preceptor is not only someone who is advanced on the spiritual path, or even just someone who has reached the fully enlightened state. A Guru, in the Upanishadic (teachings of the Indian Upanishads) sense of the word, is someone who is spiritually enlightened and who also is well versed in the scriptural teachings and methods of training aspirants according to their level of understanding. Therefore, a counselor of Yoga must first achieve a high degree of understanding and personal - spiritual emancipation since the subtleties of the mind must be well understood. The teacher must be able to be a refuge for all people, have an extensive knowledge of the teachings pertaining to his/her level of attainment, and enthusiastically pursue all forms of Yoga. The term *Guru* means one who enlightens or imparts spiritual wisdom and eradicates ignorance.

Every true mystical tradition, be it religious or non-religious, requires a traditional link because the Initiatic teaching given to those who become initiated into a tradition, needs the benefit of a preceptor who has received the teaching from a previously initiated teacher and has correct understanding of the teaching. Otherwise it would be, as an Eastern parable explains, like a blind person trying to explain to other blind people what the world looks like simply using imagination and wit. There are others, intellectuals, who come to believe that they have attained "Enlightenment" because they read the scriptures. However, upon being tested in the world of human experience, the complexes and sufferings of life resurface. Thus, a need for a comprehensive program of spiritual development is necessary to promote real and abiding transformation in the human heart.

In the beginning, the Yogic Teacher helps the individual to somehow turn the anguish, disappointment and pain experienced as a result of interaction with the world into a desire to rise above it, as symbolized by the lotus rising out of the muddy waters. To this end, a series of techniques and disciplines have been developed over thousands of years. The Yoga counselor needs to help the seeker restructure and channel those energies which arise from disappointment and frustration into a healthy dispassion of the world and its entanglements, spiritual aspiration and self-effort directed at sustaining a viable personal spiritual program or *Sadhana* or *Sheti*. In the *Shetaut Neter* system of yoga from Ancient Egypt or Egyptian Yoga, there were three levels of aspirants.

1- ASPIRATION- Students who are being instructed on a probationary status, and have not experienced inner vision. The important factor at this level is ***awakening of the Spiritual Self,*** that is, becoming conscious of the divine presence within one's self and the universe by having faith that there is a spiritual essence beyond ordinary human understanding.

2- STRIVING- Students who have attained inner vision and have received a glimpse of cosmic consciousness. The important factor at this level is ***purgation of the self,*** that is, purification of mind and body through a spiritual discipline. The aspirant tries to totally surrender "personal" identity or ego to the divine inner Self which is the Universal Self of all Creation.

3- ESTABLISHED- Students who have become IDENTIFIED with or UNITED with GOD. The important factor at this level is ***illumination of the intellect,*** that is, experience and appreciation of the divine presence during reflection and meditation, *Union* with the divine self, the divine marriage of the individual with the universal.

In order to have a better understanding of what initiation is we must look into the distant past in order to discover its purpose and use.

PERSONAL ASSESSMENT

Before proceeding with the book any further, it is important that you assess yourself so that you may begin to reflect on your current status in terms of your position in life as well as your spiritual evolution. Answer the following questions and keep them for your own record. They will serve you by helping you to understand what you feel at the present time and what direction you want your life to take.

1- How would you describe your knowledge of religion and philosophy?

2- What do you see as the greatest obstacle to your happiness and fulfillment in life?

3- What do you see as the most important need that you have?

4- What is your current or previous religious affiliation or faith?

5- What role do you feel religion or spirituality plays in your life?

6- Have you had any previous Yoga instruction? If so where and what was (is) your experience?

7- Have you received any advanced religious instruction?

8- How do you see your life?

9- What do you think of your own potential to succeed in life?

10- If you could, what would you like to do with your life?

CHAPTER 1

Yoga in Ancient Egypt

THE EGYPTIAN WORDS AND SYMBOLS FOR THE MYSTERY TEACHINGS OF YOGA

The first and most important teaching to understand in our study surrounds the Ancient Egyptian word "Sheti." Sheti comes from the root "Sheta." The Ancient Egyptian word *Sheta* means something which is *hidden, secret, unknown,* or *cannot be seen through or understood, a secret, a mystery.* What is considered to be inert matter also possesses *Hidden Properties or Shetau Akhet.* Rituals, Words of Power (Khu-Hekau, Mantras), religious texts and pictures are S*hetaut Neter* or *Divine Mysteries. Shetat* or *Seshetat* are the secret rituals in the cults of the Egyptian Gods. *Shetai* is the *Hidden God, incomprehensible God, Mysterious One, Secret One.* One name of the soul of Amun is *Shet-ba* (The One whose soul is hidden). The name Amun itself signifies "The Hidden One": *Shetai. Sheti* (spiritual discipline) is to go deeply into the mysteries, to study the mystery teachings and literature profoundly, to penetrate the mysteries. *Nehas-t* signifies: "resurrection" or "spiritual awakening." The body or *Shet-t* (mummy) is where a human being can focuses attention to practice spiritual disciplines. When spiritual discipline is perfected the true self or *Shti* (he who is hidden in the coffin) is revealed.

Thus, Sheti is the spiritual discipline or program to promote spiritual evolution which was used in Ancient Egypt. Now we can begin to discover the teachings of that spiritual program. These all fall under the broad term "Egyptian Yoga."

What is Egyptian Yoga?

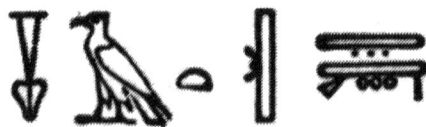

Smai Tawi
(From Chapter 4 of
the *Prt m Hru*)

The Term "Egyptian Yoga" and The Philosophy Behind It

As previously discussed, Yoga in all of its forms were practiced in Egypt apparently earlier than anywhere else in our history. This point of view is supported by the fact that there is documented scriptural and iconographical evidence of the disciplines of virtuous living, dietary purification, study of the wisdom teachings and their practice in daily life, psychophysical and psycho-spiritual exercises and meditation being practiced in Ancient Egypt, long before the evidence of its existence is detected in India (including the Indus Valley Civilization) or any other early civilization (Sumer, Greece, China, etc.).

The teachings of Yoga are at the heart of *Prt m Hru*. As explained earlier, the word "Yoga" is a Sanskrit term meaning to unite the individual with the Cosmic. The term has been used in certain parts of this book for ease of communication since the word "Yoga" has received wide popularity especially in western countries in recent years. The Ancient Egyptian equivalent term to the Sanskrit word yoga is: *"Smai." Smai* means union, and the following determinative terms give it a spiritual significance, at once equating it with the term "Yoga" as it is used in India. When used in conjunction with the Ancient Egyptian symbol which means land, *"Ta,"* the term "union of the two lands" arises.

In Chapter 4 and Chapter 17 of the *Prt m Hru,* a term "Smai Tawi" is used. It means "Union of the two lands of Egypt," ergo "Egyptian Yoga." The two lands refer to the two main districts of the country (North and South). In ancient times, Egypt was divided into two sections or land areas. These were known as Lower and Upper Egypt. In Ancient Egyptian mystical philosophy, the land of Upper Egypt relates to the divinity Heru (Horus), who represents the Higher Self, and the land of Lower Egypt relates to Set, the divinity of the lower self. So *Smai Taui* means "the union of the two lands" or the "Union of the lower self with the Higher Self. The lower self relates to that which is negative and uncontrolled in the human mind including worldliness, egoism, ignorance, etc. (Set), while the Higher Self relates to that which is above temptations and is good in the human heart as well as in touch with transcendental consciousness (Heru). Thus, we also have the Ancient Egyptian term *Smai Heru-Set,* or the union of Heru and Set. So Smai Taui or Smai Heru-Set are the Ancient Egyptian words which are to be translated as **"Egyptian Yoga."**

Above: the main symbol of Egyptian Yoga: *Sma*. The Ancient Egyptian language and symbols provide the first "historical" record of Yoga Philosophy and Religious literature. The hieroglyph Sma, ⚕ "Sema," represented by the union of two lungs and the trachea, symbolizes that the union of the duality, that is, the Higher Self and lower self, leads to Non-duality, the One, singular consciousness.

(†)

(±)

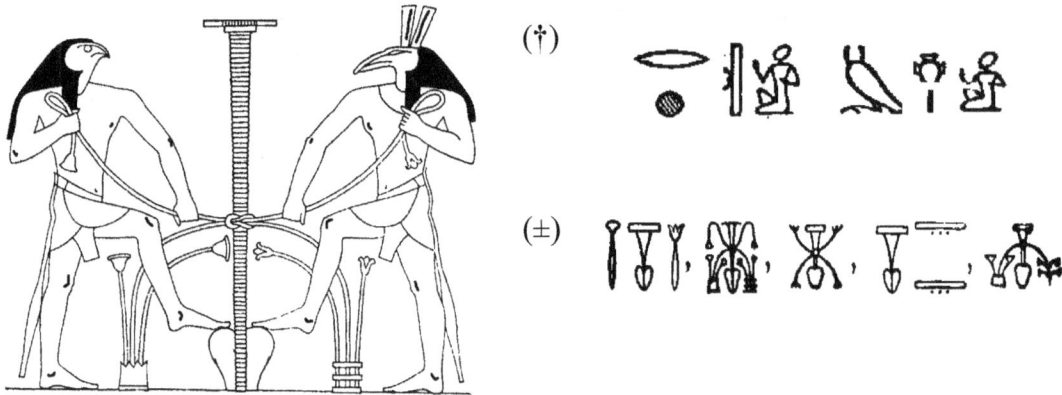

More Ancient Egyptian Symbols of Yoga

Above left: Smai Heru-Set,

Heru and Set join forces to tie up the symbol of Union (Sema –see (B) above). The Sema symbol refers to the Union of Upper Egypt (Lotus) and Lower Egypt (Papyrus) under one ruler, but also at a more subtle level, it refers to the union of one's Higher Self and lower self (Heru and Set), as well as the control of one's breath (Life Force) through the union (control) of the lungs (breathing organs). The character of Heru and Set are an integral part of the *Pert Em Heru.*

The central and most popular character within Ancient Egyptian Religion of Asar is Heru, who is an incarnation of his father, Asar. Asar is killed by his brother Set who, out of greed and demoniac (Setian) tendency, craved to be the ruler of Egypt. With the help of Djehuti, the God of wisdom, Aset, the great mother and Hetheru, his consort, Heru prevailed in the battle against Set for the rulership of Kemet (Egypt). Heru's struggle symbolizes the struggle of every human being to regain rulership of the Higher Self and to subdue the lower self.

The most ancient writings in our historical period are from the Ancient Egyptians. These writings are referred to as hieroglyphics. The original name given to these writings by the Ancient Egyptians is *Metu Neter,* meaning "the writing of God" or *Neter Metu* or "Divine Speech." These writings were inscribed in temples, coffins and papyruses and contained the teachings in reference to the spiritual nature of the human being and the ways to promote spiritual emancipation, awakening or resurrection. The Ancient Egyptian proverbs presented in this text are translations from the original hieroglyphic scriptures. An example of hieroglyphic text was presented above in the form of the text of Smai Taui or "Egyptian Yoga."

Egyptian Philosophy may be summed up in the following proverbs, which clearly state that the soul is heavenly or divine and that the human being must awaken to the true reality, which is the Spirit, Self.

"Self knowledge is the basis of true knowledge."

"Soul to heaven, body to earth."

*"Man is to become God-like through a life of virtue and the cultivation of the spirit
through scientific knowledge, practice and bodily discipline."*

*"Salvation is accomplished through the efforts of the individual.
There is no mediator between man and {his/her} salvation."*

*"Salvation is the freeing of the soul from its bodily fetters, becoming a God through
knowledge and wisdom, controlling the forces of the cosmos instead of being a slave to
them, subduing the lower nature and through awakening the Higher Self, ending the
cycle of rebirth
and dwelling with the Neters who direct and control the Great Plan."*

The Study of Yoga

When we look out upon the world, we are often baffled by the multiplicity, which constitutes the human experience. What do we really know about this experience? Many scientific disciplines have developed over the last two hundred years for the purpose of discovering the mysteries of nature, but this search has only engendered new questions about the nature of existence. Yoga is a discipline or way of life designed to promote the physical, mental and spiritual development of the human being. It leads a person to discover the answers to the most important questions of life such as, Who am I? Why am I here? Where am I going?

As explained earlier, the literal meaning of the word *Yoga* is to *"Yoke"* or to *"Link"* back, the implication being to link the individual consciousness back to the original source, the original essence, that which transcends all mental and intellectual attempts at comprehension, but which is the essential nature of everything in Creation, termed "Universal Consciousness. While in the strict sense, Yoga may be seen as a separate discipline from religion, yoga and religion have been linked at many points throughout history and continue to be linked even today. In a manner of speaking, Yoga as a discipline may be seen as a non-sectarian transpersonal science or practice to promote spiritual development and harmony of mind and body thorough mental and physical disciplines including meditation, psycho-physical exercises, and performing action with the correct attitude.

The teachings which were practiced in the Ancient Egyptian temples were the same ones later intellectually defined into a literary form by the Indian Sages of Vedanta and Yoga. This was discussed in our book *Egyptian Yoga: The Philosophy of Enlightenment.* The Indian Mysteries of Yoga and Vedanta may therefore be understood as representing an unfolding exposition of the Egyptian Mysteries.

The question is how to accomplish these seemingly impossible tasks? How to transform yourself and realize the deepest mysteries of existence? How to discover "Who am I?" This is the mission of Yoga Philosophy and the purpose of yogic practices. Yoga does not seek to convert or impose religious beliefs on any one. Ancient Egypt was the source of civilization and the source of religion and Yoga. Therefore, all systems of mystical spirituality can coexist harmoniously within these teachings when they are correctly understood.

The goal of yoga is to promote integration of the mind-body-spirit complex in order to produce optimal health of the human being. This is accomplished through mental and physical exercises which promote the free flow of spiritual energy by reducing mental complexes caused by ignorance. There are two roads which human beings can follow, one of wisdom and the other of ignorance. The path of the masses is generally the path of ignorance which leads them into negative situations, thoughts and deeds. These in turn lead to ill health and sorrow in life. The other road is based on wisdom and it leads to health, true happiness and enlightenment.

The central and most popular character within ancient Egyptian Religion of Osiris is Horus who is an incarnation of his father, Osiris. Osiris is killed by his brother Set who, out of greed and demoniac (Setian) tendency, craves to be the ruler of Egypt. With the help of Djehuti, the God of wisdom, Isis, the great mother and Hathor, his consort, Horus prevails in the battle against Set for the rulership of Egypt. Horus' struggle symbolizes the struggle of every human being to regain rulership of the Higher Self and to subdue the lower self. With this understanding, the land of Egypt is equivalent to the Kingdom/Queendom concept of Christianity.

The most ancient writings in our historical period are from the ancient Egyptians. These writings are referred to as hieroglyphics. Also, the most ancient civilization known was the ancient Egyptian civilization. The proof of this lies in the ancient Sphinx which is over 12,000 years old. The original name given to these writings by the ancient Egyptians is *Metu Neter,* meaning "the writing of God" or *Neter Metu* or "Divine Speech." These writings were inscribed in temples, coffins and papyruses and contained the teachings in reference to the spiritual nature of the human being and the ways to promote spiritual emancipation, awakening or resurrection. The —Ancient Egyptian Proverbs presented in this text are translations from the original hieroglyphic scriptures. An example of hieroglyphic text is presented on the front cover.

Egyptian Philosophy may be summed up in the following proverbs which clearly state that the soul is heavenly or divine and that the human being must awaken to the true reality which is the spirit Self.

"Self knowledge is the basis of true knowledge."

"Soul to heaven, body to earth."

"Man is to become God-like through a life of virtue and the cultivation of the spirit through scientific knowledge, practice and bodily discipline."

"Salvation is accomplished through the efforts of the individual. There is no mediator between man and his / her salvation."

"Salvation is the freeing of the soul from its bodily fetters, becoming a God through knowledge and wisdom, controlling the forces of the cosmos instead of being a slave to them, subduing the lower nature and through awakening the Higher Self, ending the cycle of rebirth and dwelling with the Neters who direct and control the Great Plan."

Yoga Practice in Ancient Egypt and the Connection to Yoga in India

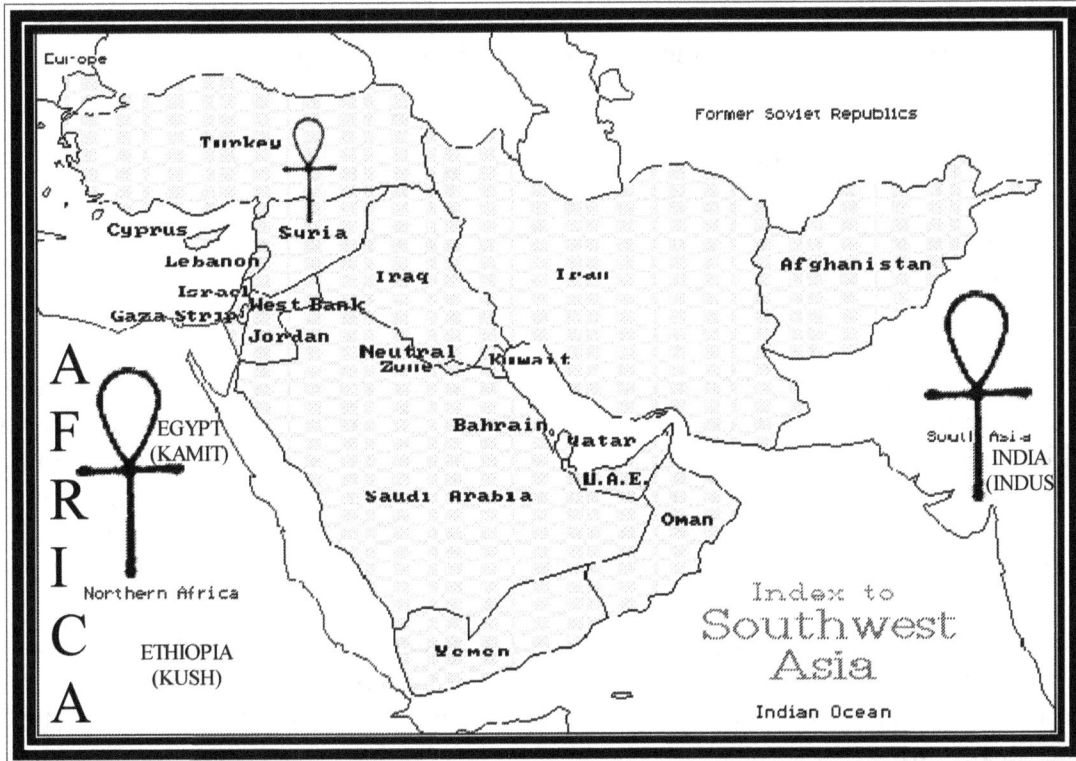

Above: Map of Northeast Africa, Asia Minor and the Indus Valley, the land area that in ancient times encompassed Ancient Egypt. The influence of Ancient Egypt was felt in the civilizations that developed in Asia Minor and in India.

Egyptian Yoga is the Basis of Indian Yoga
♀ ॐ

In ancient times, North-East Africa and Southern Asia were populated by the same cultural and ethnic group. This was confirmed by such ancient Greek historians as Herodotus and Diodorus.

> *"And upon his return to Greece, they gathered around and asked, "tell us about this great land of the Blacks called Ethiopia." And Herodotus said, "There are two great Ethiopian nations, one in Sind (India) and the other in Egypt."*

Recorded by *Diodorus* (Greek historian 100 B.C.)

During this time, the myth of Horus, the Savior who was persecuted by his uncle, was also known in India in the form of Krishna, the Indian savior who was also persecuted by his uncle. In addition to this story there are other important correlations between Egypt and India with respect to the Gods, Osiris and Shiva as well as ritual practices and myths along with their wisdom teachings. Some of these correlations were explored in the book *Egyptian Yoga: The Philosophy of Enlightenment.*

Indian tradition, like Egyptian tradition, encompasses many hundreds of deities and mythological stories. Perhaps the most popular deity in the Indian pantheon of Gods is Krishna. Krishna is an incarnation of the God Vishnu, who is a member of the Indian Trinity (Brahma, Vishnu, Shiva) which, like the ancient Egyptian Trinity, emerge from the Absolute transcendental Self. In India this Absolute Self is known as *Brahman.*

Vedanta AND Yoga philosophy IN INDIA

Vedanta philosophy originated from the ancient spiritual scriptures of India called the *Vedas* meaning "knowledge." The Vedas are related to a specific kind of knowledge, specifically, to knowledge which is heard. The ancient Sages who recorded the Vedic hymns were said to have heard them while being absorbed in transcendental realms of consciousness. Therefore, they wrote out of their divine inspiration. In essence, the Vedas were a product of the combination of the philosophy of the Aryans who had influenced India and the indigenous spiritual philosophy which already existed there.

Vedanta philosophy more specifically refers to the end of the Vedas or the scriptures commonly referred to as *the Upanishads* which constituted a revision as well as a summary or distillation of the highest philosophy of the Vedas. However, Vedanta also includes the teachings from the *Bhagavad Gita* wherein Lord Krishna expounds the various paths of Yoga in one comprehensive text for the first time. The term "Upanishad" means "to sit close to" referring to the Guru - Disciple relationship in which the student sits close to the teacher in order to be taught the mysteries of spirituality. Therefore, the Upanishads represent an evolution in the understanding of the original teaching given in the Vedas and the format in which their wisdom

BEGINNERS GUIDE TO THE PRACTICE OF NETERIAN SPIRITUALITY DISCIPLINES

is to be taught. The following segment from the *Mundaka Upanishad* details the view of the two sets of scriptures in relation to each other and the two forms of knowledge.

> *Those who know Brahman... say that there are two kinds of knowledge, the higher and the lower. The lower is knowledge of the Vedas* (the Rik, the Sama, the Yajur, and the Atharva), *and also of phonetics, grammar, etymology, meter, and astronomy. The higher is the knowledge of that by which one knows the changeless reality.*

Vedanta philosophy, as it exists in the present, is a combination of Buddhist psychology, mental and physical Yoga disciplines, Hindu mythology, and ancient metaphysical philosophy from the Upanishads. Having its original roots in the philosophy of the oneness of GOD who manifests in a myriad of ways, Vedanta achieves a balanced blend of all the philosophies and has been adapted by the present day Sages for modern day society. Modern Vedanta includes the 16 Yogas (8 major, 8 minor) of Sage Patanjali, which was an adaptation from the Buddhist *Wheel of Life*. In later times, Sage Shankaracarya expounded on the non-dualist aspect of Vedanta called *Advaita*. This exposition has had a profound effect on the refinement of the understanding originally presented in the Upanishads and in the seventh century ACE, what is regarded to be the most complete and refined exposition of Vedanta, *The Yoga Vasistha,* was written.

Summary of Yoga-Vedanta philosophy

Vedanta is based on the philosophy of Brahman and Atman. Brahman is the Absolute, omnipresent Reality which pervades the entire universe. It is the goal of the Vedantin (follower of Vedanta Philosophy) to attain personal experience and understanding of the essential being of Brahman through direct revelation. The innermost Self of the individual Vedantin is Atman and this Atman or Jiva (individual soul) is in reality one with Brahman, the universal consciousness. Brahman is beyond all material forms and consists of existence, consciousness or knowledge and bliss. Brahman, much like the Shetai, Neter, Nebertcher or Neter Neteru concept of ancient Egypt is not a deity. Brahman a conscious being, infinite and eternal, and is the origin of all that exists. Thus, as the Absolute of all things known, Brahman is incapable of being circumscribed or characterized by any one thing, concept or even by the totality of all things. Any attempt to encapsulate this divinity by saying that it belongs to a particular religion or to say that a particular philosophy can explain it would be considered idolatrous because, encompassing all and transcending all including thoughts, there are no thoughts or concepts which can fathom its depths or discern its true essence. There is only one way to "know" this Transcendental Absolute Self and that is to become one with it.

When the term transcendental is used as an appellation for the High Divinity, it implies beyond definition and beyond all concepts of the mind. This is also implied by the term Absolute. This is the highest conception of yogic philosophy in regard to the ultimate Supreme Being in ancient Egypt and India, as well as the true understanding of "God the Father" in Christianity and "Allah" of Islam.

Yoga-Vedanta holds that the true essence of humankind is Divine, not mortal - Omnipotent, not individualized. The Problem with Humanity: Individual human existence is a result of identification with one's body, sensual pleasures, desire, imaginations and passions as abiding realities due to a mind overcome by mental fetters which originate in ***IGNORANCE.***

The Solution to the Problem: The eradication of ignorance about the true Self gives rise to union (YOGA) with the Higher Self.

The Process of YOGA:

According to the teachings of *Jnana Yoga* or the Yoga of Wisdom, the process of Yoga consists of three steps:

1- ***Shravana:*** **Listening** to Wisdom teachings. Having achieved the qualifications of an aspirant, there is a desire to listen to the teachings from a Spiritual Preceptor. There is increasing intellectual understanding of the scriptures and the meaning of truth versus untruth, real versus unreal, temporal versus eternal.

2- ***Manana:*** **Reflection** on those teachings and living according to the disciplines enjoined by the teachings until the wisdom is fully understood. Reflection implies discovering the oneness behind the multiplicity of the world by engaging in intense inquiry into the nature of one's true Self..

3- ***Niddidhyasana:*** **Meditation** The process of reflection leads to a state in which the mind is continuously introspective. It means expansion of consciousness culminating in revelation of and identification with the Absolute Self: Brahman.

THE TEACHINGS TO BE LISTENED TO:

The wisdom teachings are to be heard in ***SATSANG****.* Satsanga is the discourse of a qualified teacher who explains the various scriptural teachings.

Vedanta philosophy has been called *The heart of Hinduism* since it represents the central teachings upon which the rest of Hindu philosophies are based. This is why Vedanta is referred to as the end of the Vedas. The *end* implies a distillation or extraction of the purest essence of the Vedas, therefore, the Upanishads are the principal *Vedantic* texts. Vedanta Philosophy is summed up in four *Mahavakyas* or *Great Utterances* (words of power - mantras) to be found in the Upanishads:

1- Brahman, the Absolute, is Consciousness beyond all mental concepts. The teacher explains to the student the nature of the Absolute.

2- Thou Art That. The teacher then tells the student that he/she, and in fact, that everyone is essentially this same consciousness in their innermost being.

3- I Am Brahman, the Absolute (I am GOD). This statement is to be recited by the aspirants referring to their own essential nature once they have been told *Thou art That.*

4- The Self is Brahman (The Self and Brahman are one).

Compare to the Bible:

On the essence of GOD: *"GOD is everywhere and in all things."* (Deuteronomy   4:7)

On the name of GOD: *"I Am That I Am."* (Exodus 3:14)

Jesus speaks of his own origin and identity: *"I and the Father (GOD) are ONE."* (John 10:30)

Compare the preceding statements in the Indian Upanishads and the Christian Bible to the following Ancient Egyptian scriptures (*Metu Neter,* Sacred Speech) taken from the *Egyptian Book of Coming Forth By Day* and other hieroglyphic texts:

Nuk Pu Nuk. ("I Am That I Am.")

In reference to the relationship between GOD and Mankind:

Ntef änuk änuk Ntef. ("He is I and I am He.")

In reference to the nature of God:

"The One who has made all things."
"GOD is a Spirit, a hidden Spirit, the Spirit of Spirits...The Divine Spirit."

"GOD creates but was never created."

"GOD endures without increase or diminution."

"GOD multiplies himself millions of times, and He is manifold in forms and members."

SHETAUT NETER AND VEDANTA

We will now go more deeply into the history of religion and mystical philosophy in India since our study has drawn a direct relationship between Egyptian and Indian culture. When we refer to Egyptian Yoga, we are specifically referring to the metaphysical teachings, derived from the words and ways of the gods and goddesses (Neteru) as they relate to THE GOD (Pa NETER), which lead the individual human soul to achieve a *mystical* experience of union with that transcendental Absolute Self. Mystical experience implies that the worshiper ceases the thoughts of the mind which involve personal identification with the body, ego and individuality. The individual becomes one with God by an immediate, direct, intuitive knowledge of God (Neter Neteru). This is the aim to be attained through personal religious experience in the mysteries of the *Shetai Neteru.*

Hinduism is referred to as a religion that originated in India. However, Hinduism is not a religion. The word Hindu is derived from the Sanskrit word *sindhu* ("river," referring to the Indus river). In the 5th century BCE, the Persians began to call the people of that area Hindus, which identified them as the people who lived in the land of the Indus. While most of the people of India who follow one of the indigenous religions of India are called Hindus, there is in reality no such thing as a "Hindu Religion." This is because the population of India comprises a vast array of theological views. These presently include: Buddhism, Brahmanism, Jainism, Vasudevaya* - Krishna Cult, Christianity, Samkhya Philosophy, followers of Shiva, followers of Vishnu*, Vedanta Philosophy, Shaktism, Tantrism, Yoga Philosophy, Sikhism and others. Therefore, it would be just as erroneous to label all Indians "Hindus" as it would be to call all of the people who live in the United States "Christians." For a more complete listing of traditions within Hinduism, review the section entitled Chronology of Indian Philosophy on page 25 of the book *Egyptian Yoga: The Philosophy of Enlightenment* and Appendix A: A Chronology of World Religious, Mythological and Philosophical Systems. (*related systems)

The link between ancient Egypt and India is evidenced in the Vedanta, Krishna, Tantra, and Yoga philosophies of India. Vedanta is primarily a metaphysical system of yoga philosophy which is based on the Upanishads. In the same way that the Shetai Neteru shows that the initiate who is called "The Osiris" is one with the Supreme Divinity, who is also called "Osiris", Vedanta leads the aspirant toward the understanding of the nature of the individual human soul, *Atman,* as being one with the Absolute Reality, *Brahman* (God). The Vedantic philosophy of Yoga incorporates complete disciplines of mental and physical exercises designed to lead the aspirant to transcend the sense of personal identity, clearing the way for an experience of union with the Divine Self. Tantric philosophy involves both metaphysical wisdom teachings and yogic disciplines and is considered to be the forerunner of yoga and the originator of many yogic techniques such as Mantras.

For a detailed comparative study of Indian religions, see the new book *AFRICAN ORIGINS OF CIVILIZATION, RELIGION AND YOGA SPIRITUALITY* by Dr. Muata Ashby. For our understanding it is important to distinguish between the indigenous Indian philosophies and those influences which altered the indigenous philosophies through invasions such as the Aryans. The Aryans were a group of peoples whose culture influenced the Indus Valley (c. 1500-1000 BCE) and incorporated new deities and theological ideas into the existing religious system of the indigenous native inhabitants of India who at that time previously maintained a high level of civilization from as early as 2500 BCE. Having acquired power over the Indus Valley peoples by, the Aryans created and set themselves up (c. 1000 BCE) as the head of a caste system. This caste system classified people based their function in society.

The ancient sages recognized five categories of people within all societies at all times: Those who have no aspiration in life (indigents, social outcasts), those who are bound to sense enjoyments and thus unable to apply themselves toward spiritual disciplines (Sudras), those whose goal in life is to accumulate wealth (Vaisyas), those who seek power and status (Kshatriya) and those who seek to attain enlightenment (Brahmins-meaning those who seek to know Brahman, The Absolute Supreme Being). The system described by the ancient seers was not rigid. There was no brick wall which people of different localities, skin color, sex or occupations could not cross. This is evinced by the ancient texts which speak of female sages and other saints who started life at a lower status (being worldly minded) and then later became "Brahmins" through their spiritual attainments. In a general way, these categories also represent stages within the life of each individual. You begin life being unsure of what you want to do in life. As a result you go along, indulging in the sensory pleasures of the world. At some point you recognize the need to acquire money and explore your creativity, and in striving to do so, you also seek recognition for your work. Eventually when you realize the emptiness of all your worldly endeavors, you turn to spirituality to explore the deeper meaning of life.

Much later (1,000 years) in the history of the Vedic tradition, about 200 B.C.E. With the institution of the "Laws of Manu", the leaders of the Vedic tradition that was originally started by the Aryans and their indigenous Indian followers saw an opportunity to use the classifications introduced above as a means to create a caste system to set themselves up as perpetual controllers of society and thus instituted rigid rules of social separation and racial discrimination similar to that which has been practiced in modern times in Hitler's fascist political movement in Germany, the apartheid system South Africa and the system of slavery, racism and discrimination in United States and Europe. In much the same way that Christian Popes and other religious leaders sanctioned the African slave trade and the conquest of the Americas which later led to modern forms of racism and the death of millions of Africans and Native Americans, the powerful Brahman leaders transformed society into a caste system of sexual and racial discrimination. The caste system was now set up to provide a basis for an organized system of social relationships based on the skin color and gender. They redefined the categories of society described by the ancient sages in terms of their new caste system: priests (Brahmins), warriors/nobles (Kshatriyas), merchants (Vaisyas), and laborers (Sudras). Laborers represented those in society who offered service to society through bodily labor. Merchants represented those members of society who served society through trade and commerce. Nobles represented members of society who served as society's warriors (protectors), politicians and rulers. The priests or Brahmins represented those who, claiming to be spiritually advanced, assumed the role government through a system of oligarchy (government by the few and elite members of society).

In addition, the fifth caste became known as "the untouchables." This caste was made up of the darkest skinned segment of the population who were of more direct African descent and became the least educated and provided for by society. In general, women's positions were relegated to a low status wherein they were considered as having no more value than a slave whose life was controlled by the master (men). It should be noted here that while the position of women in society and religious rituals fell with the emergence of the Aryan patriarchal system, there remained a strong sense of the female principle in the religious traditions, most prominently in the Tantric systems of religion. There were those who did not agree with the denigration of women and separation based on skin color. The Vedantic system is opposed to any form of discrimination or violence against any human being. The ancient spiritual scriptures also do not support this system of social order. Therefore it must be differentiated from Hinduism.

In modern times, Mahatma Ghandi and other great saints within the Hindu community have spoken out against the caste system and consider it to be an evil social system which has nothing to do with religion. They rightly explain that the soul is sexless and raceless and that distinctions on these basis are of a highly egoistic nature.

All human beings are composed of the same substance: energy. This point is supported by modern scientific discoveries. Therefore, regardless of appearance, all human beings are in reality alike. The differences are only due to karmic experiences which have led the soul to incarnate as a member of a particular ethnic group or sex. With this information, it is clear to understand that someone who is of a particular ethnic group or sex have been and will become members of other groups throughout their many incarnations. The teachings say that what you focus your mind on will envelop your consciousness at your time of death and propel your circumstances in your next incarnation. From this perspective, if someone puts a lot of energy into hating a particular ethnic group, it is possible that they may incarnate as a member of that group, and still being filled with hate, seek to do violence upon the ethnic group of their previous birth. In this process of reincarnation, there are unlimited possibilities. Thus, the ignorance of the soul leads it to experience countless circumstances which lead to experiences based on the desires of the mind. When these desires are based on ignorance, they lead to unimaginable forms of pain and sorrow, endlessly until enlightenment is attained.

Within that group which is referred to as "Brahmins", there are those who even to this day believe in the caste system while there are others who call themselves Brahmins because they are followers of Brahman, the Absolute Supreme Deity. There are over 600 different Christian denominations throughout the world at present. In the same way that all Christians and Christianity cannot be condemned because of the actions of certain individuals and groups, the varying philosophies of India should not be repudiated or put down due to the activities of one group.

When most people think of India, there is an image of poverty and lower technological status as compared to the western world. However, there is another image which encompasses India as a very religious land, full of religious people with a temple on every corner. In reality, India is populated by a people not so different from the rest of humanity. As such, they encompass a wide range of beliefs, both political and religious. There are some who eat meat while others are vegetarians. In fact, many Indians are becoming swept up in the frenzy for material wealth as a result of their exposure to Western culture. Many Indians, like many Westerners and members of other cultures in modern times, practice only the outer or elementary forms of religion such as regular visits to churches and Temples, but do not truly delve deeply into the mysteries of the philosophy which would lead them to understand how to promote real social order and spiritual enlightenment. For those who are ready to ask more serious questions and to intensify their practice of Yoga, there is a well established system of initiation to direct them along the spiritual path.

The wise aspirant should put aside his/her preconceived notions and seek to eradicate ALL prejudices and illusions about the world, humanity, history and divinity in order to investigate the nature of the universe and of the innermost Self. All of these questions should be investigated with a dispassionate intellectual eye, having developed the faculty of discriminative reasoning to discover for him/herself the teachings of these philosophies in order to discover the correct path for themselves. Those who simply believe in what they are taught by anyone other than an

44

enlightened spiritual preceptor are subject to error. Therefore, do not be eager to believe what your hear from even the most eloquent or knowledgeable speakers. Seek to prove spiritual truths within yourself. However, once you have become convinced of the higher level of consciousness within your chosen teacher, you should whole heartedly study and follow their teachings. Of course, *higher level of consciousness* here refers to their level of attunement to the Self, their ego-lessness, humility and intuitive understanding of the teachings, and not just the level of intellectual knowledge which they possess or appear to possess. Your actions in the mystical sciences should be governed by reason and truth, MAAT, Dharma, the Beatitudes or virtues as in all other areas.

Egyptian Yoga is the Basis of Christian Spirituality

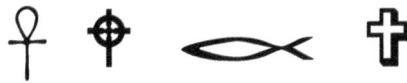

In 1945, the discovery of 52 *Gnostic* texts at Nag Hammadi, Egypt, which dated back to the time of the biblical Jesus, have redefined the manner in which the social climate during the time of Jesus is being viewed by scholars and religious theologians. Up to the time of their discovery, it was known that many sects of Christian groups existed. These groups were considered to be outcasts and heretics by the Roman Catholic groups. Many existing scriptures of the time were claimed by their proponents to have been inspired by Jesus. The *Gospel of Thomas* is one of the most important Gnostic Christian texts. It is not written in parable form like the gospels of the Bible although it has many correlations to them. In the Gospel of Thomas, the teachings of Jesus are in concordance with the Egyptian Mysteries, Indian Tantrism and the Tao of China.

Therefore, traditional Christianity as it has come to be know by the world at large is only a portion of the true picture of Christian Philosophy. By the time the Roman Catholic Church had compiled and canonized the scriptures which would make up the present day Christian Bible, these works had undergone many revisions and changes. Modern scientific x-ray tests have proven that the earliest papyrus manuscripts on which the Christian texts were written were changed, erased and written over as many as 14,000 times or more. It is also known that the early councils of the Roman Catholic Bishops altered, edited and even omitted gospels and other books from the Bible. Thus, we must understand that the teachings of Christianity which have been handed down through traditional sources are not the complete nor are they the original teachings. Through the study of the origins of Christianity, it is possible to discover a more complete view of ancient mystical Christian philosophy.

The ancient Christian texts discovered in Egypt show a different side of Christianity which relates to the mystical nature of the true meaning of the symbols and practices of the faith and directly link Christianity to the mysteries of Osiris, Isis and Horus. For example, the symbols of Christianity above were used in ancient Egypt prior to the Christian era. Many other correlations between ancient Egypt, India and Christianity were discussed in *Egyptian Yoga: The Philosophy of Enlightenment*. You should keep in mind that the mystical teachings of Vedanta and Gnostic Christianity have a common origin in Egypt. Therefore, with the correct understanding, the

Egyptian Mysteries, Gnostic Christianity and Yoga-Vedanta can be studied and understood in a complementary way, each providing insights into the wisdom of the others.

Christianity centers around the story of Jesus who is an incarnation of God. Christianity developed as a new movement out of the already existing Hebrew tradition, itself also having its origins in ancient Egypt. Christian Yoga is based on Gnostic Christianity, a tradition of Christianity which involves the practice of developing Divine love for God, all humanity and nature in an effort to become Christ-like, and thereby resurrected as a new human being with Divine self knowledge. This process of resurrection implies becoming one with God through a divine marriage of the individual soul with the Absolute Spirit. This is what is meant by attaining the Kingdom of Heaven. Thus, Jesus represents the ordinary human being, the human soul, who incarnates on earth and suffers the pain of mortal life. Through spiritual practice and Christian living (selfless service and universal love), Jesus (the individual soul), becomes Christ and attains the Kingdom of Heaven.

The Mystical Plan of Christianity:

The Kingdom of Heaven

↑

Christ

↑

Jesus

The subject of Christian Yoga is a vast topic of study. It will be covered extensively in an upcoming book by Dr. Muata Ashby entitled: **"The Mystical Journey from Jesus to Christ."**

HORUS, JESUS AND KRISHNA

Lord Krishna is a God form or symbol within the Indian Hindu mythological system. He represents an incarnation of the Supreme Being or Brahman. Literally translated, the name "Krishna" means "Black" or "The Black One." Therefore, Lord Krishna and Osiris both were known as "The Black One." Krishna of India and Horus of Egypt have equivalent symbolism in that they show, through their myths, what is correct action that leads the way to salvation.

46

In the same way that Horus was persecuted after his birth by the King of Egypt, his uncle, Set, who had murdered Horus' father (Osiris), Jesus was persecuted after his birth because the ruling king feared that Jesus would take the throne which was rightfully his. Like Horus, Krishna was also viciously persecuted from the time of his birth by his uncle, the king, because he was also prophesied to be the righteous king who would end the injustices of the existing king. The evil King Kamsa, Krishna's uncle, foresaw that Krishna would assume the kingship and defeat him, so Kamsa ordered that all male children born around the same time as Krishna be killed (this part also parallels the story of Jesus).

Like the eyes of Horus, the eyes of Krishna represent the Sun and the Moon, duality unified into one whole. Krishna was born of a virgin mother as were Horus and Jesus, to fight the forces of evil on earth. As with Horus, he contained the entire Universe in his essence, as do all humans.

Horus, Jesus Christ and Krishna are symbols of the Soul in each of us which is the innermost Self that is constantly engaged in a battle of opposites (duality) within our minds and physical bodies over good-evil, virtue-vice, light-dark, ying-yang, positive-negative, prosperity-adversity, etc.

The correspondence in the birth stories of Horus, Krishna and Jesus is only one correlation out of many which point to a common origin of these traditions. If these myths are understood literally, then it would be odd to discover exact stories which match in almost every detail in different lands. The chances of this occurring is remote at best. However, if they are seen as mythological stories with deeper messages, then we are able to see that there is a common origin and that these stories refer not to an event which occurred long ago, but to an ongoing process which is occurring in the life of every human being even now.

The story surrounding the birth of a savior was never intended to be understood in a factual or literal sense or as referring to a single character or personality in history. There is something more important, beyond the actual facts themselves, which the ancient sages sought to convey. Principally, we are to understand that a savior is a metaphor for that principle within each of us which seeks to be saved from the clutches of egoism and to discover true peace and happiness. It is you, your deeper Self, who is the incarnating soul, and it is you who are persecuted by the world with its endless attempts to force you to conform, to give up your freedom and to succumb to the joys and sorrows, negativity and illusions of the world. But it is also you who, through your own intellect expanded by wisdom (understanding the teachings) and self-effort directed toward the divine, who can effect your own salvation and triumph over the forces of evil (selfishness, greed, hatred, lust, etc.).

Thus, myths surrounding these three saviors point to a special connection between ancient Egyptian Religion which worshipped Horus as the incarnation of Osiris, Indian Vaishnavism - Vasudeva cult which worshipped the God Krishna as the incarnation of Vishnu and Christianity which worships Jesus Christ as an embodiment or incarnation of God (the word of God) on earth.

In reference to the terms Horushood, Christhood and Krishnahood, the word ending "hood" is an appellation used here to reference the highest achievements of Horus, Jesus Christ and Krishna. The word "*Christ*" is not a name but a title, like Vice-President is a title. *"Christ"* means: *"He or she whose head is Anointed with oil"* or *"The Anointed One."* Horus, Sage, Saint, Buddha, Christ, Krishna, etc. are terms or names to describe the same thing. Horushood or Christhood refers to certain qualities exhibited by mythological or historical personalities as symbols representing the potential state of enlightenment of every sentient being in the universe.

Christs are those persons who have attained complete purification of their psychological personality. They experience cosmic consciousness, the experience of being one (identifying oneself) with everything.

So, salvation (achieving oneness with the Divine) comes from ATTAINING Horushood, Christhood, Buddhahood, etc., that is, becoming a Horus, Christ or Buddha through a life of virtue, wisdom, courage and Self-Knowledge. Those who become a Horus, Christ or Buddha have attained the consciousness that survives death and will live on after their death of the body, being free from ignorance.

THE DIVINE MOTHERS

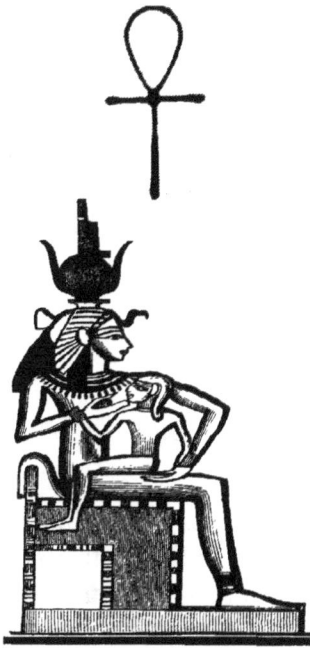

Isis nurses baby Horus:
The ancient Egyptian version of the
mother and child
(The Madonna).

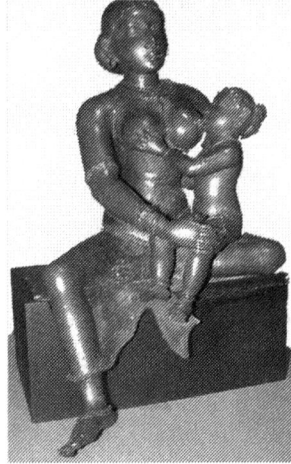

Above: The image of The Maddona from
modern India, c. 16th century A.C.E.
based on ancient Indian Mythology 600
BCE *Yasoda nurses the child Krishna.*

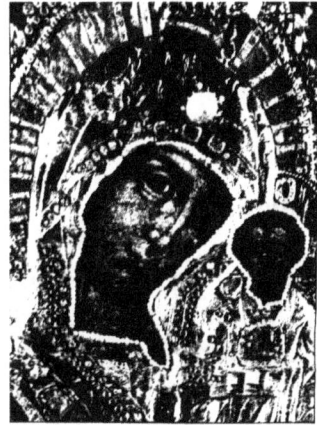

The Christian Madonna and Jesus

THE DIVINE CHILDREN

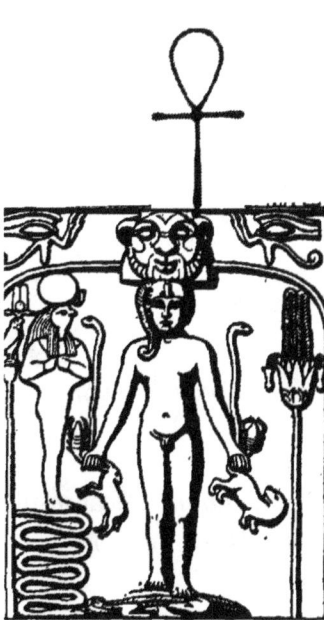

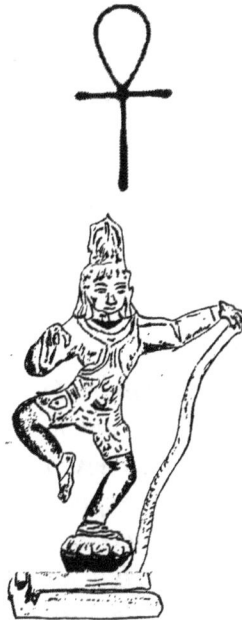

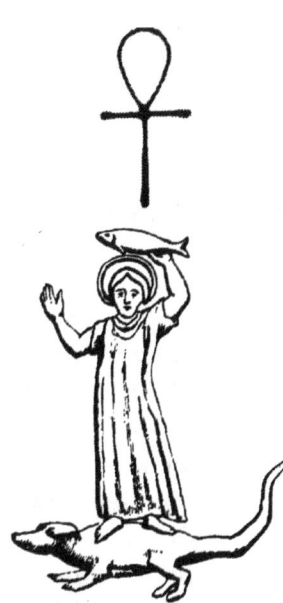

Top center: Horus the child in control of the forces of nature. At left: Krishna in the same aspect.
At right: Jesus in the same aspect.

CHAPTER II
The Initiatic Way of Education
And The Process of Initiation

INTRODUCTION

What is initiation?

Many people thing of initiation, when associated with spiritual studies, as some kind of fantastic event which will in and of itself cause a major transformation in a person's life. Initiation should be thought of less as an event and more as the process of embarking on a journey of spiritual living which will lead to spiritual enlightenment. With this broad understanding it should be clear that this entire book is initiating you, the reader, into the higher teachings of life. Every time you turn a page you are learning more and more about the world and as you do you are learning more about yourself. In this section we will discuss the process of initiation and the way in which spiritual knowledge is imparted.

From time immemorial the tradition of teacher and student has been carried on by Sages and Saints the world over. This is evident even in the world religions. Horus of Ancient Egypt was initiated into the mystical teachings by Aset (Isis). Rama (A form of Krishna) was initiated into the teachings by Sage Vasistha. Jesus was initiated into the teachings by John the Baptist. As in any other discipline of life spiritual studies require an authentic teacher. However, even the greatest teacher cannot teach a person who is not qualified to learn. Therefore, we will begin by enumerating the ten virtues of a spiritual aspirant. These imply the qualities that anyone desiring to practice spirituality needs to work on to develop.

The ancient Egyptian precepts of initiatic education

(1) "Control your thoughts,"
(2) "Control your actions,"
(3) "Have devotion of purpose,"
(4) "Have faith in your master's ability to lead you along the path of truth,"
(5) "Have faith in your own ability to accept the truth,"
(6) "Have faith in your ability to act with wisdom,"
(7) "Be free from resentment under the experience of persecution" (Bear insult)
(8) "Be free from resentment under experience of wrong," (Bear injury)
(9) "Learn how to distinguish between right and wrong,"
(10) "Learn to distinguish the real from the unreal."

THE QUALITIES OF AN ASPIRANT

The first qualification necessary for a spiritual aspirant is that he or she must have the *initiative* or primary interest in advancing spiritually. It is no coincidence that the word "initiative" and the word "initiation" convey a similar connotation. You must be the one to take the first step toward your own spiritual emancipation. You must be the one to approach others of higher spiritual development so that you may begin to discover the path which you wish to follow toward your eventual freedom from all worldly pains and sorrows. In short, it is you who must put forth the effort which will effect your own liberation from the bondage of illusion and ignorance which grips the masses of people all over the world. Having discovered this initiative within yourself, you are qualified to receive spiritual instruction.

The ancient spiritual texts of all traditions state that it behooves an aspirant to seek out the true wisdom which alleviates the pain and sorrow of human existence while elevating the human spirit. If the wisdom one holds has not produced an improvement in one's quality of life, then it is possible that the teaching or its practice is wrong. In the task of spiritual practice there is no mediator between oneself and one's higher Self. However, a guide is needed to show the way to discover the true Self in much the same way as any other human endeavor. Someone who is knowledgeable about the spiritual path can help in advising and teaching others. Take for example a concert pianist or an N.B.A. basketball star. Both of these professionals perfected their skills through correct teaching and practice, beginning from a point of utter ignorance to the level of spontaneous performance. In order to excel at spiritual development, one must apply the correct technique and practice daily. This is the path of Yoga, exercising conscious effort every day to unite oneself with the higher Self.

Yoga, the union of the individual human consciousness with the universal consciousness, can occur without any special instruction from a religious or a spiritual preceptor. This is known as the path of nature or as it is better known, the school of hard knocks. It involves repeated incarnations, pain and suffering, to teach you the futility of trying to find abiding happiness in the world rather than within yourself.

Although much of the Egyptian teachings have diffused into the world religions, in the course of time they have been misinterpreted and reconfigured so that there is great confusion and misunderstanding as to their true meaning. This has created a situation in which many present day clergy speak the teachings but do not have a clear understanding of how to apply them in their own lives to transcend the pain and suffering of existence, let alone, be able to enlighten their followers as to how to evolve spiritually.

Yoga is a tradition which has established a long proven record of success in teaching those who desire to discover the Self. The traditional approach to yoga instruction has been broken up into three stages. These are: 1-Listening, 2- Reflection and 3- Meditation. In a broad sense, you will be instructed in this same manner throughout this book series. First you will receive the teaching, then you will be assisted in reflecting on that teaching and incorporating it into your life. You will then be instructed on how to intensify your reflective movement and gradually reach a meditative state of concentration on the divine.

Every true mystical tradition, be it religious or non-religious, requires a traditional mystical link because initiatic teaching given to those who become initiated into a tradition, needs the benefit of a preceptor who has received the teaching from an enlightened teacher and has correct understanding of the teaching. Otherwise it would be, as an Eastern parable explains, like a blind person trying to explain to other blind people what the world looks like simply using imagination and wit. There are others, intellectuals, who come to believe that they have attained "Enlightenment" because they read the scriptures. However, when they are tested by natural human situations of adversity, they cannot control their emotions or find mental peace. Some, immersed in the subtle ignorance and egoism of the mind don't even realize their misunderstanding of the teachings and of their own attainment or spiritual level.

Others study the teachings with earnestness and great seriousness and find that they cannot realize the subtlety of the teachings in order to effect their Enlightenment. They find that they cannot control their minds, emotions or desires as the teachings suggest and thus are unable to discover the deeper meaning of the teachings.

An example of the inability to control the mind is the cigarette smoker. He or she "knows" that smoking is poisonous and yet they are unable to stop. Why? Because their self-knowledge is superficial (egoistic) and they have not discovered the wellspring of will and inner fulfillment within themselves so they continue to search for fulfillment outside of themselves through objects which seem to gratify their needs. In reality, these external habits that seem to bring pleasure are in reality leading to greater pain and disappointment. i.e. asthma, heart disease and lung cancer along with greater restlessness and mental unrest.

Still, others seek to escape the world as they know it by immersing themselves in work, drugs or other intense distractions. An example of this type of personality is someone who needs constant activity so as not to feel lonely or bored. This personality is constantly searching for action by turning on the television, calling someone, gossiping or having some other interaction. If this attitude becomes intensified, this personality seeks to agitate him/herself constantly by always finding something to be upset or argumentative about. Unless there is a fight or other intense emotion present, this personality feels lost. Those who suffer from this defect have developed an intense dependency on sense perceptions and emotions. They cannot feel right unless there is some activity present, be it positive or negative. Even if there is no trouble, they will create trouble, so as to agitate their minds and feel "alive."

A sage does not live a life based on the sense perceptions nor on the desires of the mind and body. He or she has discovered the illusoriness of the senses, the emptiness of desires and the futility of trying to fulfill them in the realm of time and space. Those who are advancing on the spiritual path have discovered that they do not need to lean on sense perceptions to feel alive, nor on events to make themselves feel happy. They have begun to discover that sustenance and happiness comes from within. It is there that all desires are truly fulfilled. For this reason, proper initiation into a teaching and learning under the instruction of an enlightened master or a senior student who is in association with a master is necessary in order to develop the correct understanding and practice of the teachings.

While the teachings may seem explicit to the highly intellectual mind, there are nuances of misunderstanding which will occur. This is why association with an authentic teacher is essential on the spiritual path for those who are serious about their spiritual development. Any other learning process is subject to error and confusion which will lead to disappointment and frustration. The initiatic teachings exist as an alternative to ordinary worldly thinking.

Christianity, having originally been an initiatic mystery religion, was no different in its approach of the transference of the teachings from teacher to student. Long before the establishment of Christianity as a religion, water was used in ceremonies to initiate new followers into the philosophy of mystery religions. Prior to entering a temple in Egypt and other countries, people would bathe as a symbol of inner purification. Christianity adopted this ritual and it was used at the initiation of Jesus by John the Baptist. This ritual act served to link Jesus to a tradition into which he would later initiate his disciples as well. But what was this initiatic relationship all about? What was its purpose and how was this purpose to be accomplished? These are very important questions for anyone seriously considering treading the spiritual path. Therefore, it is appropriate here to discuss what aspiration really means and what an authentic teacher is.

THE QUALIFICATIONS OF AN ASPIRANT

"When the student is ready, the master will appear."

"Those who understand or believe will be persecuted and ridiculed."
—Ancient Egyptian Proverbs

When a person begins to wonder about the origin of the universe, the purpose of life, the cruelty of life, the inability to be truly happy in the world and the transitoriness of all things, such a person may be ready to inquire about the deeper truths of her/his own existence and to seek answers to such questions which have plagued them for perhaps many lifetimes.

The reason that most people accept the injustices, cruelties and sorrows of the world is that they tend to overlook the obvious illusoriness of relationships and the fleeting nature of sensory pleasure. There is lack of inquiry into the nature of pain so people go on believing that they will eventually find happiness in the world. They believe that pain is just a "normal" part of human life and as such must be accepted and dealt with as best as possible when it occurs or that they just need to be more careful to avoid painful situations in the future. They almost never entertain questions about the unreality of the world and life in general and when they do, they might turn to others who are as intensely involved in the world and by so doing, become once again distracted with the burdens of life.

"Passions and irrational desires are ills exceedingly great; and over these GOD hath set up the Mind to play the part of judge and executioner."
—Ancient Egyptian Proverb

A spiritual aspirant or initiate may be defined as: anyone seriously seeking spiritual development and chooses to enter (be initiated) into a lifestyle directed toward spiritual realization rather than perishable worldly attainments. But what is this lifestyle? What is required to make the goals of spiritual life become reality? Who is qualified to practice yoga and what does it mean to be a serious yogi(ni)?

The *Shiva-Samhita* (III.16-19), an Indian yoga scripture, states that the most important quality which an *adhikarini* or "qualified person" (one who is ready to learn Yoga) must have or strive to attain is *vishvasa* or a "positive frame of mind." This is followed by moderate diet, sense restraint, impartiality, and veneration of the teacher.

People who have trouble coping with life sometimes seek help through counseling with psychologists, priests, pastoral counselors or friends. In the case of a Yoga counselor or a Yogic Spiritual Preceptor (Guru), the benefits of such an association are a step beyond those of ordinary psychology and psychotherapy which seek to integrate one's personality into the accepted "norms" of the mainstream society and which considers anyone who does not adhere to such standards to be abnormal. From the perspective of yoga philosophy, much of the accepted "normal" behavior is really insane behavior which has been accepted as "normal." For example, it is accepted as "normal" to gossip, to use profanity, to become angry at others, up to a point. It is all right to scream at someone, but if you hit them then you could be sued. When that point is crossed, then measures are taken by society in an attempt to curb such behavior. In this sense, the mind of the ordinary human being is conditioned by what society promotes and what the desires and thoughts in the mind compel the person to do. From this perspective of what most people have come to know and for the most part, accept as "normal" human behavior, yoga pushes the aspirant to become "super normal." It pushes the aspirant to rise beyond his/her current level of so-called "normal" mental conditioning to conquer anger, hatred, greed, impatience, sadness, discontent and the improper use of words within him/herself.

> *"When emotions are societies objective, tyranny will govern regardless of the ruling class."*
>
> *"Indulge not thyself in the passion of Anger; it is whetting a sword to wound thine own breast, or murder thy friend."*
>
> —Ancient Egyptian Proverbs

Yoga is a process of reversing the conditioning effect which ordinary human life has on the mind. Everything which affects the mind conditions the mind; this is the nature of the mind. Ignorance of the Self is the primary and most important concern in yoga because ordinary human life intensifies ignorance, and thereby human pain and suffering as well. Yoga un-conditions the mind in order that the aspirant may attain unity with his/her Higher Self and achieve supreme freedom and supreme peace in the state of Horushood (Godhood, Christhood or Kingdom of Heaven, Liberation, Moksha, Enlightenment), instead of being trapped in the confines of the ego-self. In this sense, the practice of yoga conditions the mind so it experiences expansion while worldly conditioning and egoism results in mental contraction, dependency on the world and intensification of pain and suffering.

In the beginning, the Yogic Counselor must help the individual to somehow turn the anguish and pain experienced as a result of interaction with the world, into a desire to rise above it, as symbolized by the lotus rising out of the waters. To this end, a series of techniques and disciplines have been developed over thousands of years. The Yoga counselor needs to help the seeker restructure and channel those energies which arise from disappointment and frustration into a healthy dispassion of the world and its entanglements and spiritual aspiration and self-effort directed at sustaining a viable personal spiritual program or *Sadhana*.

The ancient Egyptian Mystery system is called *Shetaut NETER* meaning the knowledge of the hidden or secret (Shetaut) way of the Gods and Goddesses (*NETER*). Shetaut is also the name of the Absolute, the hidden and transcendental Supreme Being which sustains creation and is synonymous with the terms or names *Amun* and *Nebertcher*. In the *Shetaut NETER* system of yoga, there were three levels of aspirants.

1- **The Mortals**: Students who were being instructed on a probationary status, but had not experienced inner vision.

2- **The Intelligences**: Students who had attained inner vision and had received a glimpse of cosmic consciousness.

3- **The Creators or Beings of Light:** Students who had become IDENTIFIED with or UNITED with the light (GOD).

The teachings surrounding the cult of ISIS give important information concerning the conduct necessary to be an initiate in the mysteries of spiritual development (YOGA). The *Veil of Isis* is the veil of ignorance which blocks divine awareness from human perception. The following teaching reveals the nature of Isis, who in this aspect represents the all-encompassing Divine Self.

"I Isis, am all that has been, all that is, or shall be;
and no mortal man hath ever unveiled me."

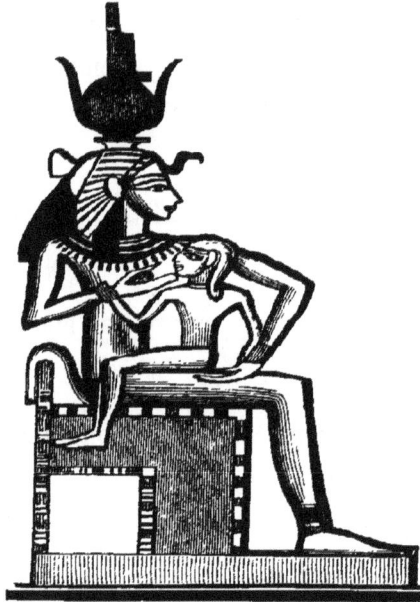

*Above: Isis nurses baby Horus (who is the
incarnation of Osiris):
The ancient Egyptian version of the mother
and child (The Madonna), and the initiation
into the teachings of Egyptian Yoga (Shetaut
Neter).*

A devotee of ISIS is: *One who ponders over sacred matters and seeks therein for hidden truth.* It is not enough to just hear the ancient myths or to understand them at an intellectual level. The aspirant must go deep within him/herself to discover the subtle ideas being conveyed. *Plutarch* describes the character of an initiate of Isis as:

> *He alone is a true servant or follower of this Goddess who, after has heard, and has been made acquainted in a proper manner (initiated into the philosophy) with the history of the actions of these gods, searches into the hidden truths which lie concealed under them, and examines the whole by the dictates of reason and philosophy. Nor indeed, ought such an examination to be looked on as unnecessary whilst there are so many ignorant of the true reason even of the most ordinary rites observed by the Egyptian priests, such as their shavings* and wearing linen garments. Some, indeed, there are, who never trouble themselves to think at all about these matters, whilst others rest satisfied with the most superficial accounts of them: They pay a peculiar veneration to the sheep,** therefore they think it their duty not only to abstain from eating flesh, but likewise from wearing its wool. They are continually mourning for their gods, therefore they shave themselves.*

*In the *Papyrus of Nes-Menu*, there is an order to the priestesses of Isis and Nephthys to have "the hair of their bodies shaved off." They are also ordered to wear fillets of rams wool on their heads 𓇋𓏏𓏤 as a form of ritual identification with the hidden (Amun) mystery. Wool was also used by the Sufis, followers of esoteric Islam. The name "*Sufi*" comes from

"Suf" which means "wool." The name Sufi was adopted since the ascetic‡ followers of this doctrine wore coarse woolen garments (sufu).
**sacred to Amun.
‡an *ascetic* is one who practices severe and austere methods of spiritual practice.

One particular statement in reference to the teachings, *...the hidden truths which lie concealed under them....,* begs the question: What are these "hidden truths" which are "concealed" within the "history of the actions of the gods?" The following statement from the Yoga Vasistha elucidates on this question, introducing us to the esoteric or metaphysical level of religion as opposed to the ritualistic-mythological level.

"O Rama, Gods and Goddesses and other deities with name and form are representations created by Sages for those whose intellect is weak as a child's..."
Yoga Vasistha Nirvana Prakarana Section 30

The elaborate system of "Gods and Goddesses" as well as the symbols representing a "Supreme Being" are merely metaphors created by the ancient Sages for those who are not spiritually mature (possessing a highly developed sense of intellectual subtlety) to understand that God transcends all thoughts, symbols and concepts of the mind. Until the intellect (*Saa*) is developed, the symbols are used but when spiritual sensitivity dawns, the hidden or esoteric meaning of the symbols is revealed, leading the initiate to greater and greater levels of inner awareness or Enlightenment.

Isis represents the Supreme teacher (preceptor) of the mysteries. Having attained spiritual knowledge by listening to the teachings of Isis, the task of the initiate is continuously reflected upon them until the veil of ignorance (egoism) is lifted. Through the process of continued intellectual refinement (reflection on the teachings), the veil is torn away. Thus, the mortal consciousness (symbolized by the veil) is transcended and Isis is realized in her unveiled form. In order to behold her unveiled form, ordinary human perception cannot be used. This is why *no mortal man* has unveiled her. Only those who have become like Isis (divine in consciousness) can see her. Through gradual intellectual refinement attained through the process of reflection and meditation, the mind of the initiate becomes transformed. Thus, the initiate sees with Divine eyes and not with mortal ones. He or she is now beyond birth and death (mortality).

Unveiling Isis is unveiling your true Self. One must go beyond the "mortal" waking, dream-sleep and dreamless-deep-sleep states of consciousness to discover (unveil) one's true nature. Over five thousand years before the rise in prominence of the cult of Isis and Osiris in Greece and Rome, the Egyptian *Pyramid Texts* described the process of spiritual transformation through the mythology surrounding the *Eye* of Horus and its return to the initiate following its theft by Set (see ***Egyptian Yoga: The Philosophy of Enlightenment***). In later times, the struggle against Set was carried on in the mysteries of Isis which lasted until the year 394 A.D. when the Temple of Isis at *Philae* was closed by Christian Zealots who had taken over Egypt and Ethiopia. The process of initiation and spiritual awakening may be further defined as follows.

57

In the Indian system, the categories of students are classified by the characteristics that are favorable and unfavorable for spiritual disciplines. The serious aspirant should study these well in order to understand what is required for the successful practice of spirituality and to promote them within himself or herself.

The *Yoga Sutra* (III.7), the textbook of Classical Yoga, lists the following impediments on the yogic path: illness, languor, doubt, heedlessness, sloth, dissipation, false vision, non-attainment of the higher levels of the spiritual path, and instability in a given level of attainment. These are also called distractions (*vikshepa*) of consciousness, and the *Yoga Sutra* (I.29) prescribes the practice of mantra[2] recitation (*Japa*) and contemplation (*bhavana*) of the sacred syllable *OM* for their swift removal. The *Linga Purana* includes: lack of faith, suffering, and depression. This work states that such obstacles can be removed through constant practice and devotion to one's teacher. The *Bhagavata-Purana* includes *siddhis* (psychic paranormal powers) as mental distractions.

The *hatha-yoga* work *Shiva-Samhita* (V.10 ff.) states that the weak aspirant (*mridu*) is unenthusiastic, foolish, fickle, timid, ill, dependent, rude, ill-mannered, and un-energetic. He is considered fit only for *mantra-yoga* or the recitation of empowered sounds (*mantra*).

The mediocre aspirant (*madhya*) is endowed with even-minded-ness, patience, a desire for virtue, kind speech, and the tendency to practice moderation in all things. He/she is considered capable of practicing *laya-yoga*, or dissolution of the mind through meditative absorption.

The exceptional aspirant (*adhimatra*) is someone who shows such qualities as firm understanding, aptitude for meditative absorption (*Laya*), self-reliance, liberal-minded-ness, bravery, vigor, faithfulness, willingness to worship the "lotus feet" of the teacher, and delight in the practice of Yoga. This reference to the lotus feet of the teacher refers to the understanding that the teacher, having attained God-consciousness or Self-realization, is indeed God incarnate and therefore his/her feet should be venerated as Gods feet. (see Fig. 1)

The extraordinary aspirant (*adhimatratama*) who may practice any type of yoga, demonstrates the following virtues: great energy, enthusiasm, charm, heroism, scriptural knowledge, the inclination to practice, freedom from delusion, orderliness, youthfulness, moderate eating habits, control over the senses, fearlessness, purity, skillfulness, liberality, the ability to be a refuge for all people, capability, stability, thoughtfulness, the willingness to do whatever is desired by the teacher, patience, good manners, observance of the moral and spiritual law, the ability to keep his struggle to him/her self, kind speech, faith in the scriptures, the readiness of the divine, knowledge of the vows in his/her particular level of practice, and the active pursuit of all forms of yoga.

"I, GOD, am present with the holy and good, those who are pure and merciful, who live piously and give up their body unto its proper death. To them, my presence becomes an aid, straightway they gain inner vision, knowledge of all things, and win my love by their pure lives, and give thanks, invoking my blessings and chanting hymns, intent on the me with ardent love. It is I, who will not let the operations that befall the body work to their natural end. I'll close all

---

[2] Hekau in ancient Egyptian Terminology

the entrances, and cut the mental actions off which base and evil energies induce. Mind-less ones, the wicked and depraved, the envious and covetous, and those who murder or do and love impiety, I am far off, yielding my place to the Avenging Demon, who rusheth on them through their senses."

—Ancient Egyptian Proverb

The TEN VIRTUES of the Egyptian Initiates, presented earlier, contain three injunctions concerning faith. One of them concerns your faith in the teacher which also includes the teaching itself and the other two refer to you as the spiritual aspirant.

(4)"Have faith in your master's* ability to lead you along the path of truth,"
(5)"Have faith in your own ability to accept the truth,"
(6)"Have faith in your ability to act with wisdom,"

*The ultimate master is Osiris, the Higher Self within you.

"The self chooses the proper instruction for self."

—Ancient Egyptian Proverb

Even though your present mental capacity may seemingly be unable to understand the subtleties of the wisdom teachings, you must develop the faith that you are innately capable of conquering all the obstacles because deep down you are a divine personality endowed with boundless resources. When this faith deepens into realization, it is this "knowing" that you are endowed with all the resources within yourself to achieve Enlightenment which becomes the basis for your cultivation of contentment and peace in your personality. There is no need to be jealous or envious of others. When you see someone with a good quality, aspire to acquire that quality within yourself. You have the power to do so. When you see someone with a negative quality, recognize it and search yourself to see if you have any similar qualities and work to eliminate them within you. Once you have learned to examine yourself and maintain a watchful eye on your actions and thoughts, you will develop subtlety of intellect which will lead you toward greater and greater self control and spiritual sensitivity. If you spend time focusing on the negative qualities in others, soon you will find your personality abounding with these very qualities. It is the nature of the mind to imitate that which it focuses on, therefore, always try to focus on the positive in others. You should know the virtues well and reflect on them daily, drawing strength from your inner spirit.

A common reaction in people who are ignorant of spiritual truths and who are very much engrossed in their egos is that when they come into contact with those who have made superior spiritual achievements, they tend to look for any kind of imperfection in order to pull that person down. This could be because they internally feel ashamed of their lower status, are jealous, have been conditioned by society to ridicule and put down those above them or they misunderstand the teaching. This type of an attitude is a major obstruction on the spiritual path because unless you are very advanced, you will need guidance. It can be avoided by studying the teachings and maintaining humility, inner reflection and watchfulness of your thoughts and desires at all times.

Once faith in the teaching, the teacher and yourself is established, there must also be humility. Humility must be contrasted from humiliation. Humiliation is a sentiment which is experienced when one allows oneself to believe that one is a miserable ego-personality rather than the Supreme Monarch of all that exists. You as your true Self cannot be degraded since "you" are the basis for all that exists.

> *"HUMILITY is a greater virtue than defying death; it triumphs over vanity and conceit; conquer them in yourself first!"*
>
> —Ancient Egyptian Proverb

Thus, you can only feel humiliated when you see yourself as the body that is being ridiculed or put down. Therefore, strive to identify with your higher Self rather than your ego-self.

Always assert:

I am not this perishable body, I am a divine personality. These people see only my body. They cannot see my true Self which is also their Higher Self. They either praise or put me down according to their own egoistic feelings. They are acting out of their own level of ignorance. Therefore, I should not allow their statements to determine the way I feel about myself."

> *"Searching for one's self in the world is the pursuit of an illusion."*
>
> —Ancient Egyptian Proverb

As an aspirant, you must always assert that you are one with the divine and that insults cannot hurt you and thus, you should recognize an insulting remark for what it is, an expression of ignorance, and restrain yourself from responding in kind. This act shows neither weakness nor dullness of mind. To the contrary, it shows great strength and self-control and from a practical level, it tends to disconcert and diffuse the attempts by others to hurt or upset you, for you can only be hurt if you allow yourself to be susceptible to the insults of others. When you follow this course, you are diffusing the fetters of anger and pride which had control over you because you are not letting them take control of you.

> *"When you answer one who is fuming, turn your face and control yourself.*
> *The flame of the hot hearted sweeps across everything.*
> *But those who step gently, their path is a paved road."*
>
> —Ancient Egyptian Proverbs

You must realize that both insults and praises are whimsical comments by others which are changeable according to their feelings. You must strive to care only about the praises or criticism given by your spiritual preceptor or from the precepts of moral conduct given in the scriptures. In this manner you will eventually gain the fortitude of an immovable rock against the arrows of insults from others and also, from the negative feelings and thoughts of your own mind. You will be secure within yourself regardless of whatever anyone might say or what situations you experience in life. This kind of fortitude can only come from your progress on the spiritual path through a life which is based on ethical values rather than material or sensual values. Your emotions will lose their grasp over you and this will allow mental peace and calm to become the major feature of your being. As this occurs, your intellectual and intuitional capacity will increase and this will lead to a higher understanding of the teachings and their practice. This process will eventually open up the intuitional faculties of the mind wherein you will gain experience of your own divinity.

"See that prosperity elate not thine heart above measure; neither depress thine mind unto the depths, because fortune beareth hard against thee. Their smiles are not stable, therefore build not thy confidence upon them; their frowns endureth not forever, therefore, let hope teach thee patience."

—Ancient Egyptian Proverb

While it is important to bear insult and injury, there should be a distinction between bearing insult and injury and allowing oneself to be physically or mentally abused. You should be able to bear comments by others who are trying to denigrate you or cause fear in you. However, bearing injury does not imply that you should accept negative conditions. You should use your God given talents in an effort to improve your living conditions and to provide for your personal safety. If someone was trying to injure your body, either by accident or intent, you should make every effort to avoid this. However, even if you meet with the cruelest enemy, you should strive to see that enemy as an expression of God's creation who is acting out of ignorance and spiritual immaturity. In this way, even in the most distressing situations you will be able to maintain your peace of mind and communion with the divine, for the only way that you can be injured is if you identify yourself with your physical-ego self and forget about your Higher - Divine Self. The real "you" is beyond pain, suffering and death. You must assert that any comments directed toward you are being directed toward your body and not the real you. Then you will be practicing intensive yoga at all times, be it in prosperity or adversity. You must understand that when people curse at you, they are cursing your ego, and you are not the ego so what reason is there to become upset?

When you encounter adversity, you should direct your mind to reflect on the teachings of Yoga spirituality. Allow yourself to develop dispassion toward those desires within you which brought you to your current condition. Allow yourself to fully experience the folly of your error and let the profound realization of your error enter your heart. This practice will gradually cleanse you of the mental impressions which pushed you to attempt to gain a certain object or circumstance which you now discover to be empty or un-fulfilling. Allow this flow of mind to move toward the wisdom of the teachings: there is nothing in the world of human experience that can fully satisfy you. Allow yourself to recognize the extent to which you are attached to your ego-personality. When prosperity arrives, do not become attached to it because you know it is fleeting. Instead, praise the Divine for allowing you to have a positive situation which you can use to promote harmony and peacefulness of mind for the study and practice of the teachings.

There can only be insult and emotional injury where there is an ego to be bruised. When you are constantly worried about the approval of others or when you are constantly accepting the insults of others and taking them personally, you are in effect saying: I (this body and mind) am good or I am bad according to what these people are saying - or just as my thoughts suggest. You must develop a philosophy of life wherein you are guided by the higher, more sublime vision of your own divinity. When you give prominence to ethical values and make your sensual and egoistic desires subservient to the ethical principles, you develop all of the good qualities needed for spiritual aspiration. When you give prominence to the sense enjoyments and the ego, then you are creating more entanglements in life and more restlessness in the mind which lead you away from spiritual realization and further into the mire of human existence.

Throughout this book, we will explore the ancient Egyptian teachings of *MAAT* which are the progenitors of the Indian *DHARMA* and the Christian *BEATITUDES*. All of these philosophies serve to engender an ethical vision of life and produce harmony for individuals and for society. Thus, they are looked upon as the foundation of spiritual development.

You are not the body but the spirit within that gives it life. You must develop faith in your own ability to discover the path which leads to self-discovery through your studies and association with those who are more advanced than yourself. You should not make it a habit to spend time with those who are ignorant of mystical philosophy, those who are worldly minded or those who are afflicted with low morality or criminal behavior. However, those who are worldly minded, who come to you for advice have recognized your developing spiritual qualities and should therefore be received by you with humility and compassion in their time of need. In helping others in this way, you are allowing yourself to be the conduit of divine inspiration. In essence, you have become an instrument for divine work and in doing this work, you become more aware of your own divinity. In any case, you should never take upon yourself (your ego) the credit for the deed, but you should acknowledge your own divine essence as the real doer. Your body and mind are just instruments of your soul.

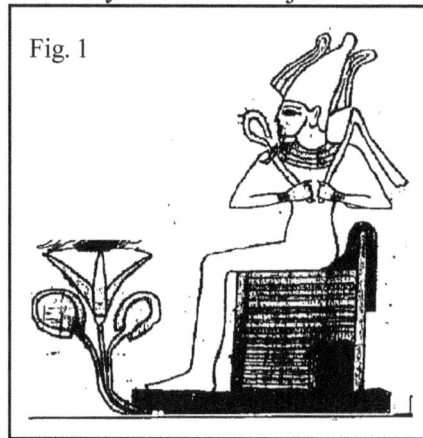

Fig. 1

In reference to the veneration of a spiritual teacher, the mythology behind the "Lotus Feet" of the master was not only used in India, as you have just read (in the section on the *exceptional aspirant*), but also in ancient Egypt. Look at figure 1. This picture of Osiris is a reproduction of the one which appears in the Hunefer Papyrus. You can see that the Lotus comes out of the Primeval Waters upon which Osiris sits as commander. Now look at figure 2. This picture is an actual rendition of the Papyrus of Ani. In this picture the lotus springs forth out of the feet of Osiris. Thus, Osiris is the first known Supreme Being of the Lotus Feet. The "feet of the master" is a major issue in Christianity as well. The phrase "fell at his feet" appears six times in the Bible, showing the importance of humbling the ego in the presence of a holy personality from whom one wishes to draw spiritual grace.

In John 13 of the Christian Bible, Jesus exhorted his disciples to follow his example in humility as he washed their feet. This was a major lesson in humility because they considered him to be the most holy personality. If the most holy personality could wash the feet of those who are supposedly not holy and exalted, what does this mean? Jesus explains that indeed they have called him Lord and Master and he has washed their feet, so they should be humble to wash each other's feet. Jesus shows by example that no job one performs is unimportant or belittling. This is the kind of humility and self-effacement which must be developed by an aspirant. Most people if asked to stand at the door way and wash the feet of their guests would feel humiliated.

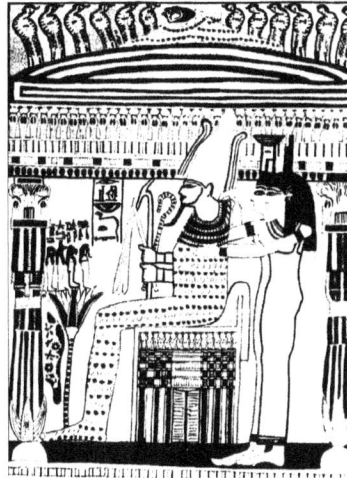

Fig 2

An aspirant must develop humility if he or she wants to truly learn from a Spiritual Preceptor. In today's society, people have a tendency to develop arrogance and pride in themselves and in their knowledge. With such an attitude, they cut themselves off from the possibility of learning something new. They try to examine everything intellectually including spiritual personalities. This intellectual examination or evaluation of things is often subjective rather than objective. In their arbitrary frame of mind, people tend to develop a debating nature which is directed toward finding faults rather than toward understanding. They examine philosophers, and always finding something wrong with them, are never able to discover which philosophy is the correct one to assist their spiritual growth. If you approach a teacher with the attitude "I already know all of this stuff, but let me see what this person has to say anyway," you will not be able to learn because your mental frame of mind is closed to learning; you are prejudiced. When you have discovered someone who inspires you and engenders faith in you, then you must humble yourself to that person. In other words, you must bow to their Lotus Feet. Only then can spiritual education truly begin in earnest. Only then can there be a true teacher-student or Spiritual Preceptor-Disciple relationship.

The ego, with its cravings and desires, is the primary obstacle to spiritual realization. The practice of humility is the most secure way to prevent the development of the ego-sense. By constantly putting down the ego-sense whenever it arises by performing selfless acts of kindness and service to others, the mind becomes filled with thoughts and feelings of a universal rather than an egoistic nature. These universal thoughts lead to the experience of universal or God consciousness rather than individual consciousness.

The story presented in John 13 is not unique. There is a similar story in the ancient Hindu epic Mahabharata, where Krishna, the "Lord and Master", purposely takes on everyday duties such as stable duties, kitchen clean up, as well as washing the feet of his followers. Therefore, the practice of humility and selflessness extends to the most ancient times and carries with it a most illustrious history. Humility reduces the pressure and urgency of cravings on the mind which egoistic feelings foster. When the pressure of egoism is lifted from the mind, the light of wisdom is able to illumine the mind and dispel its illusory desires and cravings. These desires and cravings are no longer necessary because the mental thoughts which clouded the true Self have given way to your discovery of inner fulfillment wherein all desires are truly satisfied.

63

How do you know when you are growing spiritually? When the troubles of life no longer feel insurmountable, when you become slower to anger, when you begin to discover a higher vision of yourself, when you begin to discover inner peace and contentment and when you no longer depend on the events of the external world for your happiness, these are some indications that you are moving toward self-discovery. This is the goal which the art and practice of Yoga in Life is directed to.

When you are living in the world, you are continually being challenged. Everyone is being continually tested, however, those who are practicing yoga develop a special sensitivity and are able to have a greater sense of spiritual awareness of the process. They are able to see the challenging situations of human life as opportunities to further purify their heart. Most of those who face life without training in yoga philosophy see life as an uncertain realm of arbitrary events with no deeper meaning. Their sole purpose is to seek happiness by acquiring pleasant circumstances and material riches and this attitude intensifies their struggle as well as the pain of disappointment when they fail. An ordinary person not initiated into yoga would see an adverse condition in life such as the loss of a material object as a motive for grief, anger or cursing, etc. An initiate would see it as an opportunity to control the emotions and to develop insight into the fact that human life is illusory because at any moment anything can be taken away, even one's life. Also, an initiate would realize that what appears to be a prosperous condition or a harmonious condition between people or human relationships can change at any moment to a situation of enmity and disappointment. Therefore, there is no point in grieving over something that is lost or allowing oneself to become agitated over the praises or curses from others, rather it is more important to discover what is real, cannot be lost and is not subject to variations based on feelings or emotions, the Self within.

The tests of an aspirant relate to the following questions: Have you controlled your anger? your fears? your lusts? your emotions? your desires? It is on the basis of such evaluation that you judge your spiritual progress, and not on the basis of visions during meditation or psychic experiences etc. When you face life with the teachings of yoga, then you are as if equipped, with a suit of armor which insults, annoyances, and egoistic values cannot penetrate. You begin to discover an inner peace which surpasses both outer pleasures and pains as well as internal desires of the ego. This occurs in degrees, but when you are sincere and repeatedly practice the teachings, even though you may fail many times before succeeding, you will progress.

It must be clearly understood that the primary qualification of an aspirant is belief in the teachings. If you at least believe that you are a soul wandering in ignorance of your true nature through many incarnations, at least intellectually, then there is hope for your being able to practice yoga successfully. However, those who are strongly of the opinion that the world is the only reality, that the body is their Self and when the body dies they cease to exist, are not fit to receive the teachings of yoga. Such people are compared to buffaloes or hippopotamuses because their minds are so dulled by their sense perceptions and ignorance that the only idea they have of existence is what their senses perceive. You would not try to teach music to a buffalo would you? In the same way, even the greatest teachings of spirituality would be wasted on such people. Therefore, the scriptures clearly state that these unqualified people should not be taught any advanced forms of spiritual philosophy. Rather they should be encouraged to develop moral character, virtue and ritualistic practices of religion. They should be taught the mythological stories of religion until they are ready to be instructed in the higher metaphysical teachings. Also, those at this level will benefit from the recitation or repetition of words of power. This practice will have the effect of purifying the mind.

There is one important aspect of spiritual aspiration. As you tread the path of spirituality, you must engage in the service to your spiritual preceptor. This means that you should assist in the endeavors of the spiritual preceptor, the dissemination of the teachings, the promotion of yogic principles in all areas of life, the promotion of peace and non-violence against human beings, animals, or nature and other duties outlined in the scriptures. This service has the effect of purifying your heart by expanding your sphere of activity to encompass the entire world and not just your individual ego. Also, it places you in a position to learn the deeper aspects of the teachings and to develop spiritual qualities as you associate with one who is more advanced than yourself. If you are not associated with a particular spiritual preceptor, you should look to God who is the Supreme Preceptor of all preceptors and in the same manner, render service to the Divine Self in the same way as you would to a spiritually advanced person who is "close to God" as discussed earlier.

WHO IS A TEACHER

"When the ears of the student are ready to hear, then come the lips of wisdom to fill them with wisdom."

"The lips of the wise are as the doors of a cabinet; no sooner are they opened, but treasures are poured out before you. Like unto trees of gold arranged in beds of silver, are wise sentences uttered in due season."

"The lips of Wisdom are closed, Except to the ears of Understanding."

—Ancient Egyptian Proverbs

When you are growing spiritually you will recognize those who are spiritually advanced. You will be led to them in a mystical way and you will receive the teaching which you need at that time. First you need to begin to purify yourself and make yourself into a good student because only then will you recognize a good teacher. Then you will be fit to receive teachings and to put them into practice because only then will you be ready to understand them.

Spiritual development does not occur in a flash or through a magical touch. It occurs with incremental practice of the teachings as you gradually integrate them into your life through your own self-effort and your level of self-effort determines your level of success. Once you learn the correct methods of spiritual discipline, you can then choose those disciplines (meditation, selfless service, study of scriptures, etc.) which suit your personality and then gradually increase the intensity of your practice even while you carry on the normal duties of life. This process leads to peace and enjoyment of life and to spiritual Enlightenment in an integrated way.

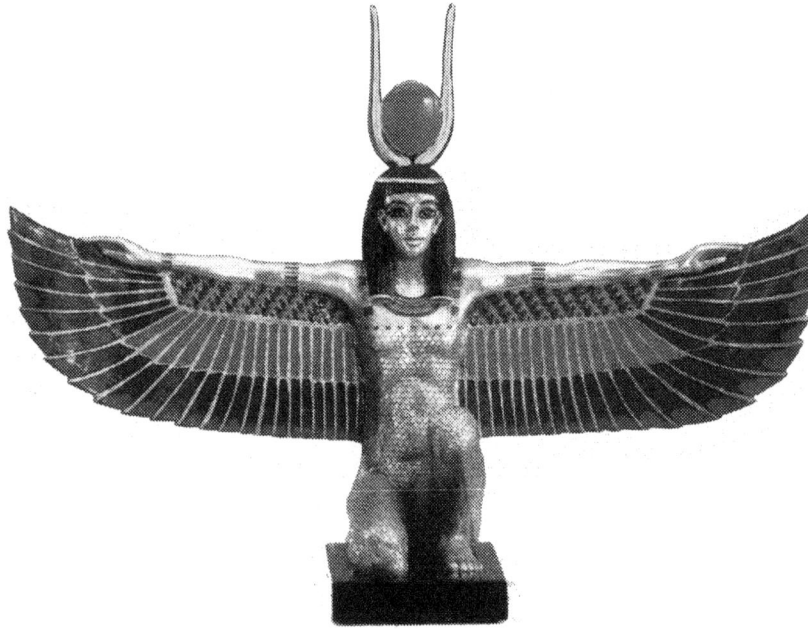

"Rekhat" (Isis – Lady of Wisdom)

Aset (Isis), The Lady of Wisdom, who initiated her son Horus into the mysteries of spiritual life and led him to enlightenment and victory against the evil and unrighteousness of Set and his demon associates. She is the supreme wisdom and power behind all priests and priestesses. See **"The Ausarian Resurrection"** by Dr. Muata Abhaya Ashby.

The need for a true teacher of spirituality cannot be overemphasized in the course of spiritual practice. An aspirant is like an athlete. He or she needs coaching and practice in order to attain mastery over the lower self. Every area of your life where you have achieved success, is because you studied and practiced, if not in this lifetime, in a previous one. Spiritual Enlightenment cannot be achieved through magic or through unnatural means. It is achieved through understanding and hard work, not ordinary work, but those activities which lead to purification of the heart.

It is possible to promote your spiritual growth through the books written by genuine spiritual preceptors. The new forms of media such as audio and video have gone even further in conveying the message of the teachings to the entire world. However, at some point, books and tapes can only go so far in explaining the fruits of the true practice of spirituality. This is because the mind can develop many misconceptions and illusions about spirituality just as in any area of ordinary worldly life. Therefore, a guide or coach who is advanced in its practice should be sought out and approached with humility and honesty to ask questions and dispel subtle forms of ignorance. This is the process of spiritual teaching called initiation. The aspirant is initiated into a philosophy and way of life which he or she needs to learn and practice by studying, reflecting and meditating on the teachings. Initiation is a conscious choice to adopt a teaching and to embark on the task of basing your life on it in order to purify your mind and body through the teaching so that you may become a conduit of the divine.

The wisdom texts and scriptures are like a painting of fire. The painting provides an image of what a fire looks like but no warmth emanates from it no matter how close you get. For that, it is necessary to have a real fire. In much the same way, books provide an idea of what is meant by the teachings, however in order to understand their subtlety, something more is needed. A true teacher is one who lives the teaching. Such a one can breathe life into the scriptures and myths to make them understood in the language of today. This is the fire of knowledge which burns away ignorance and illusions which are the cause of human suffering and misery.

There is no nobler occupation than being instructor of Yoga Philosophy, because there is no greater endeavor than relieving the burden of those who are beset by the pain and mental suffering caused by ignorance of their true Self. Also, there is no greater force to dispel the mental anguish of society than Yogic Mystical Philosophy because it gets to the root of psychological complexes in a way that Western psychology does not. Therefore, meeting an authentic teacher of Yoga Philosophy is a highly coveted event by those who have begun to recognize the deeper levels of their own being and the glory of yoga.

One of the main problems of society is the relative lack of interest in the scriptures and secondly, the relatively small number of authentic spiritual preceptors available to teach those who are interested. Many people do not find spirituality attractive because they feel they would "lose" out on life if they became seriously involved. Others see the prospect of spirituality as being too remote for their understanding. They do not realize that their attempts to experience joy from the world are doomed to failure. Further, they do not understand that they already have all they need to be truly happy so they continue to search outside of themselves. These problems arise from the intensification of their ego-body identification and the belief in the erroneous concepts about religion and yoga. Since all souls have emanated from the Higher Self and must some day return to the Self, Yoga is really the ultimate path of all souls. You may choose to procrastinate it however, by being distracted in the phenomenal world of human experiences, but you must realize that you are procrastinating the only true happiness (bliss) which exists in exchange for transient moments of joy followed by pain and suffering. The choice is yours as you are endowed with free will.

An authentic Spiritual Preceptor is not only someone who is advanced on the spiritual path or even just someone who has reached the fully enlightened state. A Guru, in the Upanishadic (teachings of the Indian Upanishads) sense of the word, is someone who is spiritually enlightened and who also is well versed in the scriptural teachings and methods of training aspirants according to their level of understanding. Therefore, a counselor of Yoga must first achieve a high degree of understanding and personal - spiritual emancipation since the subtleties of the mind must be well understood. The teacher must be able to be a refuge for all people, have an extensive knowledge of the teachings pertaining to her/his level of attainment, and enthusiastically pursue all forms of Yoga.

The teaching is often understood differently at different levels. Just as there are different levels of math, such as arithmetic, algebra and calculus, there are different levels of religious practice. The different levels of religion are the Mythological, Ritualistic and the Metaphysical levels. In much the same way, there are varying levels of aspirants who attain to different levels of religious understanding and experience at different times.

Only one who has experienced and matured to greater levels of attainment through *personality integration* can assist others in understanding those higher levels. Here, personality integration refers to the extent that the individual has realized his/her own ego-lessness and identification with the transcendental Self. One on the spiritual path intending to work with and help others, needs to understand the process of initiation and his/her own level of attainment well. Such understanding can only be gained by undergoing the process of practicing the teachings in his/her life. Many teachers (psychologists, psychiatrists, yoga instructors) are deluded as to their understanding of the mind, the philosophy described in the scriptures and of their own attainment. Sometimes, this very delusion causes their failure to cope with the afflictions of others. They are not able to maintain their own peace and serenity and are unable to show others how to deal with their own problems in an effective and lasting way. Therefore, if a teaching is given by one who does not live the teaching or by one who is mistaken about her/his own attainment, that teaching will not be effective.

An authentic teacher of yoga philosophy is someone who is advanced on the path of self-control, one who is indifferent to either positive or negative situations which arise, one who is not affected by praise or censure and is not desirous of any object in the phenomenal world. He or she has discovered inner fulfillment and is a wellspring of joy to all whom they come into contact with. They are not interested in developing relationships with students based on emotionality or other egoistic sensibilities and they are not interested in keeping disciples as servants for their own amusement or in keeping company to inflate their own egos because they have transcended all of these human frailties. They are fulfilled through their realization of their own divinity and help others out of compassion and universal love which flows through them directly from the divine source.

In this manner they help others who seek them out. Acting out the will of the divine which flows through them untouched by egoism, Sages carry out the work of enlightening others. Some aspirants become enlightened in a short time while others in a longer time. The actions of a Sage affect incalculable amounts of people because their actions ripple through the world as a wave ripples across a lake when a stone is thrown into it. By their writings, expositions, their subtle spiritual influence and by their examples as living embodiments of the wisdom, they have an effect on the course of the world and on all whom they come into contact with.

It is acceptable to have advanced yoga students (disciples), provide initial yoga instruction including introduction of exoteric and esoteric knowledge and provide support and encouragement to aspirants, but as a rule, the lower order priests and priestesses does not initiate the disciple into the subtle mysteries of advanced spirituality. This role is reserved for the fully enlightened Guru or spiritual master. A preceptor (*Sebai*) is a spiritual teacher who may or may not have the function of a *guru* or spiritual guide proper. It should be noted here that enlightened personalities are not necessarily nor exclusively to be known as "gurus" although they perform the same function. They may reside in any part of the world and are members of all ethnic groups. Further, they may exist in embodied or non-embodied form. Also, they may be either male or female.

When the *Hem* or priests and priestesses determine that the aspirant is ready to receive the more subtle spiritual instruction of an enlightened personality (*Sebai*), he/she may refer the aspirant for advanced teaching while continuing the counseling-teacher relationship. Therefore, the Upadhyaya and the Guru can complement each other. The Yoga Vasistha emphasizes the importance of teaching the wisdom of the Self as a way of raising one's spiritual consciousness. This is because, by keeping the wisdom of the Self (the Absolute, God) foremost in the mind through the continuous reflectiveness caused by the teaching process, the mind does not stray to sense objects or to other distractions. The mind therefore flows toward the Absolute essential nature, the transcendental Higher Self, at all times.

In the *Yoga Vasistha,* Sage Vasistha says: One who is ceaselessly devoted to *Brahman**, who exists for the sake of the Self, who rejoices in talking about *Brahman*, and who is engaged in enlightening others about their essential nature, he attains Liberation even in this life. III. 9:1 (*Absolute Self)

In ancient Egypt, the general term for priest or priestess was *Hem or Hemt.* Priesthoods and priestesshoods were also divided into different ranks. There was the *Keri-Eb* or high priest i.e. *Hierophant.* Some of the titles of the Keri-Eb were *"He who sees the secret of heaven"* and *"Chief of the secrets of heaven."* Then came the various levels which handled the administrative duties of the temple which included teaching the mysteries of spirituality as well as the arts, law, writing (hieroglyphics), management, etc. Some of the titles for the various levels of priests were *"The Treasurer of the God", "The scribe of God's House", "The reciter-priest", "The Mete-en-sa", Scribe of the altar"* and *Superintendent of the House of God."* Judges were also part of the priesthood. They specifically belonged to the following of Goddess *MAAT.* The largest priestesshoods belonged to the Temples of the Gods Amun, Asar, Ra and Heru, and the Goddesses *Net, Aset* and *Hetheru.* These Goddesses are also known by other names which are given according to the mystical symbolism of the teachings. These include Isis, Nephthys, Bast, Mut, Nekhebet, Uatchet, and all other forms of the Goddess.[3]

A reference to the ancient Egyptian view concerning a *Hierophant* or teacher of the mysteries comes from *Philo of Alexandria.* Philo was a mystic practitioner of the Egyptian mysteries and Gnostic Christianity. Gnostic Christianity is an outgrowth of ancient Egyptian Religion. Gnosticism includes mystical writings in Coptic and Greek language about the nature of the soul and of creation along with mystical wisdom and philosophy which lead to mystical awareness. Orthodox Christianity or the Roman and Byzantine Catholicism which survives to this day originated out of Christian Gnosticism.

In reference to the "Divine Spirit" and "Moses", Philo gives the following instruction:

"It [the Divine Spirit] is [ever] present with only one class of men—with those who, having stripped themselves of all things in genesis, even to the innermost veil and garment of opinion, come unto God with minds unclothed and naked."

"And so Moses, having fixed his tent outside the camp—that is, the whole of the body—that is to say, having made firm his mind, so that it does not move, begins to worship God and entering into the most holy mysteries. And he becomes, not only a *mystes*, but also a Hierophant of revelations, and teacher of divine things, which he will indicate to those who have had their ears made pure. With such kind of men the Divine Spirit is ever present, guiding their every way aright."

Philo directly addresses the idea of divine inspiration using Moses, whom the Bible states was an Egyptian Priest, as an example. Philo's description of the "meeting" between God and Moses is an example of the orthodox versus the Gnostic understanding and practice of spirituality. While the orthodox view presents this meeting as Moses being conscious of himself as a person looking at God

---

[3] for more details on the levels of the Ancient Egyptian clergy see the book *Egyptian Mysteries* by Dr. Muata Ashby

who is outside of himself, the Gnostic understanding is that God is communed with, by setting aside the ego consciousness. Further on, Philo states that it is when this ecstasy occurs (*having fixed his tent outside the camp*) that the true worship of God begins. It is this ecstasy which provides real insight into one's own spiritual nature and which bestows the highest ability to teach others about the mysteries of the soul.

This point is very important for a serious aspirant to understand. As a worshipper of the Divine, if you maintain yourself separate within your mind and body and hold onto your ego, you are only practicing a ritualistic form of worship. This form of superficial practice of spirituality will not bestow true knowledge on you. Rather, your knowledge will be based on the information you are able to gather from your mind and senses which are limited and conditioned.

> *"Strive to see with the inner eye, the heart. It sees the reality not subject to emotional or personal error; it sees the essence. Intuition then is the most important quality to develop."*
>
> —Ancient Egyptian Proverb

In most orthodox (adhering to traditional or established beliefs) forms of religion, the worshiper is mentally aware of him/herself as being an individual looking at another individual (God) in the form of pictures, idols, scriptural descriptions, etc. In Gnostic or mystical forms of religion (Egyptian mysteries, Vedanta, Taoism, Buddhism, Gnostic Christianity) which employ yoga philosophy and meditation techniques, the worshiper is directed to cease the thoughts of the mind which involve personal identification with the body and ego and thereby become one with the Absolute by an immediate, direct, intuitive knowledge of God, the ultimate reality. This intuitive knowledge refers to a personal religious experience in Gnosticism. A contrast should be drawn here between the mystical-ecstatic experience (just defined) and the ritualistic religious experience. The ritualistic or surface level religious experience is often accompanied by heightened emotions, visions and other phenomena, however there is no transcendental vision of the Absolute and no transcendence of the ego-self. In other words, an ecstatic religious experience at the level of the mind and senses does not show you that you are not the body, mind and senses and does not reveal your true Self.

Lastly, it would be an exceedingly great error for someone to claim to be a realized spiritual master if they are not. This is because the psychic illusion that would be created within their own mind would hamper their own spiritual movement. However, the imitation of spiritual personalities and their behavior is permitted and even promoted to the extent that it is grounded in reality and honesty. The idea is that we are what we feel, act, believe and think. Therefore, as we feel, act, believe and think in a particular way, we become like onto that. Thus, it is all right to emulate the qualities of a Sage because this process helps to control the ego and develop sagely qualities. Generally, self-realized masters do not go around proclaiming their enlightenment. Rather, it is more the case that their disciples are drawn to them because of their teachings and example. The advancing aspirant can know who is an advanced personality due to his/her own increasing purity and wisdom. Therefore, in order to recognize a true teacher, you need to develop your own intuitive faculties. This is accomplished by studying the teachings and by developing serenity and strong moral character.

The Role of the Teacher

The teacher does not become sentimentally involved with students, feel sorrow for those who do not follow the teachings or elation over those who do. The teacher, having discovered the source of pain and suffering, seeks to eliminate it wherever it may be, through the force of wisdom which, like the Eye of Ra, burns away all ignorance in its path. Where there is wisdom there can be no ignorance and therefore, no pain and suffering, just as there can be no darkness in a room where the light has been turned on. However, the teacher does not seek to violate anyone's freedom of will. Those who wish to be under the guiding influence of the teacher must do so out of free will, since not even a teacher of the highest power can remove their pain and ignorance if they do not want to become enlightened. Therefore, a teacher makes him or herself a conduit, an instrument for the Divine through which the Divine may enlighten others when they are ready. In the mean time, nature (Neters) through the unseen mysterious force of Meskhenet (karma) guides souls who are not ready to receive the teaching of the advanced Spiritual Preceptor. The path of nature is the path of spiritual growth through many life times and requires the experience of many sorrows, disappointments, disillusionments and violence. However, these events are planned by nature to awaken the deeper need of the soul to seek spiritual enlightenment through wisdom rather than through the world of sense enjoyments and complicated karmic entanglements.

The teacher, by becoming an example and transcending the pain and sorrow of human existence, can then express true compassion for humanity. So the most effective way to help humanity is to help yourself to become enlightened. Then the obstacles which trouble most people will not affect you in the least. Your wisdom and realization will be as an armor which protects you against the miseries of the world. Even the most sincere social workers cannot help humanity to the fullest if they themselves are suffering from the maladies of human existence. If you do not know how to swim in the ocean of the world of human experiences, you cannot save others from drowning. The large number of psychologists and psychiatrists who experience problems such as stress and commit suicide is an example of this. Therefore, unless you are above being affected by the human condition by working to overcome it in yourself through yogic science, you cannot assist those who are affected by that condition.

While there is always a value to any action an ordinary person takes to uplift society (value to society and to themselves), the most effective way to change the world is to begin changing yourself. As Jesus said: *seek ye first the kingdom of Heaven, and his righteousness; and all these things shall be added to you.* While continuing to work for the betterment of humanity, you must not take on the burdens of the world upon your shoulders. You must trust and have faith in the plan of NETER (God) who works through the Neters (the Neters-mysterious divine forces of nature and the cosmos). You must honestly understand that your own need to help society and rectify injustice is an expression of your own need to achieve wholeness and this wholeness cannot be found in the world from an egoistic perspective. If you do not trust in nature's ability to help others, it is like saying that you do not trust in God, that God's creation (the world) is imperfect and unjust. This would be an expression of your own ignorance.

> *"Salvation is accomplished through the efforts of the individual. There is no mediator between man and his / her salvation."*
>
> —Ancient Egyptian Proverb

You cannot assist others who do not want to be assisted or who are not qualified to receive the teachings of mystical spirituality (Yoga philosophy). You can only work to purify your heart and to promote the same in others by your example and be prepared for the time when they will seek your assistance. This does not mean that you cannot or should not engage in projects to help others. To the contrary, such projects can help you to develop purity of heart by providing experiences and opportunities for you to practice selflessness, self-control, dispassion, detachment, etc. and thereby promote effacement of the ego. The key is in the attitude with which you perform your duties. If you engage in actions with an attitude of egoistic attachment, pride, selfishness, repulsion or regret, you will intensify the fetters which bind you to human existence. This attitude would be like rejecting God's plan for your spiritual development. If you treat all of your experiences as opportunities to do divine work by allowing your soul to express itself through your mind and body when serving others and developing the latent talents within you, then your experiences will lead to inner fulfillment and mental serenity which will open the path of self-discovery. This is the true purpose of social work.

Every day, Nature (God) provides you with opportunities to purify your heart. All situations in life are carefully planned tests for you to practice developing divine virtues: humility, selflessness, detachment, positive state of mind, fearlessness, joy, etc. The teachings of Maat show you how to achieve these goals through your actions in daily activities. In reality, you enter the Hall of Maat to be judged every day of your life. The world of human experiences is the Hall of Maat. From a higher perspective, this entire universe is the Hall of Maat.

"GOD is truth (Maat), and GOD has established the earth thereupon."
—Ancient Egyptian Proverb

Therefore, you should strive to understand the way of *Maat* in order to come into harmony with the way of the universe. When you consciously commence this process, you will begin to discover the true joy of life and those around you will benefit in a most profound and mysterious way, perhaps even without your knowing it. If you allow yourself to be guided by the teachings of wisdom, you will be entering the stream of light which flows from the Divine, from the highest to the lowest. Having done this you will have enlisted the help of the greatest power that exists, your own Higher Self. Then, wherever you go and whatever you do will be blessed with the Divine essence. This is the way of Maat which puts the forces of nature at your command to do divine work. When you consciously decide to align yourself with the forces of wisdom as opposed to the forces of ignorance and egoism by changing your life through the ancient practices of mystical spirituality, you have initiated yourself on the path to enlightenment and salvation. Thus, initiation is a deeply personal and serious matter which you need to reflect upon. True transformation can occur only if you are sincere and honest with yourself and if you follow the practices as instructed. Therefore, spiritual life is not easy in the beginning but it is most rewarding in the end. It confers the greatest goal of life, eternal bliss which is not perishable like worldly attainments.

Good Association Part 1

One of the most important ways of promoting awareness and constant reflection is keeping the company of wise teachers or Sages. In ancient Egypt, the Temple system served the purpose of instructing aspirants in the wisdom teachings and then allowing them back into the world on a regular basis in order to test their level of understanding and self control by practicing the teachings when confronted with ordinary, worldly minded people. The Temple was a place where the initiate could go on a regular basis to receive instruction and counseling on the correct application of the teachings in day to day life. The idea is reflected in the *Stela of Djehuti-Nefer*:

"Consume pure foods and pure thoughts with pure hands, adore celestial beings, become associated with wise ones: sages, saints and prophets; make offerings to GOD..."

The association with Sages and Saints (Good Association) is seen as a primary way to accelerate the spiritual development of the aspirant. Again, this is because it is the nature of the mind to imitate that which it focuses on. An important definition of the symbols associated with *Sma* ⌡ or Sema is *to render clear or visible* ⌡🐍🐍👁. In ancient Egypt, the *gathering, assembly or reunion* was called *Smait* ⌡🐍○— and *Smai* ⌡🐍ıı is a name for the Temple, the gathering place. In Egypt, the priest assumed the role of preceptor, *Sbai* ⟨★⌡ıı🏠🐍, leading the initiate to understand the teachings of the hieroglyphs, to purification of the mind and body and eventually to intuitional realization through the practice of mental exercises and the application of the wisdom teachings. In ancient hieroglyphics, this is symbolized by the scenes where deities such as *Horus, Djehuti, Anubis, Hathor, Isis*, etc. lead the initiate to meet Osiris (his/her Higher Self). In India, this process is known as *"Satsanga"* where the aspirant receives teaching from the *Guru* (Spiritual Preceptor) on a continuous basis. In Buddhism the process is known as *Sanga*. In Christianity this idea was reflected in the relationship between Jesus and John the Baptist and later between Jesus and his disciples. Keeping the company of wise ones is an important and powerful tool for spiritual development because the nature of the unenlightened (ignorant) mind allows it to make subtle mistakes which can lead the aspirant astray from the correct interpretation of the teachings. Thus, receiving the teaching is the real force which causes transformation through a baptismal ritual and not the ritual itself.

Therefore, the teacher, guru, priest, etc. who is "close" to God (enlightened) as it were, is seen as greater than God because he or she can lead the aspirant toward God (knowing who and where God is and how God is to be discovered). Otherwise it would be a very difficult, long and arduous process for the aspirant to realize the truth. It would take millions of incarnations, wherein untold sufferings would occur in the process of gaining experiences which would teach the proper way to discover the Self.

Your journey through this volume will impart one most important point about true spirituality, namely, that true spirituality is universal spirituality. This means that if you discover the truth about your own religion, you will have discovered the truth about all other religions therefore, true religion is a religion of the heart. You must always keep in mind that you are transcendental, immortal and eternal and as such, you are endowed with all the qualities necessary to achieve the highest level of spiritual realization regardless of your background or country of origin.

Another important point is to try to become the best possible disciple you can while still performing your every day duties of life. Once you honestly set in motion the mystical process of your own spiritual aspiration, you will one day encounter more advanced personalities from whom you can learn and progress further in your understanding. In every city, state and country, there exist more advanced personalities who can lead you further along your path of self-discovery. Have you known anyone who is able to control their emotions? Have you known anyone who has lived through a bad situation such as the loss of a loved one or a serious illness and has moved forward with composure, without losing enthusiasm for life? Have you met anyone who has been like a pillar for others, whom others go to in times of trouble or need? If you have the good fortune to know someone like this, get close to them and ask them to show you how they came to possess those advanced spiritual qualities. Ask their permission to spend time with them so that you may benefit from their knowledge and experience in living. You may find that some people are well developed in some areas but not in others. Learn what you can and emulate their virtuous characteristics. If you get to a point where you feel there is no more to learn from that person, continue seeking and you will discover the steps which lead upward on the ladder of spiritual aspiration.

There is no greater blessing than to meet Sages and or Saints who have attained Christ Consciousness, Nirvana, Buddhahood, Horushood, Salvation, Liberation, etc. themselves while at the same time being well versed in the written teachings. They can best help you to understand the subtlety of the teachings and lead you to greater and greater awareness and comprehension which will lead to your own mystical realization in a shorter time than through any other method. They cannot transform you into a spiritual personality; you must do that yourself. However, they can direct you on the correct path and point out your mistakes if you are willing to listen. You need not specifically search for someone who is Enlightened in your own religion. You may continue to follow your own religion while still learning the subtlety of spiritual discipline and yoga science as these apply to all religions equally. You should not become distracted by different religions or teachers, rather set your attention on the highest goal, Enlightenment, then all else will fall into place.

A disciple who does not practice the teachings of their spiritual preceptor with the notion that the preceptor will provide for his/her spiritual development is like a person who expects to become physically fit by merely going to a gymnasium without doing any exercise. The preceptor provides the mental food in the form of the wisdom teachings and then it is up to you to take this food, consume it, digest it, absorb it and allow it to become part of your being.

Since your innermost self (God) is your Supreme Preceptor, all of the situations you find yourself involved with are divinely inspired to provide for your spiritual education. The same Divine Self is instructing you through the spiritual preceptor and it is this same Divine Self which aids your reflecting and understanding process.

How to Approach a Spiritual Preceptor

There are many orders of priests and priestesses but the Seba is the imparter of mysteries to the initiates. This is a special personality, someone who has achieved Divine Consciousness, which is the goal of all spiritual efforts. Those personalities have chosen to maintain the initiatic tradition and instruct new aspirants who will become initiates and eventually priests and priestesses as well as Preceptors. Gaining an insight into who they are and how to approach them is of paramount importance in achieving the higher goals of spiritual development. You may begin by reading the books of those personalities so as to have a partial communion with their minds and then you will want to meet them in person in order to truly understand what you have read!

There are many people who do their own research and believe they have discovered the "mysteries" and thus they go around teaching others and sometimes even starting new religions but in the end their lack of authenticity emerges in the form of egoism, unrighteousness, inability to handle crisis, inability to resist worldly temptations, inability to show others the path to spiritual realization beyond slogans, exuberant rantings or emotional appeals. Many preachers use exciting methods to talk about their scriptures and may even sound authentic but the excitement soon dies down and the aspirant is left without a viable understanding or path to follow. Also, many self-styled spiritual leaders are not interested in showing others a higher path because then they would loose their source of income. An authentic Spiritual Preceptor is not interested in developing cults, slaves, servants or keeping people at an ignorant level.

An authentic teacher is and should be treated as a precious resource, even more so than millions of dollars in the bank. Why? Because that person will free you from untold mysteries over many future lifetimes and they will lead you to enlightenment in this lifetime so that you can truly enjoy whatever wealth you have. Even if you are poor you will also be led to enjoyment of life since the successful aspirants transcend all good or bad conditions in the world.

You should approach the preceptor with humility and not insolently. As soon as the authentic teacher hears arrogance, conceit, self-importance, vanity, snobbishness, etc., their lips close and the flow if the enlightening stream of the river to enlightenment ceases to flow towards you. Even if you egoistically sought to attend their class you would not understand or benefit from the teaching. Respect, humility deference and obedience are keys to approaching a preceptor. Without these your relationship cannot exist. For this reason you should practice Maat and get rid of the gross (overt) impurities (anger, hatred, greed, jealousy, lust, envy, etc.) in your personality. The preceptor will show you how to get rid of the more subtle (unconscious) impurities so that you may progress in the teaching.

(4)"Have faith in your master's ability to lead you along the path of truth"
-Ancient Egyptian precept for the initiates.

Also, never take the preceptor for granted. Never treat or refer to the preceptor as you would a "friend" or a "buddy" or as "one of the guys." Also, as the preceptor is elevated in consciousness but operating through a physical body, there will possibly be human occasional error or faults in areas outside of the teachings. An ignorant aspirant would look at this with the idea that enlightenment means absolute perfection in everything and in this manner dismiss the teacher as inadequate and thus loose out on the benefits that would otherwise be derived from the association. Therefore, as in ordinary relations, there should never be gossiping about faults or petty foibles or minor eccentricities.

"It takes a strong disciple to rule over the mountainous thoughts and constantly go to the essence of the meaning; as mental complexity increases, thus will the depth of your decadence and challenge both be revealed."

-Ancient Egyptian Proverb

Ordinary friendships, based on egoism, are burdened with egoistic desires and expectations. A preceptor is not interested in fulfilling your egoistic desires but rather in dispelling these. Therefore, if you do not have the understanding as to what is the nature and purpose of the initiatic affiliation your relationship on that basis is doomed and you will be the one leaving the relationship without transforming, without growing and enlightening yourself. Never treat the preceptor as an ordinary person who like others has an "opinion" you can accept or disregard. If you want to be a "free spirit," to exercise "free will" you have no need of the preceptor. If you are a sincere aspirant you will have no need to exercise free will to commit sinful acts or unrighteous schemes, nor will you need to reserve the right to hurt others or delude yourself. Therefore, your free will can be surrendered to the Divine without a second thought or reservation. Once you are secure in the authenticity of the person you have chosen as your teacher you must realize that that person is a representative of the Divine on earth and should be accorded the same respect and admiration as a facilitator who will help you on the path. You have come to that person because you recognize your ignorance and the elevation of the teacher. Therefore, cease all thoughts of pride and self-importance. Otherwise you are only toying at being an aspirant and have no chance to be a real initiate. As you check out a teacher yes you should be cautious and slow to ally yourself, but once you choose to do so your allegiance should be complete and unreserved, unconditional and wholehearted. The unrighteous and therefore, limited ways of relating thwart the spiritual process of the teacher disciple relationship and will render it fruitless. They cause rifts in the mind of the aspirant and prevent them from pursuing the teaching in the correct manner. Sometimes as children, they may keep themselves from facing the preceptor after they have made some transgression, due to pride and shame. At these times when life humbles the aspirant it is even more important that they should trust in the teacher who will never rub their noses in it or turn them away. A preceptor is like the sun, who witnesses the good and the bad but yet remains aloof, dispassionate but yet in touch. So the preceptor understands how tough it is to make it through the gross and subtle temptations, fancies, notions and desires of life and is thus prepared to forgive all. Even though a transcendent master is beyond personal hang-ups, desires, attachments and so on an aspirant should never disrespect the preceptor, steal from the preceptor (objects or knowledge) or speak out of turn or test the patience of the preceptor. Some aspirants, due to ignorance, believe they can go around taking knowledge from different teachers without giving anything in return. So they remain unchanged because they do not give themselves, their allegiance, trust and support to the cause of the teacher. Therefore, they never get the opportunity to form a long-term relationship with the teacher which they need in order to develop deeper understanding of the teaching. Their understanding remains superficial and thereby they develop delusions of grandeur as advanced initiates and in reality they are setting themselves up for a great fall.

"Sacrifice the first portions of the harvest, that your strength and faith to bring about what you desire may be increased; give the FIRST portion, to avoid danger of worldly

indulgence; Give that you may receive. Fulfill the requirements of the universal law of equilibrium"

-Ancient Egyptian Proverb

Every aspirant must offer their ego, pride and ignorance on the divine altar of wisdom. They must sacrifice the egoistic notions, and vanity in order to attain insight and wisdom. They must pledge their service to the preceptor in the form of physical, mental and spiritual support and devotion. Further, an aspirant should not hesitate to beg the preceptor's forgiveness for any transgression. While the preceptor is not personally bothered by transgressions or insolence, etc. the preceptor's voice is silenced in the presence of such ignorant aspirants and this hurts them severely, allowing the cycle of ignorance pain and suffering in life and reincarnation to continue unabated. Disrespect and callousness as well as ill manners and rudeness are symptoms of spiritual immaturity, i.e. ignorance. Spiritual teachings to such a personality will be as effective as a instructing a dog or a cat on the finer principles of brain surgery. This unrighteous way of relating closes the door to real spiritual instruction. And this closing has been the fault of the aspirant. Take care to not be two faced and burn your bridges, thinking that you have attained some higher level and no longer need your teacher or discovered a better teacher, and thus disrespecting the old. The old brought you to the new you think you have arrived at and is therefore worthy of the same respect and gratitude that was supposed to have been there all along. While the teacher exists in transcendental bliss regardless of the aspirant's righteous conduct or lack thereof the aspirant is severely affected by their actions. Even the subtlest unrighteous act is a pathway to strengthening of the ego and egoism leads to impaired intellect and degraded feeling. Unrighteous behavior reverberates in the consciousness of an aspirant and forms negative impressions in the mind that clout understanding and may take lifetimes to erase. Therefore, take care to make sure that your relationship with the preceptor is righteous if not in the beginning, certainly in the end. But there is only one true ending if it can be referred to as such and that is the attainment of enlightenment. Does a river end when it joins the ocean? In like manner the true end of the road of the teacher disciple relationship is the aspirants attainment of enlightenment but this is not the end but a merging of the aspirants consciousness with that of the teacher, the beginning of conscious experience of the transcendental spirit and here begins also the journey of the aspirant who has now become a preceptor and this is the initiatic tradition, which reaches back to the far reaches of time all the way back to the first aspirants, those who learned from God (Djehuti) directly and became preceptors to those who followed next and so on up to the present.

You must treat a Spiritual Preceptor even better than you treat someone you love. Ordinary love affairs are fraught with strife, love and hate periods sprinkled with passionate moments and dashes of exuberant flights of fancy. People develop possessiveness and attachments and call these love and also they fall in out of love as if it were a disease. This of course is not true love. True love transcends even the capacity to feel anger or disdain. If you truly love something you stick with it through thick or thin and there is no "falling out" of it. It is an upward and expanding movement that is all encompassing and eternal. So unless you have loved in this way do not believed that you have truly loved for loved anything. Your relationships are only training you for the true love and you must learn that from the preceptor.[4]

You must attempt to never loose your temper in the presence of the preceptor and never treat the preceptor unrighteously or with resentment. You must learn to receive whatever the teacher says and

---

[4] See the book *Egyptian Tantra Yoga*

apply it in your life. Many aspirants have learned to do things "their own way" instead of following instructions from the teacher. You may question for deeper understanding but not to challenge in order to get out of your duty or to discredit what has been said so that you may feel justified in disobeying the edict. That is the path of the weak minded and the ignorant. Never attempt to put emotional guilt trips on elevated personalities. These are immature attempts and getting the desires of your ego and they will be impotent in the face of the elevated preceptor. Gossiping about the preceptor or any other person is also a sign of degraded consciousness and will eventually lead you away from the teacher as well as true spiritual knowledge. Bouncing around from one teacher to another is also a way to go astray, as you cannot find water if you dig several superficial wells, but rather a single deep well. Therefore, even though you may read the books of many teachers or see many teachers there should be one special one with whom you may develop a rapport that will cause the flow of divine wisdom to move in your direction. Therefore, seek out a teacher who has a personality that is in harmony with your own. That is, if you are an intellectual person, look for a teacher who emphasizes the wisdom aspect of the disciplines. However, while you may have a special resonance in some aspect of the teachings there should always be practice of the other disciplines so that you may develop your entire personality and not be like the fanatical ignorant masses. Also, you must strive to never say you will do something for the teacher and then not do it or develop excuses. All of these things and more are for the world and will not bring you the favor of the preceptor. Favor is attention and when you have this the lips of the preceptor move for you as they will not for others and you will receive the grace of insight into Divine Consciousness that is the objective of all aspirants the world over.

Aspirants should take care to pay their dues. This means that at no time should they allow themselves to believe that they have achieved anything on their own or without the assistance of mentors and teachers. There are many unrighteous writers who take the writings of others and give no credit to them and even act as if they themselves wrote the information. In like manner some aspirants conduct discourses on the teachings and do not give the proper credit for what they have learned and thereby develop egoism as they dazzle others with their "wisdom." However, as they fatten their own ego they are actually leading people to a place that they will not be able to lead them beyond and here is where stagnation in the teachings commences. Some preachers rely on drama or exuberant performances while giving sermons. This distracts people and may even make people believe that these preachers or lecturers know what they are talking about but the listeners will not be able to transform themselves because the teaching is dishonest and incomplete. If an aspirant does not pay homage to the teacher they are committing an injustice and the higher wisdom will escape them even if it be presented to them or even if they come across it in a book.

Approach with a spirit of service and do not practice the mysteries as a part-time dabler. In order to progress you must work diligently and learn how every waking moment is to be dedicated to the Divine. This is the only way to succeed in dispelling the veil of ignorance. The world is a very powerful force with the ignorant mind and an aspirant must fight hard to overcome the yoke of worldly consciousness. Only complete dedication and service towards the Divine will open the doors of the House of Asar (palace of enlightenment). Therefore, you must understand that being an initiate means complete devotion to spiritual life and this translates to reverence and service towards the Spiritual Preceptor. Never allow the preceptor to do work that you can do since their time should be reserved for the higher dissemination of the teachings. So again, in serving the teacher you are facilitating the teachers time and availability to teach you and others. The teacher may not always ask for help because he/she wants to give you room to act on initiative. Thereby the initiatic process cannot be one-sided. The aspirant who hopes to become an *initiate* needs to *initiate* the contact with the teacher and have the *initiative* to make good use of the teaching.

You may find a Spiritual Preceptor who has all the qualifications to lead you, someone who is not only elevated but also who is capable of teaching you how to elevate yourself, for the two capacities are not the same nor are they always found in the same personality. A person may be elevated but not versed in the scripture or the ways to develop aspirants. Therefore, if you feel a burning desire to grow spiritually and you have dealt with your worldly responsibilities so that you can be free to pursue the teaching seek out a teacher. That person may be in your hometown but if not you must go to them and touch the floor with your face before them and humbly ask for their permission to be accepted as a student. First though, develop a keen understanding of what it means to be an aspirant and become familiar with and practice the disciplines of Maat which purify the heart. Do not present to God a dirty vessel. Wouldn't you wash a bow before placing food in it as an offering to God? In the same manner, your presentation of your personality before a preceptor as if to God herself. Therefore, be clean in your body, mind and soul to the best of your ability, then, even if you have to go around the world to meet and work with your teacher the trip will not be a waste of time but a glorious start on the golden road to enlightened experience.

THE TRADITION OF INITIATION

Those who are seriously interested in pursuing spiritual life should follow the instructions given in the previous section, seeking to purify themselves so as to become proper vessels to recognize and understand the teacher when he or she arrives. There is a tendency sometimes to engage in the flights of emotionality and in the psychic contacts that can be made when you begin to discover the inner dimensions of the mind. Sometimes aspirants believe they have encountered genuine divine personalities not realizing that these are expressions of their own mental creations as in a dream. Others believe that since they have experienced certain psychic "energies" or have developed certain psychic abilities, that this in and of itself constitutes spiritual enlightenment.

You must clearly understand that psychic phenomena do not necessarily signify or accompany spiritual enlightenment such as we are discussing here. Spiritual enlightenment is nothing short of mystical union with God. Therefore, while people may exhibit great feats of psychic nature or amazing control of bodily functions such as living without food for weeks or months or holding the breath for hours, etc., these are not to be automatically equated with spirituality and indeed may not have anything to do with spirituality in regard to the particular person who possesses such powers. Nevertheless, a spiritually enlightened personality may possess some such powers or may not. In any case, only one who is a genuinely advanced or an advancing spiritual personality can discern the difference. Thus, you must strive to purify yourself and dispel the illusions and misconceptions in your mind as to what constitutes true spirituality so that you may be led to the true spiritual teacher. Seek out those who exhibit compassion, patience, dispassion, equanimity of mind and selflessness. These are advanced psychic powers although they are not normally considered in this way. A stark contrast can be seen between ordinary egoistic human beings who think of providing for themselves and the pleasures of the body at the expense of others (the ignorant and worldly minded), and the more spiritually advanced individuals. The qualities of the ignorant, discontent, desire, hard-heartedness, distraction, mental agitation, restlessness, selfishness, etc., lead to experiences of pain, disappointment and frustration in life whereas the qualities of a spiritually advancing personality, selflessness, contentment, peacefulness, detachment from worldly possessions and relationships, etc., lead to greater levels of inner peace and self-discovery. These allow the mind to sink to deeper and deeper levels revealing the true nature of one's own being.

In the spiritual realm, you may encounter the divine in the form of God, Goddess, or an archetypal divine being. You may also experience this realm as wholeness, light, freedom, an awakening, etc. You need to understand that as you tread the path of initiatic science, you will need to gradually let go of all your mental concepts and notions of spirituality. This means that whatever you discover is to be understood as a relative reality because it is being perceived through the mind and senses which are limited.

If you do not have a specific spiritual preceptor who is versed in the spiritual disciplines of Yoga, the most important idea you need to keep in mind is your conviction to attain the highest. You must honestly and ardently ask for assistance and guidance while offering all of your activities and feelings to the Divine. As you learn about the various yogic paths, you will begin to develop a feeling for which course suits your personality. This is the reason why there are so many paths of yoga (devotional, wisdom, action, life force development, etc.). The process of becoming established on your personal path may involve a lot of ups and downs, trial and error, however you must be assured that if you follow through you will eventually reach the goal you have set.

Thus, self-initiation involves your decision to make the mystic path of yoga your life's endeavor. You must develop a strong desire to discover who you are and what the world is and you must have a deep rooted conviction that it is possible for you to understand and apply the principles and disciplines of yoga to your life, regardless of your life situation. At some point you may want to become formally initiated by a particular spiritual preceptor. This means that you have decided to come into closer association with the teaching as espoused by that teacher and that you are desirous of aligning yourself with the spiritual tradition of that teacher.

There are teachers who specialize in certain aspects of yoga disciplines. For example, a spiritual preceptor may focus on yoga through the wisdom teachings. This implies, studying, reflecting and rationalizing in order to develop a subtle intellect which will be able to discover the spiritual truth. Another spiritual preceptor may focus on developing and disciplining the physical body through physical exercises and breathing exercises in order to achieve the same goal. Another may focus on prayer, and another on meditation, etc. However, if you find a preceptor who is well versed in Integral Yoga, which is the combination of these main yogic paths, you should not need to search further for other teachers.

In the mean time, apply yourself to the teachings to the best of your understanding and if possible, associate with others who are honest seekers on the path of self-discovery. Finding those around you who are sincerely interested in practicing yoga for spiritual development can be a powerful means to spiritual growth. When people come together, their energies are multiplied toward the task which they have chosen to undertake. This is also true of spiritual practice. Therefore, those who meet and help each other can keep the enthusiasm and level of interest up in positive as well as hard times. Also, in a group setting, the subtle vibrations are more strongly attuned to the study process which in turn helps the process of concentration and understanding. The group learning process is a powerful practice which helps toward the goal of purification of the heart, especially when it is conducted under the guidance of a spiritual preceptor.

The Ritual of Initiation

Rituals are a powerful process which can lead the mind toward spiritual thoughts and aspirations or toward pain and sorrow in life. People cling to ignorance by constantly seeking for pleasure and fulfillment in the world of time and space through human relationships, wealth, possessions, etc. Examples of negative rituals are: going to the video store, watching television, gossiping, partying or going to the movie theater in search of excitement. In the course of ordinary life you may experience these but if you rely on them as a source of pleasure and happiness you are bound for disappointments. All of life's activities are ritualistic to some degree. Every day we repeat many actions such as eating, sleeping, going to work, school or watching television. Other activities are less frequent but just as ritualistic; these include marriage, childbearing, etc. The basis of society's rituals is custom and habit. Society teaches and socializes young individuals into the activities it deems acceptable and thereby societal rituals develop. Rituals can be bad or good according to the level of spiritual realization within the individual as well as the society as a whole. If a society allows exploitation of some of its members, then rituals and customs develop which affirm that belief system. When society developed the materialistic view of life and discounted the spiritual values, material values became part of the general culture. Thus, pursuing material wealth and the experience of sensual pleasures have become the most commonly practiced rituals in modern day society. This is reflected in business, government and in the family way of life at all levels of society. These rituals are all performed toward perishable goals and thus can never satisfy the inner need of the soul. This movement constitutes a movement in ignorance which leads to further ignorance. While religious rituals are also in the realm of human activity, if performed with growing levels of understanding and devotion toward the Divine, they will lead to greater and greater peace and self-knowledge. Therefore, the Sages and Saints have enjoined several rituals, prayers and words of power to help spiritual aspirants turn the mind toward spiritual realization rather than toward perishable worldly attainments which will inevitably lead to disappointments, pain and sorrow.

With this in mind, the following initiation ritual is presented for those who have not yet come into personal contact with a living spiritual preceptor and who would like to begin formal spiritual practice in the mystical system of yoga on their own until such time as they come into contact with a spiritual preceptor.

First, locate an area of your home where you can perform spiritual practices such as yoga exercises, prayers and meditations and not be disturbed. This area will be used only for yoga practice.
Now gather the basic materials needed to create your own altar. An altar is a place of worship which contains certain artifacts which hold specific spiritual symbolism that lead to spiritual awareness. The following items are to be considered as a basic listing of items. You are free to choose other items which resonate with your spiritual consciousness.

1- Small **table**
2- **Candle** - The candle holds deep mystical symbolism. It contains within itself all of the four elements of creation: fire, earth (wax in solid form), water (wax in liquefied form), and air. All are consumed in the burning process and all of them come together to produce light. This singular light represents the singular consciousness which shines throughout the entire universe. This light is the illumination which causes life to exist and it is the reason and source

of the human mind. This light is life itself and life is God. Therefore, God is ever-present in the candle, in the universe (nature) and in your heart and mind.

3- **Incense** - Incense invokes divine awareness through the sense of smell. When you perform spiritual practices and use a special incense consistently, every time that you smell the incense you will have divine thoughts and feelings even if you are not in the regular area of meditation. Therefore, select a fragrance which appeals to you and reflect within yourself that this is the fragrance of God in the same way as a flower emanates fragrance. Visualize that you are smelling divinity itself.

4- **Ankh** - The Ankh is one of the most universal symbols expressing eternal life, the union of opposites and it was, and is used by the world religious traditions (ancient Egyptian religion, early Christianity, Indian religion and others.

5- **Sculpture**, picture or other symbol of a Deity (as a symbol of the Supreme Being). This may be an ancient Egyptian Deity such as Horus, Isis, etc., or a Christian Icon such as Jesus or Mary, an Eastern icon such as Buddha (Buddhist), or Krishna, Rama or Saraswati of the Vedantic-Hindu tradition, etc. Choose an icon according to your spiritual inclination. This will help you to develop devotion toward the Divine and will hasten your progress in yoga. This is called worship of God with name and form. As you progress you will be instructed on how to worship the Divine in an abstract way without using any names or forms.

6- Small **audio cassette recorder** (to lead your spiritual sessions).

7- **Audio Recordings** of prayers, meditations, exercises, discourses from authentic Spiritual Preceptors.

8- For the first time initiation it is recommended that you reserve **one hour at four A.M.** and that you fast from 6 P.M the night before. This is also a good practice to continue during your regular morning worship and meditations.

9- After reading this manual completely, **select a Hekau** - Mantra (words of power) which resonates with you. If you do not feel a special connection to a particular hekau or if you would prefer to wait for a period of time to allow yourself to become acquainted with the philosophy and the presiding deities of the hekau, simply use "Om" for now. Om is a universal word of power which was used in ancient Egypt and is used extensively in India by yogis. Om or AUM* is related to the word Amun from ancient Egypt and Amun is related to the Amen of Christianity. Therefore, Om is generally useful for spiritual practice. Om* is also not related to a particular deity but is common to all. It is also the hekau-mantra of the 6th energy center at the point between the eyebrows known as the ancient Egyptian *Arat* or Uraeus serpent and the *Third eye of Shiva* in India. You will use hekau for chanting during your worship periods, and at idle times during the day. You will use it from now on to dig deeply into the unconscious regions of your mind as a miner uses a pick to cut into a mountain in search of gold. *(see *Egyptian Yoga: The Philosophy of Enlightenment* for a more detailed description of AUM and Om)

10- Recite the auspicious hekau-mantras for commencing your spiritual practice. These are given on page 76-78 of this volume. Each prayer should be recited four times. This quadruplicate format is a symbolic way to propitiate the divine forces which control the four quarters of the phenomenal universe and the heavenly realms. There are four directions which the mind is aware of (East, North, West and South) in the physical plane as in the astral. The prayer is directed toward the purification of the mind and body which will allow your spiritual practice (movement) to be unobstructed in earth as well as in heaven. It is a propitiation to the Divine that you should not be confined to the temporal world of time and space, and physical body and ego self consciousness, so that you may go beyond the ignorance of ordinary human existence and thereby discover the truth of your true nature as one with the Supreme Self.

11- Play the Morning Worship and Meditation audio tape (available from C.M. Books, P.O. Box 570459, Miami Fl. 33257). Other tapes containing Indian chants of Mantras (words of power) are also available. These tapes help you to attune the mind toward the Divine through specific utterances, chants, prayers and songs which lead to Enlightenment. Osiris and Isis of ancient Egypt, and Krishna and Shiva of India are Deities whose main form of worship include the chanting and singing of devotional words of power (Hekau-Mantras). Therefore, chanting the names of God and prayers which describe and glorify the attributes of God as well as the message of self-knowledge are most important elements in the practice of true mystical worship of the Divine.

The sacred music of ancient Egypt was so potent, inspiring and compelling that it lives on in the Christian Coptic music tradition of modern day Coptic Church in present day Egypt. It is believed by anthropologists that the primary characteristics of modern Coptic music were adopted from the music of ancient Egyptians. These characteristics include the use of triangles and cymbals, and a strong vocal tradition. The Copts are regarded as the genetically purest direct descendants of the ancient Egyptians due to their lack of intermarrying with the other Egyptians who are of Arab descent. The whole of the Coptic service is to be sung. The singing is alternated between the master chanter, the priest, and a choir of deacons. This technique of chanting was also used in ancient Egypt during the processions and recitals of the mystery rituals.

12- From this day forward, resolve to practice the teachings presented here. See yourself as one of the chosen few initiates into the divine spiritual life.

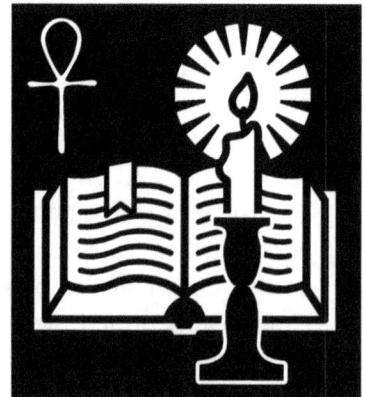

Initiation With a Spiritual Preceptor

In essence the entire program of study in Yoga is an initiatic ritual. However, a specific ritual of initiation is additionally efficacious since it serves to establish a subtle connection between teacher and disciple which fosters greater understanding through personal contact. It allows the aspirant to develop a devotional feeling toward the teacher and the teachings which relate to the *Self.* It engenders a mystic force towards spiritual aspiration even when done alone. Essentially, initiation is an expression of a person's personal conviction and desire to engage in a lifestyle which will lead to spiritual transformation. It is a commitment to a process of learning spiritual teaching and its practice. The initiation ritual performed with a Spiritual Preceptor also fosters a mystic link between an aspirant and his or her hekau and everything else related to the spiritual practice because it causes a deeper mental impression of their divine nature. This is especially important in the practice of chanting or hekau repetition. The hekau acts to cleanse the heart (mind) and it sets up positive vibrations which calm the mind and awaken spiritual feeling. Chanting elevates the mind and lifts it to transcendental levels.

The initiation ritual is usually accompanied by certain ceremonial rites and specific instruction on how chanting works and the procedure for uttering words of power. A specific hekau is given to an initiate based on the individuals spiritual inclination, attitudes and level of evolution. Initiations may be performed for individuals or for groups. A spiritual aspirant will be drawn to a Spiritual Preceptor on the basis of internal spiritual sensitivity. At some point in life a person will look for someone who can understand him or her and lead them on the spiritual path.

In ancient times those desiring to learn from a spiritual teacher would come to them with humility and reverence. They would bring fruits or firewood to help sustain the teacher and his or her efforts in disseminating the teaching. In Ancient Egypt the people and the government would support the Temples so that the spiritual upliftment of the country might be insured. Therefore, when you approach a teacher bring an offering. This may be a symbolic object but realizing that it represents your inner desire to grow spiritually and respect for the teachings you will receive. Also, come with patience and a spirit of joy. Then you will discover the true meaning of what the teachings really mean. This does not happen overnight. Fanaticism is not a part of real spiritual evolution. It is a hindrance. True spiritual evolution occurs in degrees. There is a Yoga parable given to illustrate this point. An aspirant went to a spiritual preceptor and asked for initiation into the teachings. The preceptor said "Alright, come to the temple and study the scriptures, attend my lectures and practice what I tell you." The aspirant said "Oh no, I don't have time for that. I want liberation from this miserable world now. Why will you withhold the teachings from me?" The preceptor replied "Very well, I will give you initiation into the teachings this evening. I will come to your house this evening but you must prepare the special food offering to your preceptor." That evening, the preceptor came and was greeted by the aspirant. The aspirant had set everything up and offered the preceptor a seat. The aspirant brought the food offering to the preceptor and the preceptor took out a bowl for the aspirant to put the food into. The aspirant was about to place the food in the bowl when he noticed that it was full of muck and insects so he said: "Please oh venerable sir, let me wash your bowl and then I will place the food into it." The preceptor replied: "No, that's alright, I will eat from this bowl the way it is." The aspirant was astonished and replied: "How can you expect me to put your food into that dirty bowl, I cannot do that." The preceptor replied: "How can you expect me to teach you the highest spiritual wisdom if you will not cleanse the vessel of your mind?" Immediately the aspirant understood the teaching and fell at the feet of the preceptor and pledged to follow his instruction from then on. The aspirant should realize that any endeavor in life requires instruction. Many fall under the delusion that the spiritual path can be accomplished without the help of a spiritual preceptor. All means should be used to learn but there is no better way than attending classes and receiving instruction from an authentic spiritual teacher. Then only through humility and total devotion is it possible to truly advance.

What are You Being Initiated Into?

Those who wish to become *Shemsu Neter* (followers of the Kamitan (Ancient Egyptian) spiritual teaching, are initiated into *Shetaut Neter* and *Smai Tawi*. Shetaut Neter is the religion and its mythic teachings based on the varied traditions centered around the different gods and goddesses. Smai Tawi are the yogic disciplines, techniques or technologies used to transform a human being. These disciplines promote a transformation through a movement that purifies the personality and renders it subtle enough to perceive the transcendental spiritual reality beyond time and space. This is a movement from ignorance to enlightenment, from mortality and weakness to immortality and supreme power, to discover the Absolute from whence the gods and goddesses and all Creation arose. This is a movement towards becoming one with the universe and the consciouness behind it which is eternal and infinite. This is the lofty goal of initiation. So those who tread this path must be mature and virtuous as well as strong, physically, mentally and emotionally. The purpose of the religion and disciplines is to promote purity of heart and virtue and these lead to higher realization and spiritual enlightenment. Therefore, the next section will present an overview of Shetaut Neter and how it relates to Smai Tawi. The following section will present an overview of the Smai Tawi disciplines. For details on these areas see the books:

For Shetaut Neter see the book *The Book of Shetaut Neter* by Muata Ashby

For SMai Tawi see the books related to the particular discipline

> Wisdom Discipline: *The Mysteries of Isis* by Muata Ashby
> Meditation Discipline: *Meditation The Ancient Egyptian Path to Enlightenment* by Muata Ashby
> Action Discipline: *The Wisdom of Maati* by Muata Ashby
> Feeling Discipline: *The Path of Divine Love* by Muata Ashby
> Life Force Discipline: *The Serpent Power* by Muata Ashby

The Fundamental Principles of Neterian Religion

NETERIANISM
(The Oldest Known Religion in History)

The term "Neterianism" is derived from the name "Shetaut Neter." Shetaut Neter means the "Hidden Divinity." It is the ancient philosophy and mythic spiritual culture that gave rise to the Ancient Egyptian civilization. Those who follow the spiritual path of Shetaut Neter are therefore referred to as "Neterians." The fundamental principles common to all denominations of Neterian Religion may be summed up as follows.

What is Neterianism and Who are the Neterians?

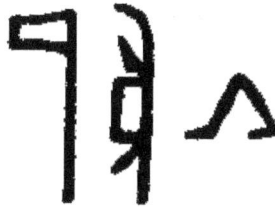

"Shemsu Neter"

"Follower (of) Neter"

The term "Neterianism" is derived from the name "Shetaut Neter." Those who follow the spiritual path of Shetaut Neter are therefore referred to as "Neterians."

Neterianism is the science of Neter, that is, the study of the secret or mystery of Neter, the enigma of that which transcends ordinary consciousness but from which all creation arises. The world did not come from nothing, nor is it sustained by nothing. Rather it is a manifestation of that which is beyond time and space but which at the same time permeates and maintains the fundamental elements. In other words, it is the substratum of Creation and the essential nature of all that exists.

So those who follow the Neter may be referred to as Neterians.

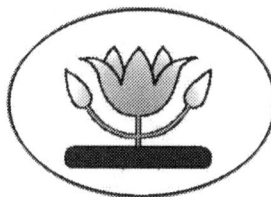

87

Neterian Great Truths

1. *"Pa Neter ua ua Neberdjer m Neteru"* -"The Neter, the Supreme Being, is One and alone and as Neberdjer, manifesting everywhere and in all things in the form of Gods and Goddesses."

Neberdjer means "all-encompassing divinity," the all-inclusive, all-embracing Spirit which pervades all and who is the ultimate essence of all. This first truth unifies all the expressions of Kamitan religion.

2. **"an-Maat swy Saui Set s-Khemn"** – "Lack of righteousness brings fetters to the personality and these fetters lead to ignorance of the Divine."

When a human being acts in ways that contradict the natural order of nature, negative qualities of the mind will develop within that person's personality. These are the afflictions of Set. Set is the neteru of egoism and selfishness. The afflictions of Set include: anger, hatred, greed, lust, jealousy, envy, gluttony, dishonesty, hypocrisy, etc. So to be free from the fetters of set one must be free from the afflictions of Set.

3. **"s-Uashu s-Nafu n saiu Set"**   -"Devotion to the Divine leads to freedom from the fetters of Set."

To be liberated (Nafu - freedom - to breath) from the afflictions of Set, one must be devoted to the Divine. Being devoted to the Divine means living by Maat. Maat is a way of life that is purifying to the heart and beneficial for society as it promotes virtue and order. Living by Maat means practicing Shedy (spiritual practices and disciplines).

Uashu means devotion and the classic pose of adoring the Divine is called "Dua," standing or sitting with upraised hands facing outwards towards the image of the divinity.

4. **"ari Shedy Rekh ab m Maakheru"** - "The practice of the Shedy disciplines leads to knowing oneself and the Divine. This is called being True of Speech."

Doing Shedy means to study profoundly, to penetrate the mysteries (Shetaut) and discover the nature of the Divine. There have been several practices designed by the sages of Ancient Kamit to facilitate the process of self-knowledge. These are the religious (Shetaut) traditions and the Sema (Smai) Tawi (yogic) disciplines related to them that augment the spiritual practices.

All the traditions relate the teachings of the sages by means of myths related to particular gods or goddesses. It is understood that all of these neteru are related, like brothers and sisters, having all emanated from the same source, the same Supremely Divine parent, who is neither male nor female, but encompasses the totality of the two.

The Great Truths of Neterianism are realized by means of Four Spiritual Disciplines in Three Steps

The four disciples are: Rekh Shedy (Wisdom), Ari Shedy (Righteous Action and Selfless Service), Uashu (Ushet) Shedy (Devotion) and Uaa Shedy (Meditation)

The Three Steps are: Listening, Ritual, and Meditation

SEDJM REKH SHEDY

L I S T E N

- ***Sedjm REKH Shedy - Listening* to the WISDOM of the Neterian Traditions**

    - Shetaut Asar   – Teachings of the Asarian Tradition
    - Shetaut Anu   – Teachings of the Ra Tradition
    - Shetaut Menefer   – Teachings of the Ptah Tradition
    - Shetaut Waset   – Teachings of the Amun Tradition
    - Shetaut Netrit   – Teachings of the Goddess Tradition
    - Shetaut Aton   – Teachings of the Aton Tradition

ARI SHEDY

R I T U A L

- ***Ari Maat Shedy* – Righteous Actions** – Purifies the GROSS impurities of the Heart

    - Maat Shedy   – True Study of the Ways of hidden nature of Neter
    - Maat Aakhu   – True Deeds that lead to glory
    - Maat Aru   – True Ritual

UASHU (USHET) SHEDY

- ***Ushet Shedy* – Devotion to the Divine** – Purifies the EMOTIONAL impurities of the Heart

    - Shmai   – Divine Music
    - Sema Paut   – Meditation in motion
    - Neter Arit   – Divine Offerings – Selfless-Service – virtue -

UAA SHEDY

M E D I T A T E

- ***Uaa m Neter Shedy* -** 𓂝𓃀𓃀𓃀𓃀 **Meditation** Experience the Transcendental Supreme Self. The five forms of Neterian Meditation discipline include.

    - Arat Sekhem, - Meditation on the Subtle Life Force
    - Ari Sma Maat, - Meditation on the Righteous action
    - Nuk Pu-Ushet, - Meditation on the I am
    - Nuk Ra Akhu, - Meditation on the Glorious Light
    - Rekh – Khemn, - Meditation on the Wisdom Teaching

89

Summary of The Great Truths and the Shedy Paths to their Realization

Great Truths

Shedy Disciplines

I

GOD IS ONE AND IN ALL THINGS MANIFESTING THROUGH THE NETERU

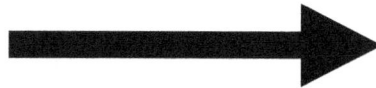

I

Listen to the Wisdom Teachings (Become Wise)
Learn the mysteries as taught by an authentic teacher which allows this profound statement to be understood.

I I

UNRIGHTEOUSNESS BRINGS FETTERS AND THESE CAUSE IGNORANCE OF TRUTH (#1)

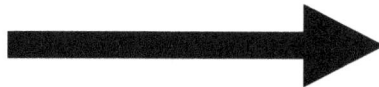

I I

Acting (Living) by Truth
Apply the Philosophy of right action to become virtuous and purify the heart

I I I

DEVOTION TO GOD ALLOWS THE PERSONALITY TO FREE ITSELF FROM THE FETTERS

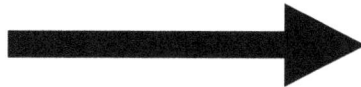

I I I

Devotion to the Divine
Worship, ritual and divine love allows the personality purified by truth to eradicate the subtle ignorance that binds it to mortal existence.

I I I I

THE SHEDY DISCIPLINES ARE THE GREATEST FORM OF WORSHIP OF THE DIVINE

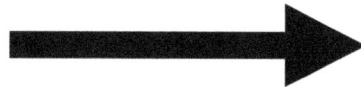

I I I I

Meditation
Allows the whole person to go beyond the world of time and space and the gross and subtle ignorance of mortal human existence to discover that which transcends time and space.

Great Awakening
Occurs when all of the Great Truths have been realized by perfection of the Shedy disciplines to realize their true nature and actually experience oneness with the transcendental Supreme Being.

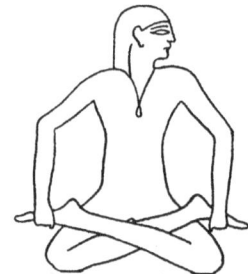

The Spiritual Culture and the Purpose of Life: Shetaut Neter

"Men and women are to become God-like through a life of virtue
and the cultivation of the spirit through scientific knowledge,
practice and bodily discipline."

-Ancient Egyptian Proverb

The highest forms of Joy, Peace and Contentment are obtained when the meaning of life is discovered. When the human being is in harmony with life, then it is possible to reflect and meditate upon the human condition and realize the limitations of worldly pursuits. When there is peace and harmony in life, a human being can practice any of the varied disciplines designated as Shetaut Neter to promote {his/her} evolution towards the ultimate goal of life, which Spiritual Enlightenment. Spiritual Enlightenment is the awakening of a human being to the awareness of the Transcendental essence which binds the universe and which is eternal and immutable. In this discovery is also the sobering and ecstatic realization that the human being is one with that Transcendental essence. With this realization comes great joy, peace and power to experience the fullness of life and to realize the purpose of life during the time on earth. The lotus is a symbol of Shetaut Neter, meaning the turning towards the light of truth, peace and transcendental harmony.

Shetaut Neter

We have established that the Ancient Egyptians were African peoples who lived in the north-eastern quadrant of the continent of Africa. They were descendants of the Nubians, who had themselves originated from farther south into the heart of Africa at the Great Lakes region, the sources of the Nile River. They created a vast civilization and culture earlier than any other society in known history and organized a nation that was based on the concepts of balance and order as well as spiritual enlightenment. These ancient African people called their land Kamit, and soon after developing a well-ordered society, they began to realize that the world is full of wonders, but also that life is fleeting, and that there must be something more to human existence. They developed spiritual systems that were designed to allow human beings to understand the nature of this secret being who is the essence of all Creation. They called this spiritual system "Shtaut Ntr (Shetaut Neter)."

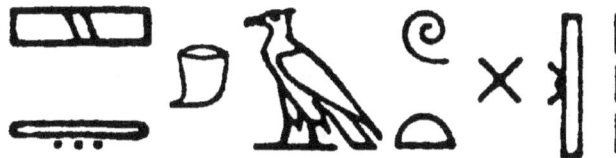

Shetaut means secret.

Neter means Divinity.

91

Who is Neter in Kamitan Religion?

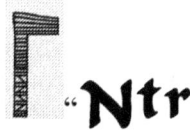

Ntr

The symbol of Neter was described by an Ancient Kamitan priest as:
"That which is placed in the coffin"

The term Ntr, or Ntjr, comes from the Ancient Egyptian hieroglyphic language which did not record its vowels. However, the term survives in the Coptic language as *"Nutar."* The same Coptic meaning (divine force or sustaining power) applies in the present as it did in ancient times. It is a symbol composed of a wooden staff that was wrapped with strips of fabric, like a mummy. The strips alternate in color with yellow, green and blue. The mummy in Kamitan spirituality is understood to be the dead but resurrected Divinity. So the Nutar (Ntr) is actually every human being who does not really die, but goes to live on in a different form. Further, the resurrected spirit of every human being is that same Divinity. Phonetically, the term Nutar is related to other terms having the same meaning, such as the latin "Natura," the Spanish Naturalesa, the English "Nature" and "Nutriment", etc. In a real sense, as we will see, Natur means power manifesting as Neteru and the Neteru are the objects of creation, i.e. "nature."

Sacred Scriptures of Shetaut Neter

The following scriptures represent the foundational scriptures of Kamitan culture. They may be divided into three categories: *Mythic Scriptures*, *Mystical Philosophy* and *Ritual Scriptures*, and *Wisdom Scriptures* (Didactic Literature).

MYTHIC SCRIPTURES Literature	Mystical (Ritual) Philosophy Literature	Wisdom Texts Literature
SHETAUT ASAR-ASET-HERU The Myth of Asar, Aset and Heru (Asarian Resurrection Theology) - Predynastic **SHETAUT ATUM-RA** Anunian Theology Predynastic **Shetaut Net/Aset/Hetheru** Saitian Theology – Goddess Spirituality Predynastic **SHETAUT PTAH** Memphite Theology Predynastic **Shetaut Amun** Theban Theology Predynastic	**Coffin Texts** (C. 2040 B.C.E.-1786 B.C.E.) **Papyrus Texts** (C. 1580 B.C.E.-Roman Period)[5] Books of Coming Forth By Day Example of famous papyri: Papyrus of Any Papyrus of Hunefer Papyrus of Kenna Greenfield Papyrus, Etc.	**Wisdom Texts** (C. 3,000 B.C.E. – PTOLEMAIC PERIOD) Precepts of Ptahotep Instructions of Any Instructions of Amenemope Etc. Maat Declarations Literature (All Periods)

---

[5] After 1570 B.C.E they would evolve into a more unified text, the Egyptian Book of the Dead.

Neter and the Neteru

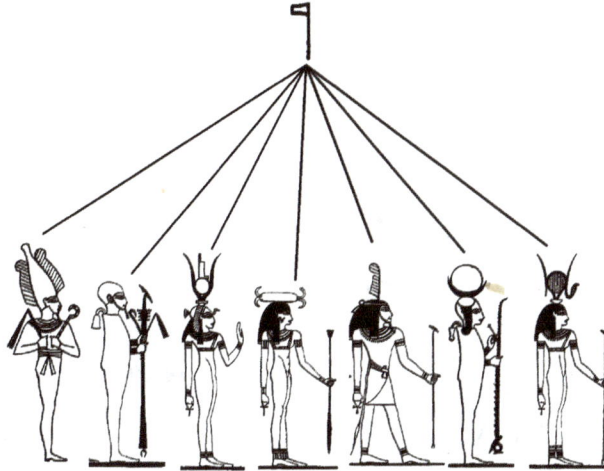

The Neteru (Gods and Goddesses) proceed from the Neter (Supreme Being)

As stated earlier, the concept of Neter and Neteru binds and ties all of the varied forms of Kamitan spirituality into one vision of the gods and goddesses all emerging from the same Supreme Being. Therefore, ultimately, Kamitan spirituality is not polytheistic, nor is it monotheistic, for it holds that the Supreme Being is more than a God or Goddess. The Supreme Being is an all-encompassing Absolute Divinity.

The Neteru

"Neteru"

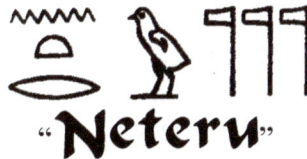

The term "Neteru" means "gods and goddesses." This means that from the ultimate and transcendental Supreme Being, "Neter," come the Neteru. There are countless Neteru. So from the one come the many. These Neteru are cosmic forces that pervade the universe. They are the means by which Neter sustains Creation and manifests through it. So Neterianism is a monotheistic polytheism. The one Supreme Being expresses as many gods and goddesses. At the end of time, after their work of sustaining Creation is finished, these gods and goddesses are again absorbed back into the Supreme Being.

All of the spiritual systems of Ancient Egypt (Kamit) have one essential aspect that is common to all; they all hold that there is a Supreme Being (Neter) who manifests in a multiplicity of ways through nature, the Neteru. Like sunrays, the Neteru emanate from the Divine; they are its manifestations. So by studying the Neteru we learn about and are led to discover their source, the Neter, and with this discovery we are enlightened. The Neteru may be depicted anthropomorphically or zoomorphically in accordance with the teaching about Neter that is being conveyed through them.

The Neteru and Their Temples

Diagram 1: The Ancient Egyptian Temple Network

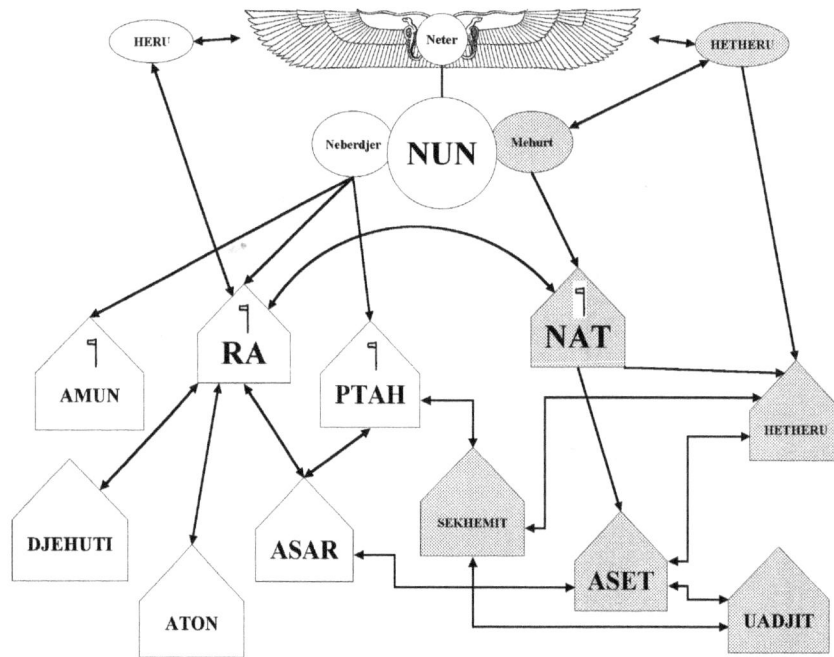

The sages of Kamit instituted a system by which the teachings of spirituality were espoused through a Temple organization. The major divinities were assigned to a particular city. That divinity or group of divinities became the "patron" divinity or divinities of that city. Also, the Priests and Priestesses of that Temple were in charge of seeing to the welfare of the people in that district as well as maintaining the traditions and disciplines of the traditions based on the particular divinity being worshipped. So the original concept of "Neter" became elaborated through the "theologies" of the various traditions. A dynamic expression of the teachings emerged, which though maintaining the integrity of the teachings, expressed nuances of variation in perspective on the teachings to suit the needs of varying kinds of personalities of the people of different locales.

In the diagram above, the primary or main divinities are denoted by the Neter symbol (⌐). The house structure represents the Temple for that particular divinity. The interconnections with the other Temples are based on original scriptural statements espoused by the Temples that linked the divinities of their Temple with the other divinities. So this means that the divinities should be viewed not as separate entities operating independently, but rather as family members who are in the same "business" together, i.e. the enlightenment of society, albeit through variations in form of worship, name, form (expression of the Divinity), etc. Ultimately, all the divinities are referred to as Neteru and they are all said to be emanations from the ultimate and Supreme Being. Thus, the teaching from any of the Temples leads to an understanding of the others, and these all lead back to the source, the highest Divinity. Thus, the teaching within any of the Temple systems would lead to the attainment of spiritual enlightenment, the Great Awakening.

The Neteru and Their Interrelationships
Diagram : The Primary Kamitan Neteru and their Interrelationships

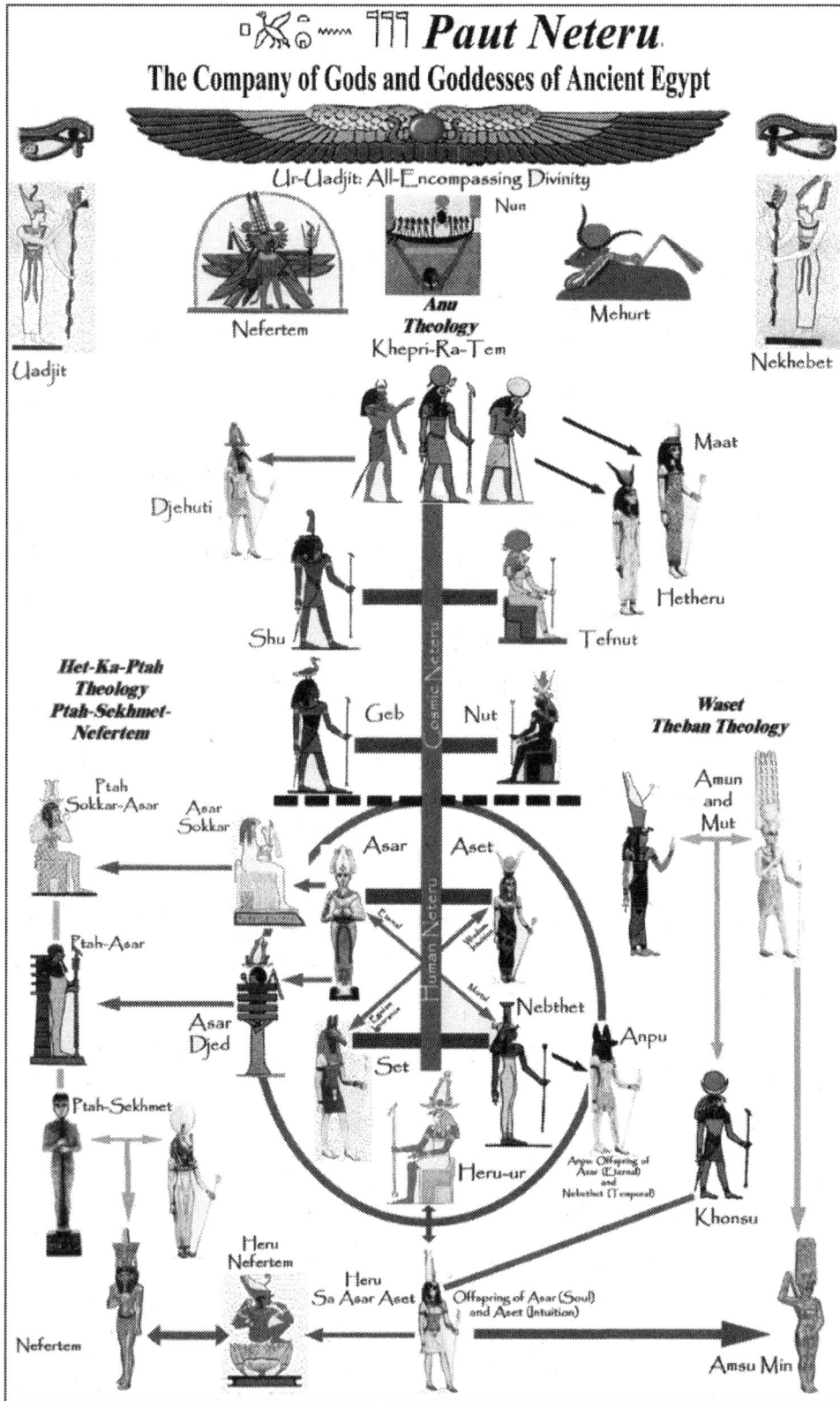

Paut Neteru
The Company of Gods and Goddesses of Ancient Egypt

Ur-Uadjit: All-Encompassing Divinity

The same Supreme Being, Neter, is the winged all-encompassing transcendental Divinity, the Spirit who, in the early history, is called "Heru." The physical universe in which the Heru lives is called "Hetheru" or the "house of Heru." This divinity (Heru) is also the Nun or primeval substratum from which all matter is composed. The various divinities and the material universe are composed from this primeval substratum. Neter is actually androgynous and Heru, the Spirit, is related as a male aspect of that androgyny. However, Heru in the androgynous aspect, gives rise to the solar principle and this is seen in both the male and female divinities.

The image above provides an idea of the relationships between the divinities of the three main Neterian spiritual systems (traditions): Anunian Theology, Wasetian (Theban) Theology and Het-Ka-Ptah (Memphite) Theology. The traditions are composed of companies or groups of gods and goddesses. Their actions, teachings and interactions with each other and with human beings provide insight into their nature as well as that of human existence and Creation itself. The lines indicate direct scriptural relationships and the labels also indicate that some divinities from one system are the same in others, with only a name change. Again, this is attested to by the scriptures themselves in direct statements, like those found in the *Prt m Hru* text Chapter 4 (17).[6]

Listening to the Teachings

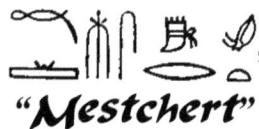

"Mestchert"

"Listening, to fill the ears, listen attentively-"

What should the ears be filled with?

The sages of Shetaut Neter enjoined that a Shemsu Neter (follower of Neter, an initiate or aspirant) should listen to the WISDOM of the Neterian Traditions. These are the myth related to the gods and goddesses containing the basic understanding of who they are, what they represent, how they relate human beings and to the Supreme Being. The myths allow us to be connected to the Divine.

An aspirant may choose any one of the 5 main Neterian Traditions.

- Shetaut Anu   – Teachings of the Ra Tradition
- Shetaut Menefer – Teachings of the Ptah Tradition
- Shetaut Waset   – Teachings of the Amun Tradition
- Shetaut Netrit   – Teachings of the Goddess Tradition
- Shetaut Asar   – Teachings of the Asarian Tradition
- Shetaut Aton   – Teachings of the Aton Tradition

---

[6] See the book *The Egyptian Book of the Dead* by Muata Ashby

The Anunian Tradition

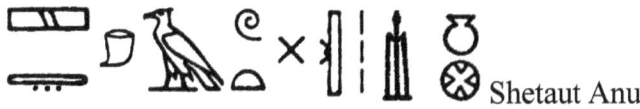

Shetaut Anu

The Mystery Teachings of the Anunian Tradition are related to the Divinity Ra and his company of Gods and Goddesses.[7] This Temple and its related Temples espouse the teachings of Creation, human origins and the path to spiritual enlightenment by means of the Supreme Being in the form of the god Ra. It tells of how Ra emerged from a primeval ocean and how human beings were created from his tears. The gods and goddesses, who are his children, go to form the elements of nature and the cosmic forces that maintain nature.

Below: The Heliopolitan Cosmogony.

The city of Anu (Amun-Ra)

The Neters of Creation - The Company of the Gods and Goddesses.
Neter Neteru
Nebertcher - Amun (unseen, hidden, ever present, Supreme Being, beyond duality and description)

Amen (Ra)   *Amenit (Rat)*

Shu   *Hathor Djehuti MAAT*   *Tefnut*

Geb   *Nut*

Set   *Osiris*   *Horus*   *Isis*   *Nephthys*

Anubis

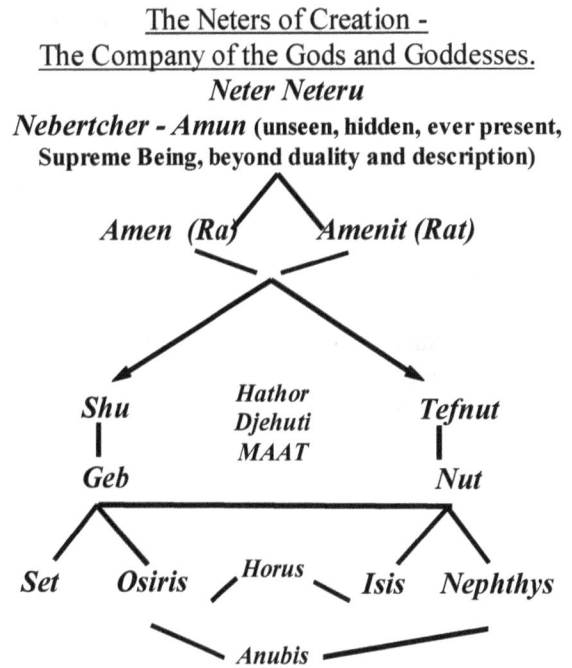

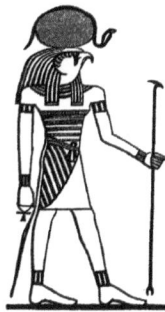

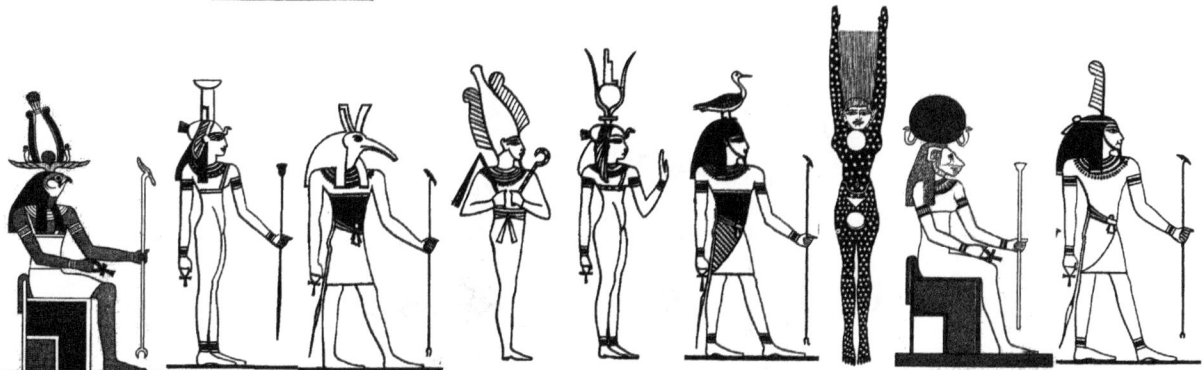

Top: Ra. From left to right, starting at the bottom level- The Gods and Goddesses of Anunian Theology: Shu, Tefnut, Nut, Geb, Aset, Asar, Set, Nebthet and Heru-Ur

[7] See the Book Anunian Theology by Muata Ashby

97

The Memphite Tradition

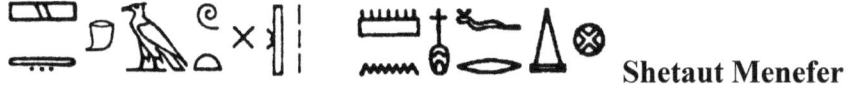

 Shetaut Menefer

The Mystery Teachings of the Menefer (Memphite) Tradition are related to the Neterus known as Ptah, Sekhmit, Nefertem. The myths and philosophy of these divinities constitutes Memphite Theology.[8] This temple and its related temples espoused the teachings of Creation, human origins and the path to spiritual enlightenment by means of the Supreme Being in the form of the god Ptah and his family, who compose the Memphite Trinity. It tells of how Ptah emerged from a primeval ocean and how he created the universe by his will and the power of thought (mind). The gods and goddesses who are his thoughts, go to form the elements of nature and the cosmic forces that maintain nature. His spouse, Sekhmit has a powerful temple system of her own that is related to the Memphite teaching. The same is true for his son Nefertem.

Below: The Memphite Cosmogony.

The city of Hetkaptah (Ptah)

The Neters of Creation - ### The Company of the Gods and Goddesses.
Neter Neteru

Nebertcher - Amun **(unseen, hidden, ever present, Supreme Being, beyond duality and description)**

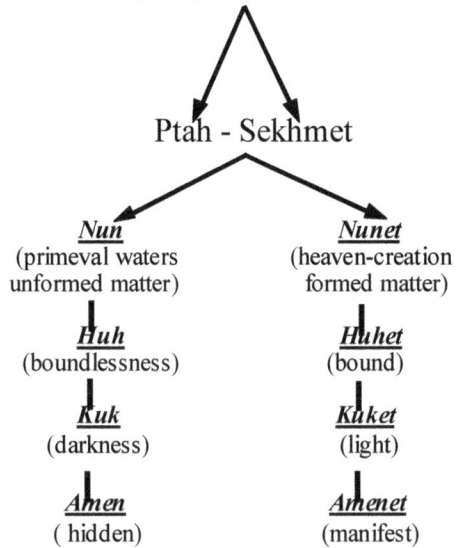

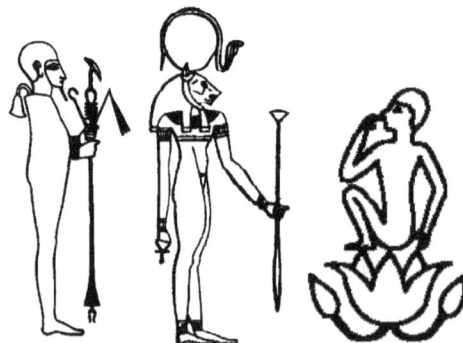

Ptah - Sekhmet

Nun (primeval waters unformed matter)	*Nunet* (heaven-creation formed matter)
Huh (boundlessness)	*Huhet* (bound)
Kuk (darkness)	*Kuket* (light)
Amen (hidden)	*Amenet* (manifest)

Ptah, Sekhmit and Nefertem

---

[8] See the Book Memphite Theology by Muata Ashby

The Theban Tradition

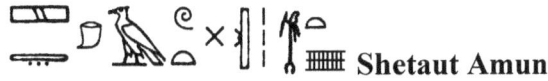

Shetaut Amun

The Mystery Teachings of the Wasetian Tradition are related to the Neterus known as Amun, Mut Khonsu. This temple and its related temples espoused the teachings of Creation, human origins and the path to spiritual enlightenment by means of the Supreme Being in the form of the god Amun or Amun-Ra. It tells of how Amun and his family, the Trinity of Amun, Mut and Khonsu, manage the Universe along with his Company of Gods and Goddesses. This Temple became very important in the early part of the New Kingdom Era.

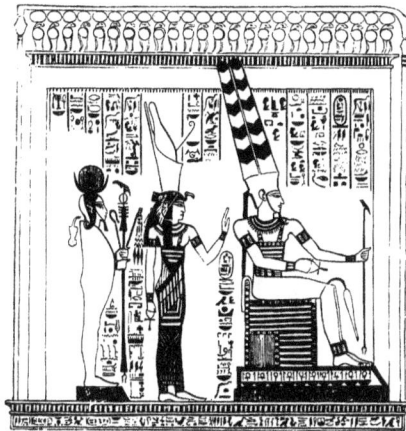

Below: The Trinity of Amun and the Company of Gods and Goddesses of Amun

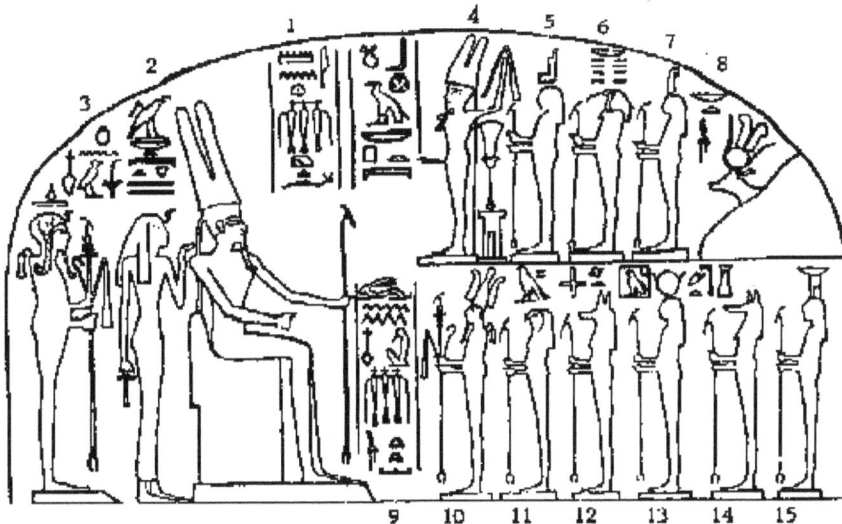

See the Book *Egyptian Yoga Vol. 2* for more on Amun, Mut and Khonsu by Muata Ashby

99

The Goddess Tradition

Shetaut Netrit

"Arat"

The hieroglyphic sign Arat means "Goddess." General, throughout ancient Kamit, the Mystery Teachings of the Goddess Tradition are related to the Divinity in the form of the Goddess. The Goddess was an integral part of all the Neterian traditions but special temples also developed around the worship of certain particular Goddesses who were also regarded as Supreme Beings in their own right. Thus as in other African religions, the goddess as well as the female gender were respected and elevated as the male divinities. The Goddess was also the author of Creation, giving birth to it as a great Cow. The following are the most important forms of the goddess.[9]

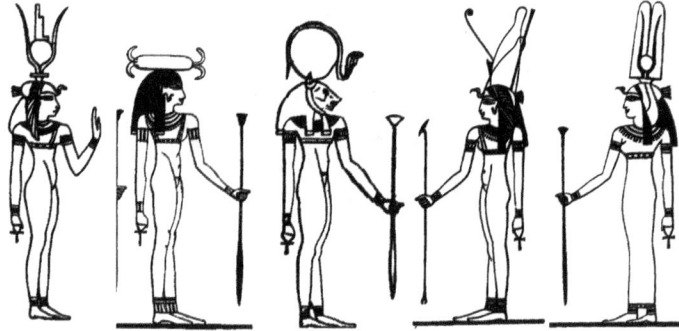

Aset, Net, Sekhmit, Mut, Hetheru

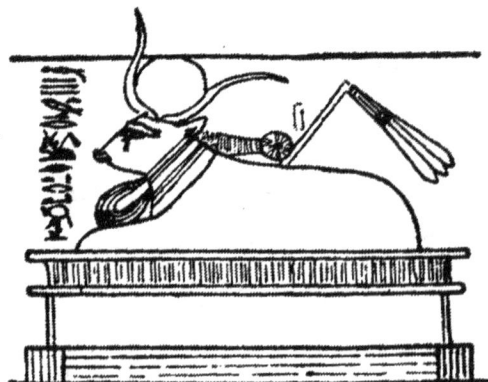

Mehurt ("The Mighty Full One")

---

[9] See the Books, *The Goddess Path, Mysteries of Isis, Glorious Light Meditation, Memphite Theology* and *Resurrecting Osiris* by Muata Ashby

The Asarian Tradition

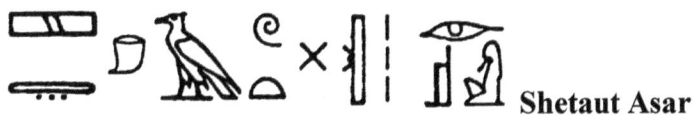 **Shetaut Asar**

This temple and its related temples espoused the teachings of Creation, human origins and the path to spiritual enlightenment by means of the Supreme Being in the form of the god Asar. It tells of how Asar and his family, the Trinity of Asar, Aset and Heru, manage the Universe and lead human beings to spiritual enlightenment and the resurrection of the soul. This Temple and its teaching were very important from the Pre-Dynastic era down to the Christian period. The Mystery Teachings of the Asarian Tradition are related to the Neterus known as: Asar, Aset, Heru (Osiris, Isis and Horus)

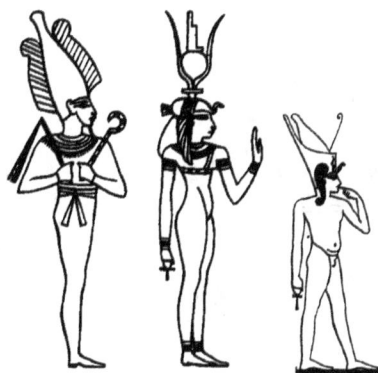

The tradition of Asar, Aset and Heru was practiced generally throughout the land of ancient Kamit. The centers of this tradition were the city of Abdu containing the Great Temple of Asar, the city of Pilak containing the Great Temple of Aset[10] and Edfu containing the Ggreat Temple of Heru.

---

[10] See the Book Resurrecting Osiris by Muata Ashby

The Aton Tradition

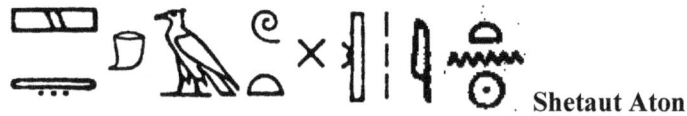 **Shetaut Aton**

This temple and its related temples espoused the teachings of Creation, human origins and the path to spiritual enlightenment by means of the Supreme Being in the form of the god Aton. It tells of how Aton with its dynamic life force created and sustains Creation. By recognizing Aton as the very substratum of all existence, human beings engage in devotional exercises and rituals and the study of the Hymns containing the wisdom teachings of Aton explaining that Aton manages the Universe and leads human beings to spiritual enlightenment and eternal life for the soul. This Temple and its teaching were very important in the middle New Kingdom Period. The Mystery Teachings of the Aton Tradition are related to the Neter Aton and its main exponent was the Sage King Akhnaton, who is depicted below with his family adoring the sundisk, symbol of the Aton.

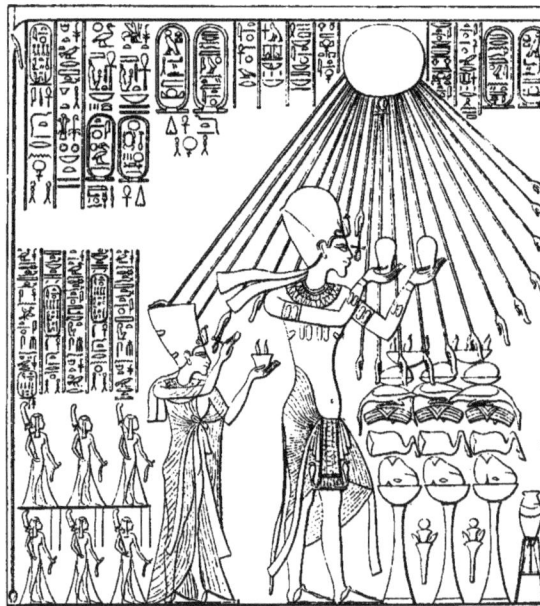

Akhnaton, Nefertiti and Daughters

For more on Atonism and the Aton Theology see the Essence of Atonism Lecture Series by Sebai Muata Ashby ©2001

The General Principles of Shetaut Neter
(Teachings Presented in the Kamitan scriptures)

1. The Purpose of Life is to Attain the Great Awakening-Enlightenment-Know thyself.

2. SHETAUT NETER enjoins the Shedy (spiritual investigation) as the highest endeavor of life.

3. SHETAUT NETER enjoins that it is the responsibility of every human being to promote order and truth.

4. SHETAUT NETER enjoins the performance of Selfless Service to family, community and humanity.

5. SHETAUT NETER enjoins the Protection of nature.

6. SHETAUT NETER enjoins the Protection of the weak and oppressed.

7. SHETAUT NETER enjoins the Caring for hungry.

8. SHETAUT NETER enjoins the Caring for homeless.

9. SHETAUT NETER enjoins the equality for all people.

10. SHETAUT NETER enjoins the equality between men and women.

11. SHETAUT NETER enjoins the justice for all.

12. SHETAUT NETER enjoins the sharing of resources.

13. SHETAUT NETER enjoins the protection and proper raising of children.

14. SHETAUT NETER enjoins the movement towards balance and peace.

The Forces of Entropy

In Neterian religion, there is no concept of "evil" as is conceptualized in Western Culture. Rather, it is understood that the forces of entropy are constantly working in nature to bring that which has been constructed by human hands to their original natural state. The serpent Apep (Apophis), who daily tries to stop Ra's boat of creation, is the symbol of entropy. This concept of entropy has been referred to as "chaos" by Western Egyptologists.

Apep

Above: Set protecting the boat of Ra from the forces of entropy (symbolized by the serpent Apep).

As expressed previously, in Neterian religion there is also no concept of a "devil" or "demon" as is conceived in the Judeo-Christian or Islamic traditions. Rather, it is understood that manifestations of detrimental situations and adversities arise as a result of unrighteous actions. These unrighteous actions are due to the "Setian" qualities in a human being. Set is the Neteru of egoism and the negative qualities which arise from egoism. Egoism is the idea of individuality based on identification with the body and mind only as being who one is. One has no deeper awareness of their deeper spiritual essence, and thus no understanding of their connectedness to all other objects (includes persons) in creation and the Divine Self. When the ego is under the control of the higher nature, it fights the forces of entropy (as above). However, when beset with ignorance, it leads to the degraded states of human existence. The vices (egoism, selfishness, extraverted ness, wonton sexuality (lust), jealousy, envy, greed, gluttony) are a result.

Set

Set and the Set animal

The Great Awakening of Neterian Religion

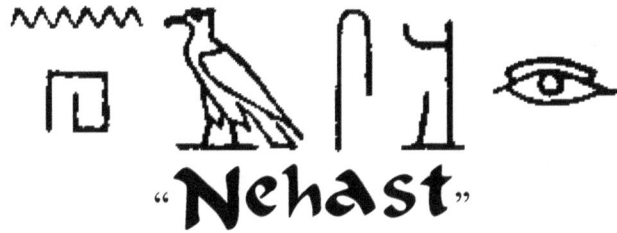

"Nehast"

Nehast means to "wake up," to Awaken to the higher existence. In the Prt m Hru Text it is said:

Nuk pa Neter aah Neter Ḩah asha ren[11]

"I am that same God, the Supreme One, who has myriad of mysterious names."

The goal of all the Neterian disciplines is to discover the meaning of "Who am I?," to unravel the mysteries of life and to fathom the depths of eternity and infinity. This is the task of all human beings and it is to be accomplished in this very lifetime.

This can be done by learning the ways of the Neteru, emulating them and finally becoming like them, Akhus, (enlightened beings), walking the earth as giants and accomplishing great deeds such as the creation of the universe!

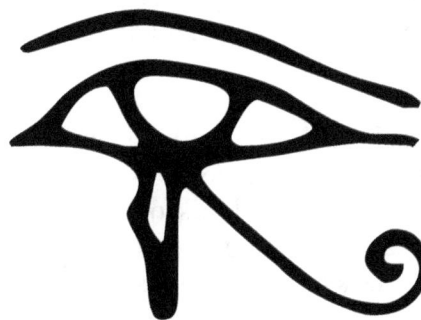

Udjat
The Eye of Heru is a quintessential symbol of awakening to Divine Consciousness, representing the concept of Nehast.

---

[11] (Prt M Hru 9:4)

CHAPTER III

THE PERSONAL SPIRITUAL PROGRAM

The daily practices to make the teachings of yoga manifest in your life.

Now that you have received some basic information about the teachings of yoga, the initiation process and the ultimate goal of enlightenment, you are now ready to proceed to setting up your own personal spiritual program which will allow you to practice the teachings of yoga in everyday life. You should begin to keep a journal detailing your experiences. Keep the journal as your personal record of inner spiritual awakening. If you review it from time to time, you will gain insights into your own progress and into the workings of your own mind.

The first stage of yoga is purification of the student both physically and mentally. Purification is accomplished through practices that promote healthy functioning of the body and mind. You will incorporate rituals, meditation and specific dietary practices into your life and record those experiences on a daily basis.

Setting up a spiritual discipline for yourself is the first step before discussing any other higher elements of mystical philosophy or wisdom because your vessel, that is to say, your mind and body, must be purified first before you can begin to achieve a mental state where you can effectively listen to and study the teachings. There are many who have heard the highest wisdom teachings but who have not benefited from them because they did not follow this first and all important instruction. Their spiritual development has been stunted because they pridefully thought that they could do it on their own by simply reading books of wisdom. This is a serious mistake when aspirants fall into the illusion of being advanced early on in their spiritual quest due to impatience and self-centricity.

Even if you have read this book and the textbook *Egyptian Yoga: The Philosophy of Enlightenment* thoroughly several times, as you develop your spiritual discipline of purification and then go back and study these books, you will discover new levels of wisdom which you had not awakened to previously. Purification of mind and body must come before or along with the study of the teachings. When these tasks are accomplished, you will discover that the wisdom teachings are being understood by you in their deeper essence, thus leading you to discover your true Self. This is a function of your own effort as well as the instruction you will receive throughout this book series or from your spiritual preceptor. In this section we will concentrate on the elementary aspects of the spiritual discipline which include:

Disease and Self Healing.
Purification of the Diet - Nutrition.
Purification of the Body - Physical exercise.
Purification of the Mind - Relaxation and Meditation

You must strive to develop the humility and desire to follow the teachings and ask for assistance when needed. You must develop faith in the initiatic tradition of mystical teaching which is passed on from teacher to disciple. This has always been the most effective method for spiritual evolution. For now, begin to develop faith in yourself and your abilities. The fact that you have pursued this course of study to seriously embark on your spiritual evolution shows that you have reached a level of spiritual maturity which qualifies you for higher spiritual attainment.

THE CAUSE OF DISEASE[12]

The spiritual Self is the source of all life including the life of each individual human personality. It is also the spiritual Self which sustains the mental and physical selves. At this level you should understand that the spiritual Self exists in the realm of nature (time and space) and also in a another dimension, the spiritual realm which is beyond time and space (movement and change), whereas, the mental and physical selves exist entirely in the realm of time and space. The body and mind, being instruments of the Soul, operate according to the laws of nature.

Contrary to the belief system which pervades modern day society that disease originates from factors outside of the body, it is the contention of yoga philosophy that the root cause of disease is ignorance of one's true nature as the Self. In the unenlightened state, you identify yourself with the mind, and through the mind and senses (which are merely an extension of the mind), with the body. When this occurs, the universal Self becomes deluded by the state of ignorance into believing in the concepts of death, disease, limitation, and individuality. Because death, disease and limitation are not characteristics of the true Self, conflict and contradiction develops deep within the unconscious mind which results in a disturbance of the mental function. This distorted or inharmonious state of mind translates into a disturbance within the Life Force Energy of the body and results in disease, because the flow of Life Force Energy (Sekhem, Prana, Chi) is blocked or otherwise disrupted throughout portions of the body. The Life Force Energy flows from the Soul to the Astral Body, which is composed of the mind and senses. Through subtle channels within the Astral body, the energy flows into the physical body and vivifies the organs. The presence of this energy is what constitutes "life." The absence of it is called "death."

The word disease itself gives a clue to this process by implying that disease results from a lack of (dis-) ease in the body. What is this ease? It is the ease of the true Self which is universal, free, all encompassing, immortal, and absolute bliss and peace (Hetep). Imagine how much dis-ease would be created if you tried to confine the ocean or the sky in a jar? How much dis-ease does a wild animal, which is used to roaming in the vast forest, experience when it is captured and placed in confinement? So when body identification occurs and the soul now identifies with concepts of individuality as opposed to universality, death as opposed to immortality, dis-ease or tension arises from within the soul level of the individual which becomes manifested in the mind as fear, anger, hatred, greed,

_____

[12] See book: Kemetic Diet

jealousy, envy and attachment. These in turn become manifested in the body as what we term illnesses and diseases, such as cancer, colds, fatigue, AIDS, and all other disease syndromes.

Thus, it is not surprising that modern medicine is finding that the most healthy activity a person can engage in is to sit quietly once or twice a day in a state of deep relaxation or meditation. Why is this? When the mind is filled with thoughts of a worldly nature, it creates ripples in the lake of consciousness, and just as the wind blows across a lake and creates ripples, the reflection of the sky is obstructed, so too the ripples created in the lake of consciousness by tension laden thoughts obstruct the reflection of the Self. When these thoughts are quieted through the relaxation or meditation process, then the Self reflects in the lake of consciousness, providing one with a feeling of expansion, a sense of peace, bliss and immortality. In this state of consciousness there is a free flow of healing Life Force Energy that maintains the body and mind healthy. This is what happens when you enter into deep dreamless sleep every night, however, because your consciousness is withdrawn during this process, you are ignorant of the experience. You only know that you feel rested and relaxed when you wake up. This is why you are told to get lots of rest when you are ill or you may feel that you are becoming ill and instinctively know that if you to go to bed early, the chances are that you will not become ill. The healing comes from embracing your true nature and letting go of your body identification by relaxing the desires of the mind and temporarily giving up worldly activities. Sleep is nature's way of providing you with this experience, however, it is not the only way to have this experience. This is where the practice of yoga comes in.

Through the process and disciplines of yoga, you are able to achieve the state where you can have this experience at all times, the state of enlightenment. The formal practice of meditation provides you with this experience initially, however, when the teachings become integrated into your consciousness, your wisdom and intuitional realization of the teachings will allow you to maintain this experience, even amidst the most chaotic circumstances. So, integral and foremost to the process of maintaining or regaining optimal physical or mental health is the practice of meditation and the other disciplines of yoga, because the ultimate state of total health is in the state of enlightenment. In yoga philosophy "true health" is termed *"Swastat"* or being established in the Self (the state of Enlightenment). Although you need to have a healthy diet, proper exercise and rest to maintain health, these factors alone can never confer total health. You must engage in spiritual practices to discover your true nature to be truly healthy. The ancient medical traditions such as the Ayurvedic system of India and The Therapeutic system of Egypt recognized this and therefore, in addition to recommending and prescribing various diets and herbs for specific illnesses, also recommended mantras and hekau repetition to calm the mind as well as the practice of meditation to promote healing.

The goal of yoga is to promote integration of the mind-body-spirit complex in order to produce optimal health of the human being. This is accomplished through mental and physical exercises which promote the free flow of spiritual energy by reducing mental complexes caused by ignorance. There are two roads which human beings can follow, one of wisdom and the other of ignorance. The path of the masses is generally the path of ignorance which leads them to negative situations, thoughts and deeds. These in turn lead to ill health and sorrow in life. The other road is based on wisdom and it leads to health, true happiness and enlightenment.

It must be understood that being enlightened does not automatically confer a state of physical health. One's state of health is also subject to the law of Karma, so even someone who is enlightened may undergo serious illnesses. There have been many enlightened sages who have developed cancer, diabetes and other illnesses. However, this does not mean that you should not endeavor to live a healthy lifestyle. Suppose, based on karma from your previous embodiments as well as this embodiment, you develop some illness. You have the choice to promote a healthy diet and lifestyle (good karma) or an unhealthy diet and lifestyle in this lifetime. Promoting a healthy lifestyle may add years to your life, whereas ignoring proper nutrition and exercise may result in your dying at an earlier age, not to mention the karmic repercussions you will still have to deal with in future lifetimes.

Promoting a healthy lifestyle is key to the practice of yoga because once you realize that your body and mind are tools to take you to the destination of absolute peace and bliss, you will want to take care of it as you would a car or some other important possession you have. In addition, unless one is very spiritually advanced, beyond identifying with the body and mind, illnesses can detract from spiritual progress because they keep the thoughts bound to the physical body. To understand this, just reflect on when you have a headache or a stomachache. Where are your thoughts drawn? Usually they are more focused on the part of the body which ails you. Therefore, promoting a healthy lifestyle through proper nutrition and exercise are also very important disciplines in the quest to attain Yoga, union with your Higher Self.

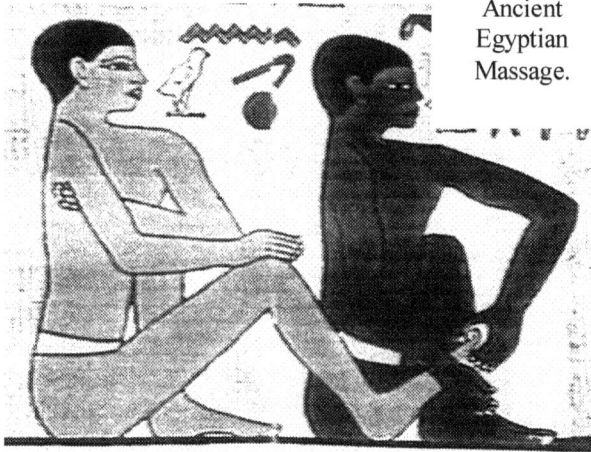

Ancient
Egyptian
Massage.

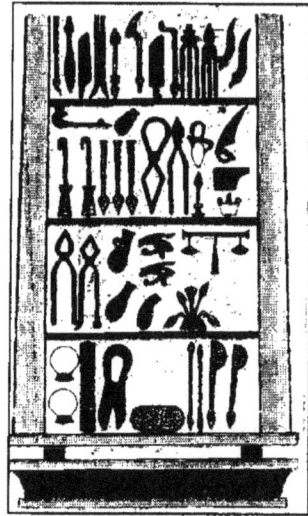

Above: ancient Egyptian
medical instruments.

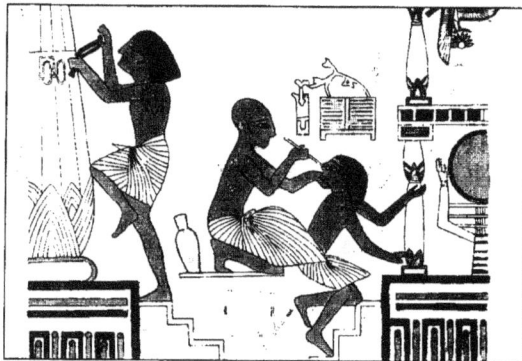

At left: an ancient
Egyptian doctor

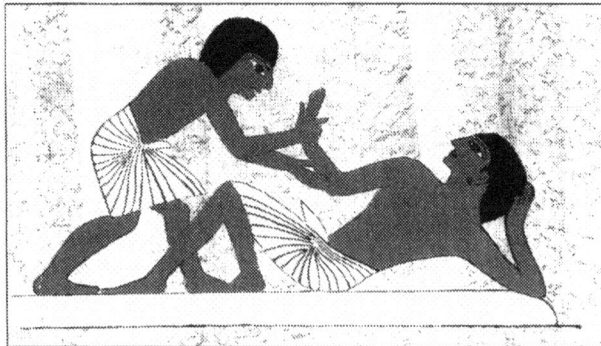

At left: Ancient
Egyptian
Massage care of the

PREVENTATIVE HEALTH AND SELF-HEALING

In the state of pristine health, the physical body of every human being exists in harmony with various bacteria, viruses and chemical processes. When the systems of the body which keep a balance become weakened, a situation of dis-ease develops. Due to ignorance in understanding (disharmony in the thought patterns), the mind has failed to lead the individual to internally create the proper substances (thoughts or solid food) which will allow for the proper energy distribution throughout the mind and body.

There are several factors involved in pain, suffering and disease, however, at their most basic level, they are all related to the mind, the state of which is a reflection of the spiritual health of the individual. The body is a creation or mold of the mind and whatever the mind creates will eventually manifest in the body and the environment of the body as well. Also, if the mind is burdened by insanity (worry, anxiety, fear, delusions, stress, schizophrenia, etc.), the energy flow from the soul to the mind to the body will be disturbed or blocked. Therefore, other than ailments caused by problems in the environment or accidents, physical dis-ease is primarily due to a mental imbalance, which in turn is due to a spiritual imbalance.

Since the body is composed of inert elements, it is the spirit, through the medium of mind (energy) and DNA, which directs and controls the elements, electrochemical composition and chemical reactions which make up the process we call life. The soul chooses the particular circumstances to incarnate into. This means that it chooses a particular set of chromosomal factors in a family along with the life-time circumstances and situations which will allow it to gain the experiences it desires and needs for its evolution.

A problem that many people encounter in ordinary human life is that there is little concern or emphasis placed on the purity of the food, both mental and physical, that is consumed. Mental food in the form of elevated thoughts and wisdom teachings are essential in maintaining healthy reason (intellectual sharpness which comes from studying the teachings) and positive mental vibrations. Nourishment in the form of solid food and exercise are prerequisites to physical health. Physical health, though not an absolute requirement for the practice of spiritual discipline, is helpful since it is more difficult to focus the mind on spiritual matters when the mind is tied up in the experiences of pain and suffering.

With this in mind, there are various modes of practice which have been devised to maintain health and to deal with ailments. However, they should not be limited to just dealing with the physical signs of disease since these are only the manifestations of a deeper psycho-spiritual root cause.

The approach to health maintenance and treatment of disease should be holistic, taking the entire human being (spiritual-mental-physical) into consideration. Also, it is important to understand that doctors and other healers do not and cannot heal others. They can only help others to heal themselves by providing information and other means to assist them in bringing their constitution back into balance. It's a good idea to have them examine and attempt to diagnose so that one may be pointed in a good direction toward understanding the problem, however, conventional medical treatments are usually directed to getting rid of the symptoms. This is what is often referred to as a "cure" by the medical profession. Sometimes it is critical to alleviate the symptoms, however, the deeper root cause of the disease should also be addressed. The drugs used in conventional medicine usually mask the symptom(s) of disease, creating the illusion that the problem has gone away when in fact, it is only suppressing the disease and pushing it deeper in the body. Hence, it is not surprising that so many people who have submitted themselves to this system of health care have developed cancer and other debilitating dis-eases.

Another drawback of many-man made drugs is that drugs themselves cause side effects that damage other organs and tissues. The only entity capable of creating a correct prescription for an ailment in the form of hormones and other chemicals released into the blood stream and immune system is the body itself. What it needs in order to do that is peace of mind, proper nutrition, and internal cleansing from poisonous substances which block its operation i.e. too much negative or too much positive emotions, unwholesome foods, overeating, negative thoughts, lack of sleep, etc.

Yoga philosophy holds that the root cause of all disease is ignorance of one's Higher Self. This ignorance leads to unnecessary anxieties and sufferings which stress the mind and body. Thus, according to yoga philosophy, a prerequisite for any healing program is that it must include methods and techniques for leading one to attain enlightenment.

The mysterious aspect of health is an area which is beyond the understanding of any science and thus falls into the realm of that which is not even discussed by the conventional medical establishment. This area includes the miraculous healings and repercussions, as well as the unexplained deaths and ailments. This area is mysterious because it encompasses many unknown factors. These include the soul of the individual and its previous involvements, previous exposure to toxic substances, deep psychological distress which may not be apparent at the conscious level, karmic entanglements of the present and from previous lives and the mission of the soul in the present incarnation. Since no two people are alike, no treatment can be exactly alike, however, there are some guidelines to health and healing which may be performed by oneself or with the assistance of others. Except in emergency or trauma cases, surgery should be the last form of treatment considered.

DIET AND HEALTH[13]

As with the healing systems of Egypt and India which encompass Naturopathic approaches to health maintenance and the natural treatment of disease, the *Therapeuts,* a Jewish sect in Egypt, were renowned for their mastery over the healing arts. For thousands of years, the temples of Egypt had been healing places where the public could go for help in spiritual as well as physical health matters. For this reason they were called *Per Ankh* or "Houses of Life." Like Hippocrates, the famous Greek physician who studied with the Egyptian doctors, the Therapeuts assimilated the healing wisdom of Egypt which included dietetics, fasting and surgery. Another similarity between the health systems of India and Egypt is that the mind-body connection and its relation to physical and mental health was well understood. The idea of the mind-body connection had been until recently, rejected by the modern day medical establishment. The ancient science of *AyurVeda* from India is similar in many respects to the therapeutic methods of preventative health care and holistic disease treatments

---

[13] see the book Kemetic Diet.

described in the *Essene Gospel of Peace* and the practices of the ancient Egyptians. In much the same way as many Hindu and Yoga sects promote vegetarianism, the Gospel of Peace emphasizes vegetarianism as a way to health. While there are a few passages in the Bible which declare that humans should eat fruits and vegetables, the Gospel of Peace devotes a great deal of attention to the subject as well as using food as a medicine.

> Genesis 1
>> 29. And God said, Behold, I have given you every herb bearing
>> seed, which [is] upon the face of all the earth, and every tree,
>> in which [is] the fruit of a tree yielding seed; to you it shall
>> be for food.

Today, there are few Christian denominations which openly and actively promote vegetarianism, since like celibacy, it is not seen as a pleasant or pleasurable practice. Rather, it is considered to be a "hard teaching" to follow by many. It should be understood that vegetarianism, in and of itself, does not make one automatically "spiritual", however, it does aid in purifying the mind and body so that spiritual disciplines may be carried out more effectively.

The Gospel of Peace describes diseases as demons and states that they are caused by sinful behavior. The sinful behavior is usually related to lifestyles which produce negative physical or mental conditions in the body. These may be: too much worry, poor eating habits or poor hygiene. The prescribed treatment given by Jesus is to balance the spiritual through prayer and meditation and the physical through vegetarianism, regular fasting and internal cleansing (enema) according to the needs of the individual and then to: *"go in peace and sin no more."* Jesus emphasizes physical purification by keeping the laws of hygiene and diet (the Earth Mother), and the spiritual by keeping the practice of prayer and devotion to the Heavenly Father.

From the Gospel of Peace:

> Follow, therefore, first, the laws of your Earthly Mother, of which I have told you. And when her angels shall have cleansed and renewed your bodies and strengthened your eyes, you will be able to bear the light of our Heavenly Father.

In the following passages, from the Gospel of Peace, Jesus expands on the parable of Genesis 1:29.

> For I tell you truly, he who kills, kills himself, and whosoever eats the flesh of slain beasts, eats of the body of death. For in his body every drop of their blood turns to poison; in his bones their bones to chalk; in his bowels their bowels to decay... And their death will become his death.

> Behold, I have given you every herb bearing seed, which is upon the face of all the earth, and every tree, in which is the fruit of a tree yielding seed; to you it shall be for meat. And to every beast of the earth, and to every fowl of the air, and to everything that creepeth upon the earth, wherein there is breath of life, I give every green herb for meat... But flesh, and the blood which quickens it, shall ye not eat.

From an ordinary standpoint, the consumption of meat is not desirable due to the fact that it causes pain to other living beings in the animal level of existence. Hurting any creature should be avoided to the extent possible since it generates discordant vibrations in the universe. These vibrations disturb the balance of nature and the mental plane of existence which in turn affects human beings and their feelings, thoughts and consequently, their actions as well. Many people dislike violence in the world, however, they are sowing it everyday by supporting the violence that is performed on animals, the violence in sports, television and in ordinary human interactions.

The body is composed of the elements of creation (earth, water, air, fire) and the four qualities of matter (hot, cold, wet, dry). If these factors are maintained in proper balance, the body will be a fit conduit to operate in the physical realm and allow the mind to perceive the subtle vibrations of the spiritual realm as well. The mind is composed of subtler elements which when purged of egoistic thoughts, is able to reflect the spiritual reality. Otherwise, the association with the grosser elements of the body renders it gross. If these factors are out of balance, the mind will be distracted with the concerns of the body (pain, illness, desire for food, etc.) and will not be able to exert self-effort toward spiritual practice in order to develop subtlety of intellect. The intellect will remain dull with the gross concerns of the physical world.

Modern physics has proven that matter is not solid but that it is in reality energy in different forms of vibration. From a yogic perspective, what is considered to be "solid" matter (the elements) is in reality condensed subtle matter. What makes it appear solid is the level of ignorance of the seer and the intensification of the belief in it as being "real." Your body appears to be solid but in reality it is as solid as a body you might experience in a dream. Due to the soul's involvement in time and space and having been taught to believe in the world of time and space as a solid reality, ordinary people reinforce these ideas through indulgence in emotions, feelings and pleasures of the senses. One of the most powerful areas of indulgence is in the consumption of foods which ground and condense spiritual energy instead of allowing it to flow freely.

Food is often used as a source of pleasure rather than necessity. Modern society advocates the consumption of good tasting, processed food even though it may contain chemicals or other substances such as sugars and salts which the body does not need in abundance. In addition to unsanitary and inhumane living conditions in which the animals are housed and slaughtered, the chemicals and processing techniques which are used by the meat industry to raise animals for food renders the meat very toxic to the human body. Over a period of time these toxins build up in conjunction with those which are already in the environment (pollution) and lead to cancers and other diseases in later years. From a spiritual point of view, the vibratory energy in meat is very grounding to the soul. This means that the elements which compose the human body are rendered "heavier", therefore blocking perception of the subtle spiritual reality and reinforcing the gross reality as being the only reality. So from a holistic perspective, the mind, body and spirit need to be taken into account when pursuing health and healing. Therefore, practices and exercises directed to all three areas need to be observed daily for optimal health.

THE DIET OF THE COMMON FOLK AND MEDICAL SYSTEM

Hippocrates (460?-377? BCE), who has been called the *father of medicine* and whose major teaching was that diet is the cause of disease, was instructed in this most important health factor by the physicians of ancient Egypt. Herodotus witnessed an elaborate system of medical science during his travels in Egypt. The following is an excerpt from his writings where he notes the general dietary practices of the ancient Egyptian people.

The Egyptians who live in the cultivated parts of the country, by their practice of keeping records of the past, have made themselves much the best historians of any nation of which I have experience. I will describe some of their habits:

1. Every month for three consecutive days they purge themselves, for their health's sake, with emetics* and clysters, in the belief that all diseases come from the food a man eats; and it is a fact - even apart from this precaution - that next to the Libyans they are the healthiest people in the world.

2. I should put this down myself to the absence of changes in the climate, for change, and especially changes of weather, is the prime cause of disease.

3. They eat loaves of Spelt - *cyllestes* is their word for them...

4....and drink a wine made from barley, as they have no vines in the country.

5. Some kinds of fish they eat raw, either dried in the sun, or salted; quails, too, they eat raw, and ducks and various small birds, after pickling them in brine; other sorts of birds and fish, apart from those which are considered sacred, they either roast or boil.

6...nevertheless they are peculiar in certain ways which they have discovered of living more cheaply: for instance, they gather the water-lilies (Lotuses) which grow in great abundance when the river is full and floods the neighboring flats, and dry them in the sun; then from the center of each blossom they pick out something which resembles a poppyhead, grind it, and make it into loaves which they bake. The root of this plant is also edible; it is round, about as big as an apple, and tastes sweet.

7. There is another kind of lily to be found in the river; this resembles a rose, and its fruit is formed on a separate stalk from that which bears the blossom, and has very much the looks of a wasp's comb. The fruit contains a number of seeds, about the size of an olive-stone, which are good to eat either green or dried.

8. They pull up the annual crop of papyrus-reed which grows in the mashes, cut the stalks in two, and eat the lower part, about eighteen inches in length, first baking it in a closed pan, heated red-hot, if they want to enjoy it to perfection. The upper section of the stalk is used for some other purpose.

9. Some of these people, however, live upon nothing but fish, which they gut as soon as they catch them, and eat after drying them in the sun.

*An *emetic* is any medicinal agent used to induce vomiting. In India, Yogis practice a similar procedure for cleansing the upper gastrointestinal tract. It is called *Jala Dhauti.* The procedure is to ingest 4-5 glasses of lukewarm water with a small amount of salt in it. Then shake up the intestines through massaging and abdominal movements and then vomit the water out using the fingers. This has the effect of removing phlegm and bile.

A- Another important point is that the sun was used for much of the cooking as opposed to stoves, and even worse microwave ovens which destroy both the gross and subtle nutritional quality of foods.

B- Many foods were eaten raw and vegetables made up a major part of the diet.

C- Wheat was not a major part of the diet. Spelt was used instead. In Indian Ayur Veda* science, wheat has been found to be incompatible with some people, causing them phlegm or congestion.

D- The ancient Egyptians lived in an area of the world where the climate was stable. This is important because their physical bodies were not subjected to drastic changes such as in those areas where seasonal temperature changes range many degrees. There are certain locations in the world where the climates change many degrees within a single day. This occurrence is jolting to the body's equilibrium and thus affects general health. This factor of the geographical climate became a primary teaching of Jesus in the Essene Gospel of Peace. Also, this Gospel describes cooking with the sun as well as the proper methods of food combining, attitude when eating and methods of internal cleansing through fasts and enema.

For a more detailed study of the teachings and practices of Kemetic (Ancient Egyptian) health and healing see the new book *The Kemetic Diet: Food for Body, Mind and Soul* by Dr. Muata Ashby.

The Teachings of the Temple of Isis and The Diet of the Initiates

While the general population was considered to be one of the most healthy groups of the ancient world, the spiritual initiates were required to keep even more strict dietary practices. The special diets of the ancient Egyptian initiates were a highly guarded secret as were the inner meanings of the myths which were acted out in the mystery rituals (***SHETAUT NETER***). For this reason, many of the special yogic practices which included a special diet and meditation were not committed to writing in an explicit fashion. Rather, they were committed to hieroglyphic form and carried on through the initiatic process. It was not until Greek historians and initiates into the Egyptian mystery schools began to write about their experiences that the more detailed aspects of the initiatic diets were available to a wider audience. The sect of Jews called the Essenes practiced an initiation period of two to three years and instituted purification diets and hygienic practices similar to those spoken about by Herodotus (484?-425 BCE) and Plutarch (46?-120 ACE). The Essenic health practices were presented in the Essene Gospel of Peace.

Plutarch, a student of the mysteries of Isis, reported that the initiates followed a strict diet made up of vegetables and fruits and *abstained from particular kinds of foods* (swine, sheep, fish, etc.) *as well as indulgence of the carnal appetite.* In the following excerpts Plutarch describes the purpose and procedure of the diet observed by the Initiates of Isis and the goal to be attained through the rigorous spiritual program. This next excerpt should be studied carefully.

To desire, therefore, and covet after truth, those truths more especially which concern the divine nature, is to aspire to be partakers of that nature itself (1), and to profess that all our studies (2) and inquiries (2) are devoted to the acquisition of holiness. This occupation is surely more truly religious than any external (3) purifications or mere service of the temple can be.(4) But more especially must such a disposition of mind be highly acceptable to that goddess to whose service you are dedicated, for her special characteristics are wisdom and foresight, and her very name seems to express the peculiar relation which she bears to knowledge. For "Isis" is a Greek word, and means "knowledge or wisdom,"(5) and "Typhon," [Set] the name of her professed adversary, is also a Greek word, and means " pride and insolence."(6) This latter name is well adapted to one who, full of ignorance and error, tears in pieces (7) and conceals that holy doctrine (about Osiris) which the goddess collects, compiles, and delivers to those who aspire after the most perfect participation in the divine nature. This doctrine inculcates a steady perseverance in one uniform and temperate course of life (8), and an abstinence from particular kinds of foods (9), as well as from all indulgence of the carnal appetite (10), and it restrains the intemperate and voluptuous part within due bounds, and at the same time habituates her votaries to undergo those austere and rigid ceremonies which their religion obliges them to observe. The end and aim of all these toils and labors is the attainment of the knowledge of the First and Chief Being (11), who alone is the object of the understanding of the mind; and this knowledge the goddess invites us to seek after, as being near and dwelling continually (12) with her. And this also is what the very name of her temple promiseth to us, that is to say, the knowledge and understanding of the eternal and self-existent Being - now it is called "Iseion," which suggests that if we approach the temple of the goddess rightly, we shall obtain the knowledge of that eternal and self existent Being.

Mystical Implications of the Discourse of Plutarch[14]:

1- It is to be understood that spiritual aspiration implies seeking the union with or becoming one with the thing being sought because this is the only way to truly "know" something. You can have opinions about what it is like to be a whale but you would never exactly know until you become one with it. God enfolding all that exists is the one being worthy of veneration and identification. This "knowing" of Neter (God) is the goal of all spiritual practices. This is the supreme goal which must be kept in mind by a spiritual aspirant.

2- In order to discover the hidden nature of God, emphasis is placed on study and inquiry into the nature of things. Who am I? What is the universe composed of? Who is God? How am I related to God? These are the questions which when pursued, lead to the discovery of the Self (God). Those who do not engage in this form of inquiry will generate a reality for themselves according to their beliefs. Some people believe they have the answers, that the universe is atoms and electrons or energy. Others believe that the body is the soul and that there is nothing else. Still

---

[14] Note: The numbers at the beginning of each paragraph below correspond to the reference numbers in the text above.

others believe that the mind is the Soul or that there is no soul and no God. The first qualification for serious aspiration is that you have a serious conviction that you are greater than just a finite individual mortal body, that you are an immortal being who is somehow mixed up with a temporal form (body). If this conviction is present, then you are stepping on the road to enlightenment. The teachings will be useful to you. Those who hold other beliefs are being led by ignorance and lack of spiritual sensitivity as a result of their beliefs. Thus, their beliefs will create a reality for them based on those beliefs. They will need to travel the road of nature which will guide them in time toward the path of spiritual aspiration.

3-4 The plan prescribed by the teachings of yoga is the only true means to effective spiritual development because it reveals the inner meanings of the teachings and it is experiential, i.e. it is based on your own personal experience and not conjecture. Otherwise, worship and religious practices remain at the level of ritualism only and do not lead to enlightenment.

5-7 The name "ISIS" represents "wisdom" itself which bestows the knowledge of the true Self of the initiate. In the Osirian Mysteries, when Set killed Osiris by tearing him into pieces, he was symbolically tearing up the soul. However, Isis restores the pieces of the soul (Osiris). Therefore, Pride and Insolence (Set-egoism) destroy the soul and Knowledge of the Self (Isis) restores it to its true nature. The Greek name for Isis is supported by the ancient Egyptian scriptures. One of the names of Isis is: *Rekhåt or Rekhit* ⌒ₒ⊜◊ ⺗ meaning "knowledge personified" and "Isis-Sothis." *Rekh* is also a name of the God in the "duat" or Netherworld who possesses knowledge which can lead the soul to the abode of the Divine, thus avoiding the fiends and demoniac personalities of the duat which lead the soul to experience hellish conditions after death. The variation, *Rekh-t* ⌒ₒ⊜⚊◊ ⺗, means Sage or learned person.

8- True spirituality cannot be pursued rashly or in a fanatical way by going to extremes. Yoga spirituality is a science of balance. It has been developed over a period of thousands of years with well established principles, which when followed, produce the desired effect of leading the initiate from darkness to light, ignorance to knowledge, an un-enlightened state to enlightenment.

9-10 The foods referred to are flesh foods (swine, sheep, fish, etc.), pulse, and salt. Indulgence in sexual activity has two relevant aspects. First, it intensifies the physical experience of embodiment and distracts the mind by creating impressions in the subconscious which will produce future cravings and desires. This state of mind renders the individual incapable of concentration on significant worldly or high spiritual achievements. Secondly, control of the sexual urge leads to control of the sexual Life Force energy, which can then be directed toward higher mental and spiritual achievement.

11- See #1.

12- There are two very important points in this line. Once again we are being reminded that good association or keeping the company of sages or other enlightened personalities is a powerful means to gain knowledge of the state of enlightenment. To this end, strive to keep good company in your family relations as well as non-family relations. Read uplifting books by the sages and the teachings of the masters. When you discover a more evolved personality, seek to maintain contact by reading their teachings and through correspondence. Do not debate with those who lack spiritual sensitivity. This form of interaction will weaken your mind. As Jesus said: *Cast not your pearls before swine, for they will trample them as they turn against you.* Trust in the Omniscient Divine Self, who knows past, present and future, who manifests as Nature to lead others on the path. Spread the teachings of yoga to those who are interested only or those whom you practice with. This kind of interaction will help you both to increase your understanding and generate a positive frame of mind.

The second important point here refers to continuous reflection and meditation on the divine which is also expressed in the opening prayer in page one of this book: *"Give thyself to GOD, keep thou thyself daily for God; and let tomorrow be as today."* It implies that one's mind should be constantly remembering the divine and glorifying the divine in all things. It means not allowing the mind to develop attachments to the fleeting events of human life be they positive experiences or negative ones. It means not allowing the negative thoughts and feelings to lead you into a pursuit of illusory pleasures of the senses which will draw you away from divine awareness and realization. It means centering the mind on self discovery and introspection at all times regardless of what your activities may be and those activities should be based solely on the principled of virtue, justice and order. This form of spiritual practice is known as "mindfulness" in Buddhism and Vedanta Philosophies.

Plutarch further reports that the Egyptian initiates:

> *...strive to prevent fatness in Apis† as well as themselves(1), for they are anxious that their bodies should sit as light and easy about their souls as possible, and that their mortal part* (body) *should not oppress and weigh down their divine and immortal part...during their more solemn purifications they abstain from wine(2) wholly, and they give themselves up entirely to study(4) and meditation(5) and to the hearing (3) and teaching of these divine truths which treat of the divine nature.* † Bull which was kept as a symbol of Osiris and Ptah.

The following dietary guidelines for spiritual and physical health are derived from the above statement.

1- Preventing "fatness"- obesity. This issue is very important even for those without spiritual aspirations. Some people who are overweight claim that they are happy and content as they are. Some scientists claim to have discovered a gene in the human system which causes a propensity to become overweight. Once again, all of your body's characteristics are due to your past karmic history of experiences and desires, not only in this lifetime but in previous ones as well. Physical weight is like a physical object which is possessed. The more you have, the more you try to hold onto, and the more stress you have trying to enjoy and hold onto "things." Desires of the body such as eating have a grounding effect on the soul because they engender the desire to experience the physical pleasure of consuming food. Desires of the body as well as strong emotions such as hate, greed, etc., have the effect of rendering the mind insensitive to spirituality. Excess weight on the body causes innumerable health problems to arise.

You can change the future condition of your body by first mentally resolving to change it and then employing the self-effort in that direction while at the same time invoking the help of the

Neters (cosmic forces - divine energies of God) to assist your quest for self-improvement. This will not be easy since the temptation of food is very great. It is related to the first energy center of the subtle spiritual body (Uraeus-Kundalini Serpent Power)[15] and it is a force which needs to be controlled in order to proceed on the spiritual path. As part of your spiritual program, begin controlling your intake of food gradually, on a daily basis. Even if you cut back a tablespoonful per day until you reach a level of intake which will support the normal weight for your body structure. Be especially watchful of yourself in respect to your habits. Do you eat out of habit, for pleasure or out of necessity? If it is out of habit or for pleasure, you must break the cycle by engaging in other activities when the desire arises. Do exercise, deep breathing, study, chant, call a fellow practitioner for support. The Serpent power will be discussed in detail in two future sections.

2- Natural wines and other naturally brewed drinks are acceptable in small quantities, however, you will notice that as you purify yourself, you will not be able to tolerate even a small amount of intoxicants. Distilled liquor is not a natural substance. It is processed into a potent form which is injurious to the body and is therefore, not suitable at all for use by those advancing on the spiritual path. The same applies to narcotics and all other "recreational" drugs. All of these distort the spiritual perception while damaging the physical body. No drug can produce a high which can be compared to spiritual bliss. Therefore, resolve to leave all drugs behind and become intoxicated with spiritual feelings and aspiration.

3,4,5- Once again, the main format for spiritual education is:

> 3- Listening to the teachings.‡
> 4- Constant study and reflection on the teachings.‡
> 5- Meditation on the meaning of the teachings.‡

‡Note: It is important to note here that the same teaching which was practiced in ancient Egypt of **Listening** to, **Reflecting** upon, and **Meditating** upon the teachings is the same process used in Vedanta-Jnana Yoga of today. See page 15.

Chapter 30B of the *Book of Coming Forth By Day* states:

> *This utterance (hekau) shall be recited by a person purified and washed; one who has not eaten animal flesh or fish.*

Chapter 137A of the *Book of Coming Forth By Day* states:

> *And behold, these things shall be performed by one who is clean, and is ceremonially pure, a man who hath eaten neither meat nor fish, and who hath not had intercourse with women* (applies to female initiates not having intercourse with men as well).

In the Mysteries of Osiris and Isis, Set represents the lower human nature and Horus the Higher. Set kills Osiris and usurps the throne which rightfully should belong to Horus, Osiris'

---

[15] see audio tape lecture Serpent PowerI - URAEUS YOGA: Workshop and Cleansing Meditation - I.

son. In various renderings of the characteristics of Set, it is stated that Set is promiscuous. Most interestingly, both Horus and Set are vegetarians. Their favorite food is *lettuce*. Therefore, we are to understand that vegetarianism increases the potential for spiritual advancement and for the vital sexual force. With this understanding, it is clear that control of the sexual urge to conserve potential spiritual energy and purification of the diet are necessary practices on the spiritual path which enable the aspirant to achieve increased spiritual sensitivity. When practiced correctly, the conserved energy can be transformed into spiritual energy by directing it through the various energy centers in the body until it finally reaches the center of intuitional vision (Eye of Horus-Udjat).

A most important point to remember when beginning practices for the purification of the body is that they should be implemented gradually, preferably under the supervision of an experienced person. If these changes result in an inability to perform your daily duties, then they are too extreme. The key to advancement in any area is steady, balanced practice. There must always be a balance between the practical life and the spiritual. In this way, spiritual advancement occurs in an integral fashion, intensifying every area of one's life rather than one a particular area exclusively. All areas must be mastered, secular as well as non-secular, in order to transcend the world process (illusion of time and space and the ego-self).

Since the physical body and all worldly attainments are changeable, fleeting and ultimately perishable, it would be wise to pursue a way of life which directs the mind toward understanding the Self and not to pursue health as an end in itself, but as a means to your own growth and spiritual evolution, which will continue even after the death of the your physical body if you have not attained enlightenment up to the time of physical death. The holistic development of an individual must be directed to achieving a state of consciousness which is not dependent on the physical body for peace and comfort. The body is an instrument which you have created through your thoughts to allow you to pursue the goal of enlightenment and thereby experience the fullness of life.

The Recommended Daily Schedule for Yoga Practice

A practitioner of Yoga must be able to integrate the main practices of yoga into daily life. This means that you need to begin adding small amounts of time for Prayer, Repetition of the Divine Name (Hekau), Exercise (includes proper breathing exercise), Study of the Teachings, Silence, Selfless Service, Meditation, and Daily Reflection. This also means that you will gradually reduce the practices which go against yogic movement as you gain more time for Sheti.

Below you will find an outline of a schedule for the beginning practice of Yoga. The times given here are a suggested minimum time for beginners. You may spend more time according to your capacity and personal situation, however, try to be consistent in the amount of time and location you choose to practice your discipline as well as in the time of day you choose to perform each of the different practices. This will enable your body and mind to develop a rhythm which will develop into the driving force of your day. When this occurs you will develop stamina and fortitude when dealing with any situation of life. You will have a stable center which will anchor you to a higher purpose in life whether you are experiencing prosperous times or adverse times. In the advanced stages, spiritual practice will become continuous. Try to do the best you can according to your capacity, meaning your circumstances. If your family members are not interested or do not understand what you are trying to do simply maintain your practices privately and try to keep the interruptions to a minimum. As you develop, you may feel drawn toward some forms of practice over others. The important thing to remember is to practice them all in an integrated fashion. Do not neglect any of the practices even though you may spend additional time on some versus others.

Practicing spirituality only during times of adversity is the mistake of those who are spiritually immature. Any form of spiritual practice, ritualistic or otherwise is a positive development, however, you will not derive the optimal spiritual benefits by simply becoming religious when you are in trouble. The masses of people only pray when they are in trouble...then they ask for assistance to get out of trouble. What they do not realize is that if they were to turn their minds to God at all times, not just in times of misfortune, adversity would not befall them. As you progress through your studies you will learn that adversities in life are meant to turn you toward the Divine. In this sense they are messages from the Divine to awaken spiritual aspiration. However, if you do not listen to the message and hearken to the Divine intent behind it, you will be in a position to experience more miseries of life and miseries of a more intense nature.

Basic Schedule of Spiritual Practice

1a- Deep breathing, using the *proper breathing technique.*
1b- Alternate Breathing exercise (10 minutes in Am and in PM),
2- Prayer (10-30 minutes in Am* and in PM),

Opening Prayer:

> *O Åmen, O Åmen, who art in heaven, turn thy face upon the dead body of the child, and make your child sound and strong in the Underworld.*
>
> *O Åmen, O Åmen, O God, O God, O Åmen, I adore thy name, grant thou to me that I may understand thee; Grant thou that I may have peace in the Duat, and that I may possess all my members therein...*
>
> *Hail, Åmen, let me make supplication unto thee, for I know thy name, and thy transformations are in my mouth, and thy skin is before my eyes. Come, I pray thee, and place thou thine heir and thine image, myself, in the everlasting underworld... let my whole body become like that of a neter, let me escape from the evil chamber and let me not be imprisoned therein; for I worship thy name..*

3-Exercise (10 minutes in am and before study time),

4-Repetition of the Divine Name in the form of your chosen hekau-mantra (10 minutes in am and in pm),
5-Meditation practice (10 minutes in Am, should be practiced after exercise, prayer and repetition of the Divine Name),

Closing Prayer after meditation or any spiritual practice:

I am pure. I am pure. I am Pure.
I have washed my front parts with the waters of libations, I have cleansed my hinder parts
with drugs which make wholly clean, and my inward parts have been washed in the liquor
of Maat.
↣

6-Study of the teachings (reading 30 minutes per day),
7-Silence time (30 minutes per day),
8-Listening to the teachings: Choose an audio recording of a yogic spiritual preceptor and listen for a minimum of 30 minutes per day without any distractions if possible. If possible, go to a yogic spiritual center (Ashram, Wat, Temple) where teachings are presented by a qualified teacher of yoga wisdom. If this is not possible, form a study group wherein the teachings may be discussed and explored.
9-Selfless service (as required whenever the opportunity presents itself),
10-Daily reflection: Remembering the teachings during the ordinary course of the day and applying them in daily living situations- to be practiced as much as possible.
*(see Morning Worship and Meditation tape)

The suggested times given above are the minimum amount you should spend on daily spiritual practices each day. Whenever possible you should increase the times according to your capacity and ability. You should train your mind so that it rejoices in hearing about and practicing the teachings of yoga instead of the useless worldly activities. Follow this path gradually but steadily.

Once you have established a schedule of minimal time to devote to practices, even if you do 5-10 minutes of meditation time per day and nothing else, keep your schedule if at all possible. Many people feel that they do not have the time to incorporate even ordinary activities into their lives. They feel overwhelmed with life and feel they have no control. If there is no control it is because there is no discipline. If you make a schedule for all of your activities (spiritual and non-spiritual) and keep to it tenaciously, you will discover that you can control your time and your life. As you discover the glory of spiritual practice, you will find even more time to expand your spiritual program. Ultimately, you will create a lifestyle which is entirely spiritualized. This means that every act in your life will be based on the wisdom teachings (MAAT) and therefore you will not only spend a particular time of day devoted to spiritual practices, but every facet of your life will become a spontaneous worship of the divine.

EXERCISE:

Physical postures and exercises were an integral part of the spiritual process in ancient Egypt. The gods and goddesses are depicted in poses which are almost identical to the poses of Indian Hatha Yoga. Yoga exercises are excellent for maintaining flexibility and strength of the body. When the muscles are tightened and flexed they secure the structure, making it work more efficient and stemming the process of deterioration while flushing out impurities as they massage the internal organs. The Qi Gong system of China has similar exercises known as Wei Dan Qi. In addition, because these exercises emphasize focusing on the breath, they draw one's consciousness internally. This internalization of one's consciousness is a necessary prerequisite for meditation, so these exercises are recommended prior to the practice of formal meditation. Thus, they are termed "psycho-physical" and "psycho-spiritual" exercises.

Exercise is also helpful in controlling the emotions. Depression, negativity and agitation in the mind are characterized by a sedentary nature. Therefore, do not allow yourself to become lethargic, apathetic, listless, or uninterested, especially in times of adversity or depression. Keep to your spiritual program in bad times as well as the good. Yoga and Tai Chi exercises are designed to have a special psycho-physical effect which releases energy blocks and develops positive flow of energy which in turn affects the mind in a positive way. The idea is to break the pattern of your established mental and emotional self and to introduce a new pattern that is directed toward peace and inner development.

GENERAL HEALTH TIPS AND BALANCED LIVING

Rest:

Continued mental agitation and stress limits the possibility for engaging in reflection which promotes integration of feelings, thoughts and ideas. Rest is an integral part of the healing process and it is a pre-requisite for proper reflective abilities. In a practical sense, this is the purpose of sleep. From a yogic perspective, the technique of deep relaxation and the discipline of meditation can promote a state of restfulness far superior to that of the sleep state.

Silence:

> *"The abomination of the sanctuary of God is: too much talking. Pray thou with a loving heart the petitions of which all are in secret. God will do thy business, hear that which thou sayest and will accept thine offerings."*
>
> —Ancient Egyptian Proverb

The practice of silence on a regular basis has the effect of allowing the individual to withdraw from interaction in the world, thereby calming the mind over time. Silence allows the individual to discover that many things do not need to be said. Inner peace awakens in those who can practice silence because the inner voice is given a chance to emerge from the mountainous thoughts and activities that externalization usually causes. Silence is seen as a mental austerity and it is considered among the practices of moral discipline and self-restraint. Silence should be practiced without making gestures to communicate with others, and at a prescribed time other than when one would normally be quiet. A specialized form of silence practice seeks to keep the body perfectly still for long periods of time (1-2 hours or more). This practice has the effect of developing strength of will as well as aiding the aspirant to remain quietly in meditative posture during the formal practice of meditation.

Being Alone

Practicing "alone time" need not be thought of as loneliness. Being alone can be an exercise in practicing being free from one's desires and attachments. These desires and attachments are the source of the mental complexes. By practicing aloneness, the mind is gradually able to conceive of life without the objects of attachment and is then able to discover its eternal companionship with the Self who is the mother of all mothers, the father of all fathers, the love of all loves, the best friend of all friends.

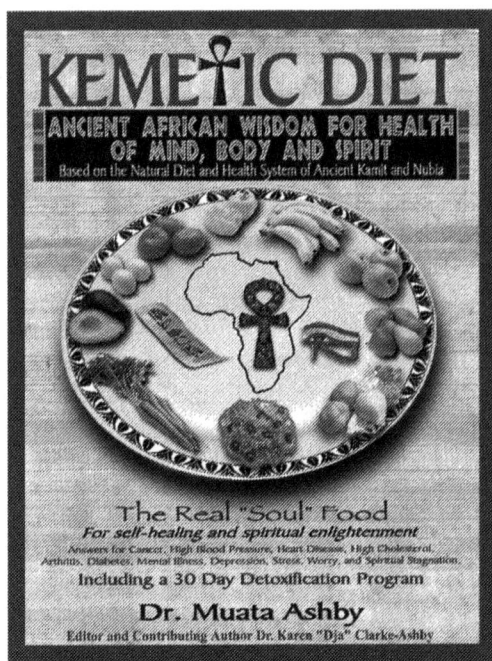

THE BOOK KEMETIC DIET

For those who wish to implement the full Kemetic program for physical, mental and spiritual health that will provide a basis for a successful spiritual practice and success in the quest for spiritual awakening. By Muata Ashby

PART II THE YOGIC DISCIPLINES AND THEIR KEMETIC ORIGINS

*THE DISCIPLINES OF YOGA THAT WERE PRACTICED IN ANCIENT EGYPT
AND THEIR PLACES OF ORIGIN IN KEMETIC CULTURE*

Kemetic Scriptural Sources of Yoga Philosophy

Most people familiar with the yogic traditions of India consider that the Indian texts such as the Bhagavad Gita, Mahabharata, Patanjali Yoga Sutras, etc. are the primary and original source of Yogic philosophy and teaching. However, upon examination, the teachings currently espoused in all of the major forms of Indian Yoga can be found in Ancient Egyptian scriptures, inscribed in papyrus and on temple walls.

The following are general outlines of yoga practices which you can apply in your life to maintain mental Health. You should make every reasonable effort to make sure that these elements are present in your spiritual program. Therefore, you should reflect on them daily and evaluate your ability to follow them. They are all designed to promote peace and harmony within you and from this space of peace and harmony, your progress in understanding the teachings and inner discovery of yourself will be promoted.

CHAPTER IIII

Introduction to The Yoga of Wisdom

In the Temple of Aset (Isis) in Ancient Egypt the Discipline of the Yoga of Wisdom is imparted in three stages:

> 1-<u>Listening</u> to the wisdom teachings on the nature of reality (creation) and the nature of the Self.
> 2-<u>Reflecting</u> on those teachings and incorporating them into daily life.
> 3-<u>Meditating</u> on the meaning of the teachings.

Aset (Isis) was and is recognized as the goddess of wisdom and her temple strongly emphasized and espoused the philosophy of wisdom teaching in order to achieve higher spiritual consciousness. It is important to note here that the teaching which was practiced in the Ancient Egypt Temple of Aset of **Listenin**g to, **Reflectin**g upon, and **Meditatin**g upon the teachings is the same process used in Vedanta-Jnana Yoga of India of today. **The Yoga of Wisdom** is a form of Yoga based on insight into the nature of worldly existence and the transcendental Self, thereby transforming one's consciousness through development of the wisdom faculty. Thus, we have here a correlation between Ancient Egypt that matches exactly in most respects.

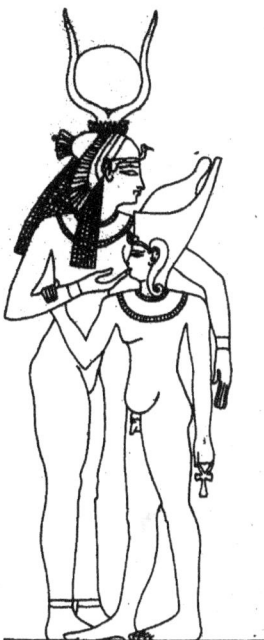

GENERAL DISCIPLINE OF THE TEMPLE OF ASET (PHILAE, EGYPT)

THE THREE-FOLD PROCESS OF WISDOM YOGA IN ANCIENT EGYPT

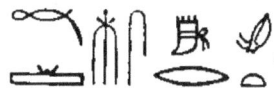

Fill the ears, listen attentively- Meh mestchert.

Listening

1 Listening to Wisdom teachings. Having achieved the qualifications of an aspirant, there is a desire to listen to the teachings from a Spiritual Preceptor. There is increasing intellectual understanding of the scriptures and the meaning of truth versus untruth, real versus unreal, temporal versus eternal.

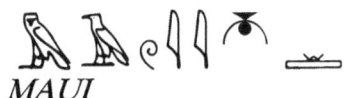

MAUI

"to think, to ponder, to fix attention, concentration"

127

Reflection

2- on those teachings and living according to the disciplines enjoined by the teachings until the wisdom is fully understood. Reflection implies discovering the oneness behind the multiplicity of the world by engaging in intense inquiry into the nature of one's true Self..

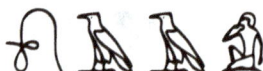

uaa

"Meditation"

Meditation

3- The process of reflection leads to a state in which the mind is continuously introspective. It means expansion of consciousness culminating in revelation of and identification with the Absolute Self: Brahman.

Note: It is important to note here that the same teaching which was practiced in ancient Egypt of **Listening** to, **Reflecting** upon, and **Meditating** upon the teachings is the same process used in Vedanta-Jnana Yoga (from India) of today.

Ancient Egyptian Proverbs of The Wisdom Path

"If you seek GOD, you seek for the Beautiful. One is the Path that leads unto GOD - Devotion joined with Wisdom."

"Do not be proud and arrogant with your knowledge. Consult with the ignorant and wise. Truth may be found among maids at the grindstones."

After the millions of years of differentiated creation, the chaos that existed before creation will return; only the primeval god[16] and Asar will remain steadfast-no longer separated in space and time.

—Ancient Egyptian *Coffin Texts*

---

[16] Referring to the Supreme Being in the form of Atum-Ra

Yoga of Wisdom

Intuitional wisdom is the objective of the various practices of Yoga but the study of wisdom teachings is the most important step in achieving intellectual knowledge which will be used to lead you to attain experiential (intuitional) knowledge. Study of the wisdom teachings is like mental food. It is this mental diet of sublime thoughts and affirmations which will give fortitude and direction to your life.

Dispassion and Detachment

"Mastery of the passions allows divine thought and action."
—Ancient Egyptian Proverb

9. Detachment, absence of the feeling of mine-ness (sense of ownership) towards son, wife, house and the like and constant equanimity of mind in all happenings whether desirable or undesirable.

10. Unflinching devotion to Me (Higher Self) through the Yoga of inseparability, abiding in solitary places, not delighting in the company of the worldly minded.

Gita: Chapter 13 Kshetra-Kshetrajna Vibhag Yogah--
The Division of Field and the
Knower of the Field.

If any [man] cometh to me, and hateth not his father, and mother, and wife, and children, and brethren, and sisters, yea, and his own life also, he cannot be my disciple.
The Bible, Luke 14:26

What does the practices of dispassion and detachment really mean in practical life? When you develop a pleasurable feeling based on your interaction with an object, you develop a longing to experience that object more. You say: "May I get more of that." This desire leads to continuous mental unrest until the object is acquired, and frustration and anger when there is no possibility of your acquiring the object. When you begin to rely on objects (anything outside of yourself, i.e., land, money, cars, people, etc.) for your happiness, saying: "When I get that then I will be happy" or "When this happens then I will be happy," you are in reality cursing yourself or dooming yourself to unhappiness. This is because there is no situation or object in this changing world of time and space which will make anyone truly happy. All things change and the human mind, once it acquires what it longed for, becomes happy---for a while, but then it grows tired of the situation and bored with the object; it then desires other objects and situations for its enjoyment. These desires of the mind are endless. This is the nature of the mind in an egoistic state and trying to satiate these desires is like trying to fill a bucket with holes in it.

When you live this way, you are in effect saying: "I don't have the inner resources to be happy; I need something outside of myself to make me happy." Your ignorance has led you to believe that happiness is to be found in objects, accomplishments or activities in the world. In reality, it is the Soul-Self which sustains all life and is the source of all happiness which you experience. In its purified form, this happiness is called bliss. Bliss is the experience of the state of enlightenment. The Neter (Self) sustains your free will, allows your mind to function and sustains the chemical processes of your body. Therefore, when you think that you are the one who sustains your daily activities, you are engaging in an egoistic illusion. It is your spirit which gives life to your body and it is the spirit which gives you strength to pursue the activities of life. So the credit for your very existence should go to your innermost Self.

Therefore, your interest in objects is misplaced. You should be interested in this Self from which you arise and are sustained. It is the Self within you which is infinite and boundless bliss. Objects have an enticing effect on the human mind because they all arise and are supported by the same blissful Self from which your very consciousness arises. This fact makes them enchanting to the human mind because the mind is always searching for what will make it happy. When you see an object, situation or person which makes you "happy", it is really the Self in that object which you are recognizing and not the object itself. However, your misguided notion that it is the object and not the Self which brings joy leads you to pursue the object which is transitory and illusory. This leads to disappointment and frustration when the objects are not within your grasp or when the situations or persons you long for do not come to you.

Wisdom dictates that you should reverence the divine essence in objects, people and situations. Strive to recognize them as expressions of the Self as you are. Don't hold onto anything or anyone, rather love others with detachment, knowing that they are transient expressions of the Self.

All things die and are reborn, therefore, if you grieve over the loss of a loved one you are grieving over something which is based on erroneous understanding. No one dies in reality; they only change forms and move on in their quest for spiritual enlightenment through many incarnations which are determined by their level of ignorance of their true Self, the Neter.

Therefore, do not become attached to anything outside of yourself and do not grieve over anything because their is no loss or gain in the Self. When you live your life according to this wisdom, you relieve the tension and pain of egoistic pursuits and open the doors of eternity.

Concentration on Opposite Moods:

"To destroy an undesirable rate of mental vibration, concentrate on the opposite vibration to the one to be suppressed."

"To change your mood or mental state, change your vibration."

—Ancient Egyptian Proverbs

Positive affirmation and concentration of the mind on the opposite mood or thought is useful in counteracting negative states of mind. Since the mind is fluid, it takes the form of its impressions or Karmas. If the individual human consciousness identifies with a specific mood or thought, it will take on that feeling as its own and thus, partake in the repercussions of that feeling. Through practice, one can learn to train the mind to think in certain ways and develop new positive mental impressions or Karmas. You must understand that all thoughts and states of mind are under your control. You can begin this practice by watching your thoughts closely. When you feel depressed, remind yourself that you, that is, your true essence (Neter, Osiris, Isis, Horus or any deity you prefer), are the source of supreme joy (bliss). Repeat mentally, *"I" am Bliss* and see how your mind changes its state. Choose a sublime teaching to study or some words of power to chant, practice yoga exercise, listen to an uplifting audio or video recording. Do not allow the mind to develop a negative state. If you distract yourself by watching a movie or going to a party, your negativity will only be suppressed and it will come out at some future time. The wonder of working with the mind is the discovery that you can control it instead of it controlling you. You do not have to be a slave to the emotional swings or cravings of the mind. You have the power because you are innately the Universal Soul. Due to ignorance, your soul has allowed the mind to rule over it with desires and cravings. As you discover the immense power within the real you, you discover the true bliss of self mastery.

WATCHING THE EMOTIONS

You will notice that when you are tense and upset, the body assumes constrictive poses and breathing becomes shallow. When this happens you need to start taking control by practicing the proper breathing technique at all times. From now on you must try to take notice of when you experience mood swings. Spiritual energy is dissipated through indiscriminate indulgence in emotional behavior. Most people are taught to vent their emotions freely in order to be healthy. In reality, the source of emotionality needs to be dealt with in order to have true mental peace and health. Otherwise, the venting of frustrations will form mental impressions which will cause habitual and uncontrollable outbursts of anger and other emotions. The true way to eradicate emotional and other psychic problems is to get to the root-cause of these problems: ignorance of your true Self. Try to make a conscious effort to control your emotional outbursts. When you notice you are out of control, stop yourself and go to a private place and practice your breathing exercises and hekau. This is the ongoing battle of Horus and Set, of positive and negative, within yourself. Each time you exercise your self effort to your capacity in each of these battles, you are building momentum to win the war of Horus over Set within yourself.

Patience and perseverance are the keys to success. Over a period of time, you will discover how your practice of yoga has changed your life for the better. Perhaps you would have argued with someone or cried for two hours in a particular situation, but now that you have been practicing yoga, you argue or cry only for one hour or not at all. Perhaps after a year of practicing yoga you discover that it takes more to get you upset now than it did a year ago. This is achieving victory over Set and success on the spiritual path. Many people judge themselves in an all or nothing manner, "I was upset a year ago and I'm still not able to control myself now, so there is no spiritual progress," and then they give up. For most people, spiritual progress occurs in degrees. At times you may notice that you are able to make giant strides in what seems to be a quantum leap. This is because you have been gathering momentum by practicing your spiritual disciplines so it is important that you continue to do so on a regular basis.

Good Association Part 2

Good Association is a form of group therapy and counseling. It is similar to the process of psychotherapy of Western psychologists, helping the individual to see the error in understanding which is causing the inability to cope with the world. The major difference between Good Association in Yoga, traditional Western forms of group therapy and individual counseling is that through the spiritual preceptor, Good Association assists and urges the individual to understand his/her transcendental true Self while traditional treatments seek to help the individual cope with life situations which produce stress and mental anguish. From a yogic point of view, ordinary human life is based on an erroneous view of existence and psychological disciplines which do not include an understanding of the human soul are also based on ignorance. Thus, treatments which are based on ignorance cannot provide effective and abiding results. From this point of view, modern psychology and modern medical science must be understood as disciplines which are only in their infancy because they have not yet acknowledged and discovered the hidden mysteries of the soul. Ordinary psychology is useful in taking extremely degraded individuals (psychotic) from the depths of abnormality and to some degree, helping them to become lucid enough to exist in the world. However, this level of existence and what modern psychology considers to be "normal" is not considered normal by yogic science. Mental abnormality exists to the degree of intensification of the ego and its accompanying complexes. The state of enlightenment or Self-knowledge is then the only state that can be called "the state of optimal mental health."

Good Association is a teacher-disciple relationship wherein yogic teachings are presented to promote spiritual and thus mental and physical health. Through continuous association with sages or other spiritually advanced personalities, the aspirant is led to discover her/his true spiritual identity. When this process occurs, the general health of the individual is improved because mental complexes and stress diminish and in so doing, the body is able to maintain itself at a more optimal level.

Note: With few exceptions, television does not provide good association. You should strive to curb your viewing time in the beginning of your program and for the next three years. A casual time spent watching an educational television show may be useful in stimulating the mind, however, when television becomes a necessity to you and you spend much of your time "glued" to it for your "entertainment", television promotes dullness of the mind and intellectual weakness which lead to spiritual insensitivity.

Also, "hanging out" with those personalities who are Setian in nature (those who are continuously affected by **anger, hate, greed, lust, impulsiveness, selfishness, brutishness force, demoniac thoughts, thugs, thievery, violence, etc.**) is detrimental to the mental peace of an aspirant, especially to a neophyte (a beginner; novice). Those who are constantly moving around, constantly argumentative and constantly agitated are afflicted with intense identification with their bodies and senses and are unaware of their divine nature.

An important feature of the state of mind which is associated with those who are virtuous or vicious is that tranquility, repose, and peace are characteristic of the virtuous while frantic movement and struggle are associated with the vicious. These same characteristics of the virtues and vices are mentioned in both the ancient Egyptian (MAAT) and Indian (Dharma) systems of moral development and the need for a state of peacefulness of mind is also emphasized as an imperative feature without which progress on the spiritual path cannot occur.

In general, a mental atmosphere of peacefulness and contentment is necessary for sublime thoughts and aspirations to emerge in the mind. Otherwise, through a life which is based on pursuing the satisfaction of the senses, there is constant desire and agitation of the mind and the individual will always be occupied with the petty thoughts and disturbances of day to day life. Therefore, the cultivation and maintenance of serenity and contentment should be a primary goal of a spiritual aspirant.

You can gradually wean yourself off of television and other negative associations by gradually engaging in them less and less until they are no longer needed. Though in the beginning you must put forth conscious effort to abstain from these practices and to engage in spiritual work, the process becomes easier and easier until there is no more effort needed to sustain your withdrawal from these activities. This is because the positive spiritual experience provides such a sense of "Self" that you will loose your dependence on the objects of the world and instinctively refrain from associations which will disrupt your growing sense of inner peace. In the mean time you must work with your mind to abstain from negative activities to the best of your ability. You must understand that you are not giving anything up. In fact, you will be gaining a closer relationship with yourself and true fulfillment of your inner desire.

The Concept of Sebai

The Sebai in Ancient Egypt

The Term Sebai means "Illuminer of the mysteries"

The highest company an aspirant can keep is with the Sabai. In Ancient Egypt the priests and priestesses were revered as enlightened councilors and spiritual leaders or sages who lead initiates to meet the Divine. There are few cases where they are canonized or considered as gods and goddesses as such. Imhotep is one such example. However, in their capacity they were charged with becoming one with the divinities during rituals in order to bring forth the glory of that divinity. Thus, in Kamitan spirituality there is more focus on the divinity as opposed to the personality of the preceptor as concerns reverence in the form of an incarnate divinity. That form of reverence and devotion was reserved for the Per-Aah or phearoah. The priests and priestesses were facilitators and enlightened guides to the mysteries. As enlightened personalities they were hailed as leaders and directors of of society.

The kind of reverence towards priests and priestesses that developed in India was unknown in Ancient Egypt. Rather, the mysteries were kept closely amongst the initiates within the temple system and the public was only allowed to participate in the holidays, traditions and public festivals. The teaching was disseminated within the temple system and it was god and the teaching which were the primary focus and not the spiritual preceptor. It was perhaps, in their wisdom that the Kemetic priests and priestesses sought to avoid the situation which has developed in modern India, that the teachings are so proliferated that there are many charlatans throughout the country, conning the common folk.

133

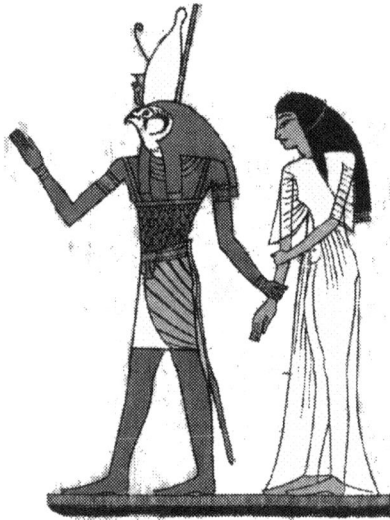

The Priest dressed as Heru, leads the female Initiate to the Inner Shrine for Initiation.

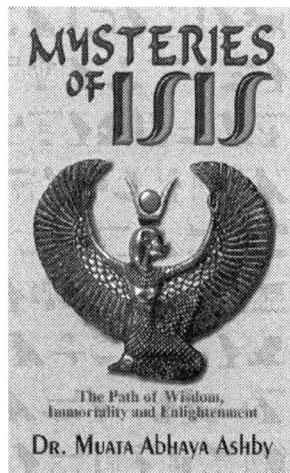

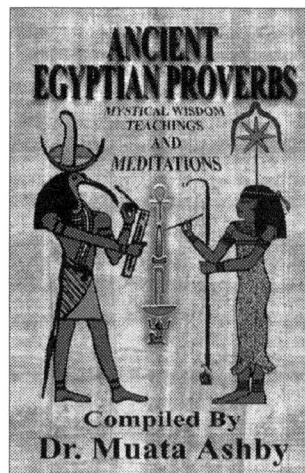

For more teachings on the path of Wisdom Yoga see the book *The Mysteries of Isis,* and *Egyptian Proverbs* by Dr. Muata Ashby

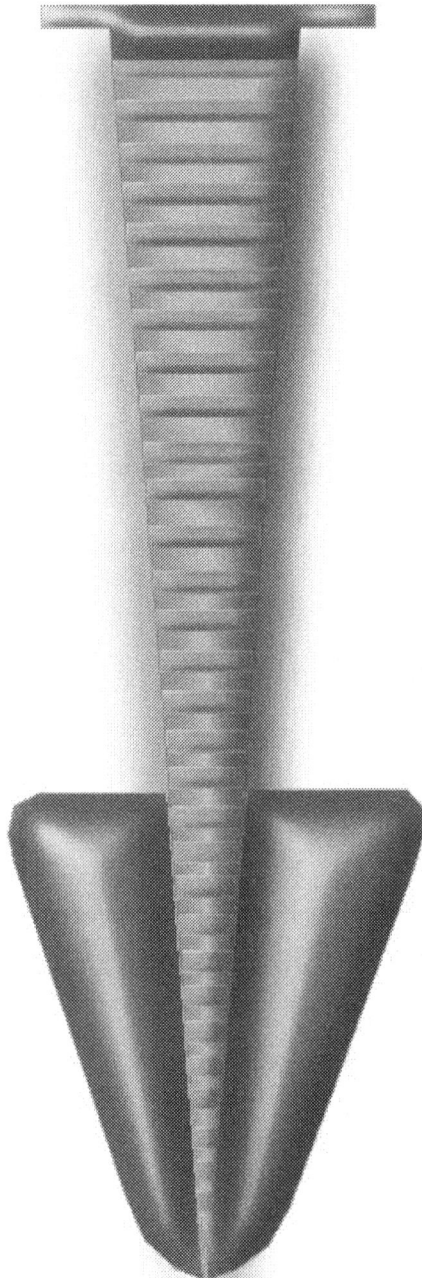

CHAPTER IIIII

Introduction to The Yoga of Righteous Action

GENERAL DISCIPLINE
In all Temples especially
The Temple of Heru and Edfu

Scripture: Prt M Hru and special scriptures including the Berlin Papyrus and other papyri.

STEPS IN THE PRACTICE OF RIGHT ACTION YOGA

1- Learn Ethics and Law of Cause and Effect-Practice right action

(42 Precepts of Maat)
to purify gross impurities of the personality
Control Body, Speech, Thoughts

2- Practice cultivation of the higher virtues

(selfless-service)
to purify mind and intellect from subtle impurities

3- Devotion to the Divine

See maatian actions as offerings to the Divine

4- Meditation

See oneself as one with Maat, i.e. United with the cosmic order
which is the Transcendental Supreme Self.

Plate 1: The Offering of Maat-Symbolizing the Ultimate act of Righteousness (Temple of Seti I)

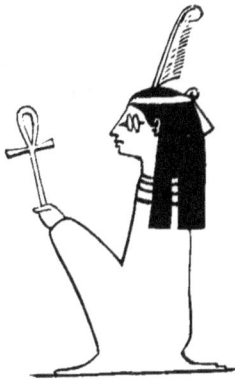

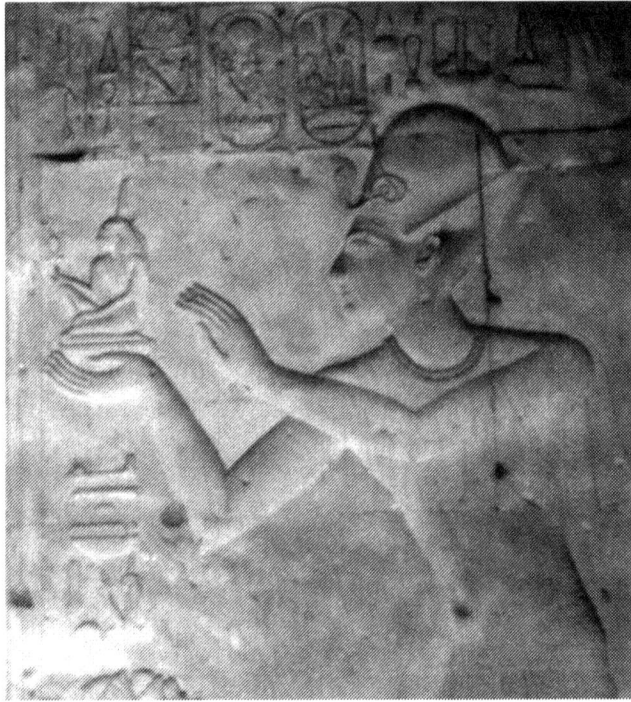

Ancient Egyptian Proverbs of The Action Path

"There are two roads traveled by humankind, those who seek to live MAAT and those who seek to satisfy their animal passions."

"They who revere *MAAT* are *long lived*; they who are covetous have no tomb."

"No one reaches the beneficent West (heaven) unless their heart is righteous by doing *MAAT*. There is no distinction made between the inferior and the superior person; it only matters that one is found faultless when the balances and the two weights stand before the Lord of Eternity. No one is free from the reckoning. Thoth, a baboon, holds the balances to count each one according to what they have done upon earth."

"MAAT is great and its effectiveness lasting; it has not been disturbed since the time of Osiris. There is punishment for those who pass over it's laws, but this is unfamiliar to the covetous one....When the end is nigh, *MAAT* lasts."

Yoga of Action:

"No one reaches the Beneficent West* (Enlightenment) unless their heart is righteous by doing MAAT." *(the land of Osiris-heaven)

"Speak MAAT; do MAAT."

Yoga of Action implies acting according to the teachings of mystical wisdom (Maat) throughout your normal day to day activities. It keeps the mind occupied with thoughts which are uplifting to the mind. It is especially useful for calming the externalized-restless mind-set and redirecting thought patterns away from dwelling on mental complexes (worries) in order to allow the mind time to integrate its higher desire to overcome the difficulties through personality integration. Mental complexes will intensify rather than resolve if dwelled upon constantly. Many people have learned through experience that when there is a difficult problem which will still be there the following day, it is better to "sleep on it." When the clouds of egoism are no longer there, such as during deep sleep or in an advanced practitioner of yoga, the rays of the Self can shine through and illumine one's consciousness with *Hetep*. Again it must be emphasized that this experience of peace is not an all or nothing experience. It occurs in degrees. You may still find yourself feeling entrapped and agitated, but now, in addition to these ego based feelings, you have an increased sensitivity to the voice of wisdom within you. This is the voice which repeats a hekau, mantra or prayers and reflects on the nature of your true essence when the ego wants to tie the mind up with worries and imaginations. You may hear this voice repeating: *"I" am fearless. "I" have all the resources within me to withstand and rise above any situation. Even this seemingly impossible situation is in line with my attaining enlightenment, and it too, like the clouds in the sky blocking the rays of the sun, will pass away.*

In the beginning stages of practicing yoga when you are not very attuned to listening to your spiritual voice, you may not experience much peace. However, as you choose to listen to that voice more and more, and indulge in prayer, hekau and the other disciplines of yoga more than you indulge yourself in egoistic practices, you will notice within yourself a river of peace, faith, security and devotion which will eventually overflow and wash away all ego based emotions from your personality. This is the victory of Horus over Set within your personality.

To the extent that you are able to control your temper, your inner war (between the Higher Self and the Lower) will not affect others around you, however, there may be an already established tendency to lash out at people around you. One should do one's best to sublimate this tendency and to remain focused on the negative and positive forces battling within oneself and work to establish Maat within one's self. This can be a difficult task when one is used to looking outside him/herself for answers and means to solve life's problems and blaming others (i.e. spouse, children, church, childhood, parents, country, political and religious leaders) for the occurrence of those problems. Situations can only affect you if it is in line with your karma for that to occur. Therefore, it is no accident or no one's fault or responsibility but your own regardless of what situation (good or bad) you may find yourself in. You may not be able to see how your actions of this life could have resulted in your current circumstance, but remember, these situations are occurring as a result of actions not only in this lifetime but previous ones. So your attitude towards dealing with all negative predicaments of life should be one of personal responsibility and forbearance. There is no need to feel bad or blame yourself or others. Blame and bad feelings are ego based viruses which infect the mind and further debilitate it. When you are typing and you make a mistake you don't spend a lot of time blaming yourself and having regrets about having made an error. You simply correct your error and carry on. The process with life should be similar. Pray for strength to endure and transcend the situation and put forth the effort to correct the error in your belief and thinking which predisposed you to have this situation manifest in your life. With patience and insight into the fact of your true underlying, boundless essence of your Higher Self, you can overcome all obstacles.

If you do not accept personal responsibility for your life, then you will never look to find that which may be in error in your thought processes and behavior which predisposed you to your experiences, and there will be no chance for you to improve your situation. If you do not learn the spiritual lesson the situation is here to teach you, you are setting yourself up to have the experience repeat itself again. This is the nature of the karmic process upon which the world process is set up. These experiences are not meant to be painful or to make you bitter. Each of these experiences give you the opportunity to practice and secure spiritual qualities such as patience, equanimity, dispassion, detachment, universal love, freedom from resentment when persecuted or wronged and all the other precepts of Maat. In doing so, you learn to view every situation in your life as your path to enlightenment. In this way, performing your practical duties of life in a righteous manner becomes one and the same with your practice of spiritual discipline. Pain and suffering is a by-product of not living a life in harmony with Maat and with an awareness of your true essence.

The yoga of action also emphasizes the performance of selfless service, termed karma yoga. When one performs selfless service, the ego loses importance and therefore, its needs and cravings become powerless illusions which can no longer afflict the mind. The highest practice of karma yoga occurs in the state of enlightenment when there is no attachment to the fruits of actions. Work is performed in harmony with one's true nature without dependency on the results, be they good or bad from a practical standpoint. Right livelihood, the practice of making a living in such a way as to benefit oneself and all other beings is practicing Maat. Yoga of Action also implies a balanced movement and scheduling of time for spiritual discipline as well as other practical duties. Extremes are to be avoided because they also cause intensification of the mental complexes. The desired movement is relaxed and deliberate intensification of self-effort according to the capacity of the individual.

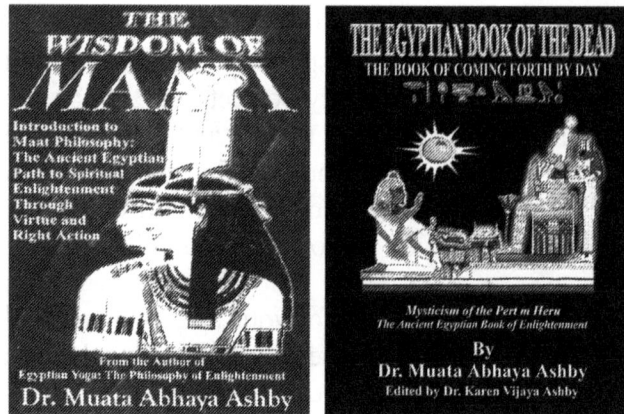

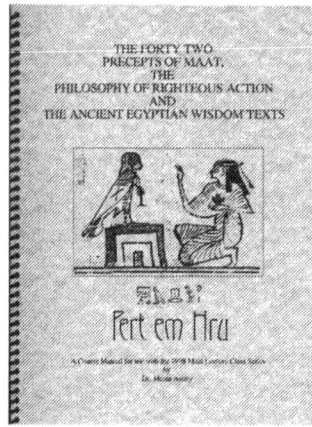

For more teachings on the path of Action Yoga see the book *The Wisdom of Maati, Egyptian Book of the Dead, 42 Principles of Maat* by Dr. Muata Ashby

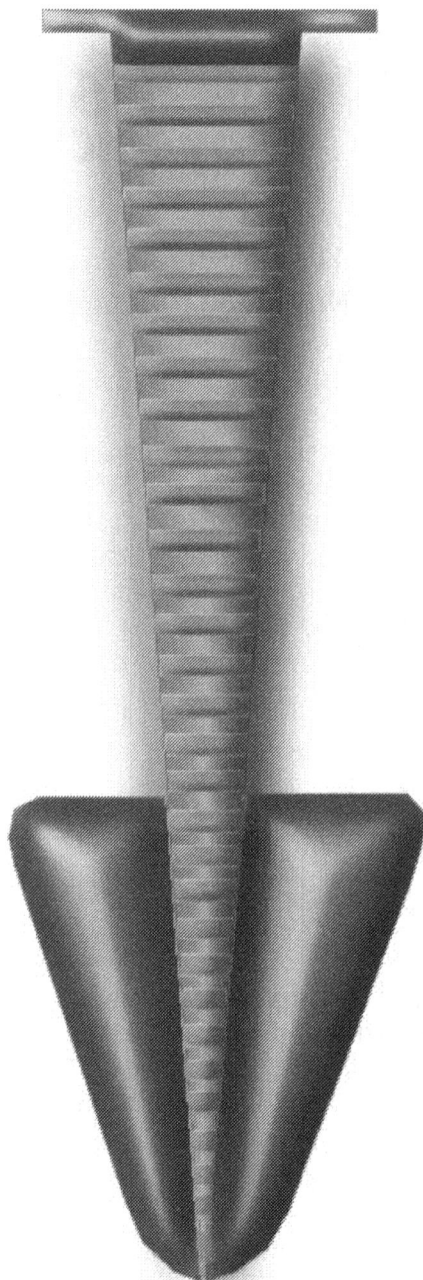

CHAPTER ||||||

Introduction to the Yoga of Postures and Movements

Egyptian Yoga Exercise Thef Neteru: The Movements of the Gods and Goddesses

The Yogic Postures in Ancient Egypt

Since their introduction to the West the exercise system of India known as "Hatha Yoga" has gained much popularity. The disciplines related to the yogic postures and movements were developed in India around the 10th century A.C.E. by a sage named Goraksha.[17] Up to this time, the main practice was simply to adopt the cross-legged meditation posture known as the lotus for the purpose of practicing meditation. The most popular manual on Hatha Yoga is the **Hatha-Yoga-Pradipika ("Light on the Forceful Yoga).** It was authored by Svatmarama Yogin in mid. 14th century C.E. [18]

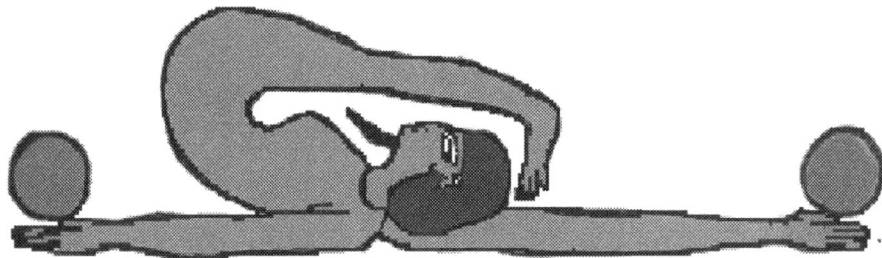

Plate 2: Above- The god Geb in the plough posture engraved on the ceiling of the antechamber to the Asarian Resurrection room of the Temple of Hetheru in Egypt. (photo taken by Ashby)

Prior to the emergence of the discipline the physical movements in India just before 1000 A.C.E.,[19] a series of virtually identical postures to those which were practiced in India can be found in various Ancient Egyptian papyruses and inscribed on the walls and ceilings of the temples. The Ancient Egyptian practice can be dated from 300 B.C.E 1,580 B.C.E and earlier. Exp. Temple of Hetheru (800-300 B.C.E.), Temple of Heru (800-300 B.C.E.), Tomb of Queen Nefertari (reigned 1,279-1,212 BC), and various other temples and papyruses from the New Kingdom Era 1,580 B.C.E). In Ancient Egypt the practice of the postures (called *Sema Paut* (Union with the gods and goddesses) or *Tjef Sema Paut Neteru* (movements to promote union with the gods and goddesses) were part of the ritual aspect of the spiritual myth which when practiced serve to harmonize the energies and promote the physical health of the body and direct the mind, in a meditative capacity, to discover and cultivate divine consciousness. These disciplines are

---

[17] Yoga Journal, {The New Yoga} January/February 2000
[18] **Hatha-Yoga-Pradipika,** *The Shambhala Encyclopedia of Yoga* by Georg Feuerstein, Ph. D.
[19] *The Shambhala Encyclopedia of Yoga* by Georg Feuerstein, Ph. D.

part of a larger process called Sema or *Smai Tawi* (Egyptian Yoga). By acting and moving like the gods and goddesses one can essentially discover their character, energy and divine agency within one's consciousness and thereby also become one of their retinue, i.e. one with the Divine Self. In modern times, most practitioners of Hatha Yoga see it as a means to attain physical health only. However, even the practice in India had a mythic component which is today largely ignored by modern practitioners.

The Yogic Postures Discipline

Most people believe that the practice of special movements or postures for the purpose of harmonizing the energies of the body, promoting health and a meditative mind began in India or China. Prior to the emergence of the discipline the physical movements in India just before 1000 A.C.E.,[48] a series of virtually identical postures to those which were practiced in India can be found in various Ancient Egyptian papyruses and inscribed on the walls and ceilings of the temples. The Ancient Egyptian practice can be dated from 300 B.C.E 1,580 B.C.E and earlier. Exp. Temple of Hetheru (800-300 B.C.E.), Temple of Heru (800-300 B.C.E.), Tomb of Queen Nefertari (reigned 1,279-1,212 BC), and various other temples and papyruses from the New Kingdom Era 1,580 B.C.E. In Ancient Egypt the practice of the postures (called *Sema Paut* (Union with the gods and goddesses) or *Tjef Sema Paut Neteru* (movements to promote union with the gods and goddesses) were part of the ritual aspect of the spiritual myth which when practiced serve to harmonize the energies and promote the physical health of the body and direct the mind, in a meditative capacity, to discover and cultivate divine consciousness. These disciplines are part of a larger process called Sema or *Smai Tawi* (Egyptian Yoga). By acting and moving like the gods and goddesses one can essentially discover their character, energy and divine agency within one's consciousness and thereby also become one of their retinue, i.e. one with the Divine Self. In modern times, most practitioners of Hatha Yoga see it as a means to attain physical health only. However, even the practice in India had a mythic component which is today largely ignored by modern practitioners. The postures below are a few of those belonging to the Ancient Egyptian Mystery System. For more information on this discipline the book *Egyptian Yoga Exercise Workout Book* by Seba Muata Ashby

Some Postures from the Egyptian Yoga Movement System

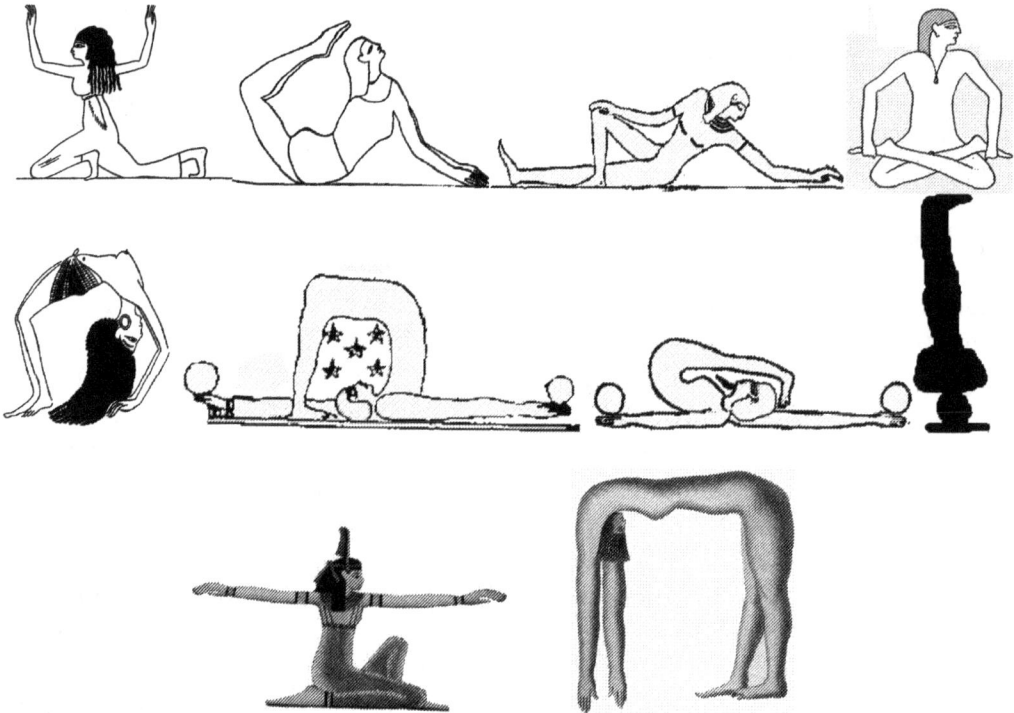

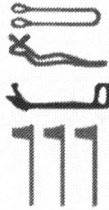

tjef neteru – movements of the gods and goddesses or

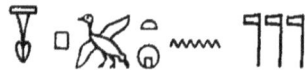

sma paut n neteru – Union with the gods and goddesses, the art of meditative movements in a ritual format to discover the power of the gods and goddesses within.

Physical Exercise:

"Her name is Health: she is the daughter of Exercise, who begot her on Temperance. The rose blusheth on her cheeks, the sweetness of the morning breatheth from her lips; joy, tempered with innocence and modesty, sparkleth in her eyes and from the cheerfulness of her heart she singeth as she walketh."

—Ancient Egyptian Proverb

Physical and mental health are the basis of spiritual health. Therefore, Yoga philosophy also includes the practice of special postures and exercises coupled with breathing techniques to promote the health of the mind and body. These exercises are psycho-physical in nature, affecting both the mind and body. These postures have an effect on one's mental attitude and physical health by stimulating, cleansing and balancing the various endocrine glands, organs and tissues of the body. Physical disturbance and preoccupation with physical illness may distract one's consciousness from higher, more sublime thoughts and aspirations. This branch of yoga is actually under the same discipline as meditation.

Recreation:

Recreation is a seldom discussed topic in philosophical treatises. It is usually seen as an "activity that is performed" in order to achieve some kind of regeneration of one's physical and psychological self. Also it is seen as a source of "fun" and excitement. The mind seeks to place itself in the most "pleasurable" environment or situations possible. From a deeper understanding of life and its purpose, the practice of many commonly accepted forms of recreation becomes inadequate because such activities have built into them, the elements of disappointment. Usually they are based on competition which pits individuals or teams against each other in a format that is designed to produce and promote conflict. Since the happiness to be derived is based upon "winning" a game, one is bound for disappointment since that cannot occur each time the activity is undertaken. If the times of disappointment are used for introspection, one will develop dispassion towards that which is illusory, painful and transient and seek to find that which is real, constant and truly pleasurable. A whole new world opens for exploration and true recreation in the spiritual realm.

True recreation is fully conscious, detached and peaceful. Only then is it possible to "feel" and appreciate the nature of one's being, of creation itself. The highest degree of recreation is therefore experienced at the point of enlightenment, when Horushood is realized. Here, every activity in life becomes "play." Life itself becomes a *"divine sport."* In Indian Vedanta philosophy this concept is called *"Leela."* There develops a continuous blissful feeling which does not pass from moment to moment as with those who move from activity to activity searching for a thrill to make them "feel alive," but existence becomes eternity, right in the very present moment. As modern physics shows, time is only a mental concept people put on intervals of eternity. The only reason why we believe time actually passes is because our minds are always concerned with the past or future events and rarely with the present moment. Raising one's spiritual awareness means becoming alive in the present, the here and now. This has been elaborated in the section on Meditation.

Recreation becomes a means to re-create one's consciousness at every moment instead of a means to forget oneself and to pass the time. It allows you to be able to deal more effectively with life's problems rather than serving to distract you for a few minutes, hours or days. Many enlightened personalities such as *Paramahansa Yogananda,* an Indian Sage who came to the West to spread the philosophy of yoga, would from time to time indulge in recreational activities. The difference is that he did not identify himself with the pleasure or illusoriness of the event. As a therapeutic practice, he advocated recreation as a means to gradually adjust the mind and body to greater and greater levels of spiritual discipline. In short, a spiritual discipline does not consist in "giving up" recreation or pleasure; it consists in understanding that the pleasure comes from within, the Self, and not from the object or activity.

Proper Breathing

Most people in the modern world do not know how to breathe properly. Most people (especially males) have learned to breathe by pushing out the chest in a "manly" or "macho" fashion. This mode of breathing is harmful for many reasons. The amount of air taken in is less and vital cosmic energy is reduced and becomes stagnant in the subtle vital energy channels, resulting in physical and mental diseases. The stagnation of the flow of energy through the body has the effect of grounding one's consciousness to the physical realities rather than allowing the mind and body to operate with lightness and subtlety.

"Belly breathing" or abdominal breathing massages the internal organs and develops Life Force energy (Ra, Chi or Kundalini). It will be noticed that it is our natural breathing pattern when we lie down on our back. Instruction is as follows: A- Breathe in and push the stomach out. B- Breathe out and pull the stomach in. This form of breathing is to be practiced at all times, not just during meditation. It allows the natural Life Force in the air to be rhythmically supplied to the body and nervous system. This process is indispensable in the achievement of physical health and mental-spiritual power to control the mind (meditation).

PROPER BREATHING: The way to promote health and control of the mind and emotions.

fig. 4

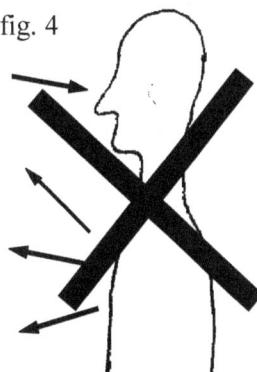

Above: Chest breathing.
Below: Abdominal breathing.

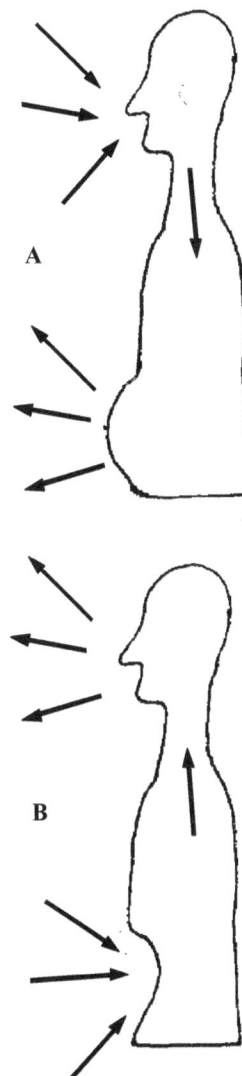

"GOD is life and through Him only Human kind lives. GOD gives life to men and women, breathing the breath of life into their nostrils."

"Be as the Sun and Stars, that emanate the life giving essence; give life without asking for anything in return; to be a sun, breath rhythmically and deeply; then as RA shall you be."

Ancient Egyptian Proverbs

ALTERNATE BREATH EXERCISE*

Prior to your practice of exercises and meditation you should practice *Alternate Nostril Breathing.* There are opposing forces (poles) of energy in all human bodies. These forces are related to mental energy, the emotions, mental and physical health. When these poles are out of balance, various mental, emotional and physical problems can arise. The study of these forces is related to the Uraeus Serpent of Egypt and the Kundalini Serpent Yoga systems of India. For now simply follow the instructions below and you will begin to feel improved health and vitality. As you study the deeper implications of the breath, more teachings will be given to enhance your practice. (Recommended text: *Sivananda Companion to Yoga*).

The opposing energy poles of the body: Uatchet (Udjat, Utchat) and Nekhebet (Ida and Pingala) can be balanced by practicing a simple alternate nostril breathing exercise. This is accomplished as follows: Using the right hand, bend the index and middle finger toward the palm while leaving the thumb, fourth and fifth (pinkie) fingers extended. Using the thumb to close off the right nostril, breath in (inhalation) through the left nostril while holding the right one closed, then close both nostrils using the fourth and fifth (pinkie) fingers to close the left nostril and leaving the other two fingers remaining bent. Release the thumb from the right nostril and exhale through the right nostril. Next breath in through the right nostril while holding the left one closed with the fourth and fifth fingers. Now close the right nostril with your thumb and retain the breath for a short time. Next, release your fourth and fifth fingers (while still holding the right nostril closed with your thumb), breathe out through the left nostril. This constitutes one cycle of the Alternate nostril breathing exercise. The ratio of inhalation: retention: exhalation should be 2:8:4 to begin, working up to 4:16:8. You may repeat a mantra, hekau while performing this exercise. Continue in this way for five minutes at the beginning and then gradually building up to fifteen minutes or longer as needed. Then practice the desired form of meditation of your choice. The alternate breathing exercise is an excellent way to balance the body's energies. The energies may also be balanced in a variety of ways, such as controlling the emotions and remaining calm, engaging one's self in activities that are in harmony with one's consciousness (hobbies, job, recreation). *(see *Egyptian Yoga Exercise Video*)

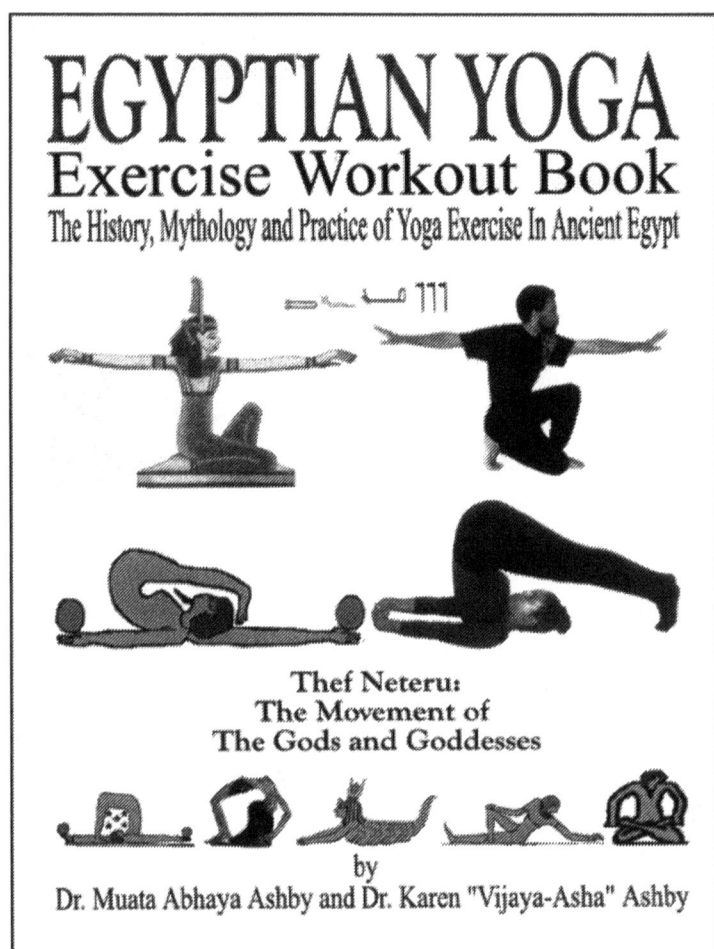

For more teachings on the path of Yoga Postures and Movements see the book *Movements of the Gods and Goddesses,* also on video by Dr. Muata Ashby

CHAPTER ||||||

Introduction to The Yoga of Meditation

KAMITAN HISTORY – 5 MAIN STYLES OF MEDITATION DISCIPLINES - *Shedi*

1. Arat Sekhem, The Path of the Serpent Power[20]
2. Ari Sma Maat, The Path of Meditation through Right Action[21]
3. Nuk Pu-Ushet, The Path of Meditation through "I Am" formula[22]
4. Nuk Ra Akhu, The Path of Meditation through Glorious Light system[23]
5. Rekh, The Path of Meditation through Wisdom[24]

3 stages in meditation

Concentration - Meditation – Superconsciousness

Mau – Uah – Syh

MAUI "to think, to ponder, to fix attention, concentration"	*uaa* "Meditation"	*Syh -* Ecstacy, religious	Swoon or subsiding during religious ecstacy - *Hed.*

---

[20] see book: The Serpent Power
[21] see book The Wisdom of Maati
[22] see book: based on the teachings of the Pert M Heru see book: Egyptian Book of the Dead
[23] see book: Glorious Light Meditation
[24] see book Mysteries of Isis

Introduction to Meditation and Hekau

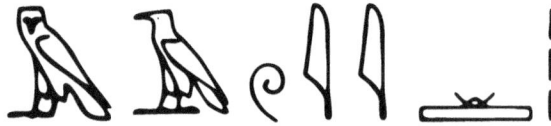

"TO THINK, TO PONDER, TO FIX ATTENTION, MEDITATION"

INTRODUCTION TO MEDITATION

Up to now we have discussed continuous awareness of the Neter Neteru as a form of perpetual meditation practice throughout the day. Now we will explore the phase of meditation as a formal practice.

Meditation may be thought of or defined as the practice of mental exercises and disciplines to enable the aspirant to achieve control over the mind, specifically, to stop the vibrations of the mind due to unwanted thoughts, imaginations, etc. Just as the sun is revealed when the clouds disperse, so the light of the Self is revealed when the mind is free of thoughts, imaginations, ideas, delusions, gross emotions, sentimental attachments, etc. The Self, your true identity, is visible to the conscious mind.

The mind and nervous system are instruments of the Self, which it uses to have experiences in the realm of time and space, which it has created in much the same way as a person falls asleep and develops an entire dream world out of his/her own consciousness. It is at the unconscious and subconscious levels where the most intensive work of yoga takes place because it is here that the conscious identification of a person creates impressions in the mind and where desires based on those impressions develop. It is these desires that keep the aspirant involved in the realm of time and space or frees the aspirant from the world of time and space if they are sublimated into the spiritual desire for enlightenment. The desire to attain enlightenment is not viewed in the same manner as ego based desires; it is viewed as being aspiration which is a positive movement.

Externalized consciousness - distracted by egoism and worldly objects. ◀ ◀ ◀ 𓂀

The light of the Self (consciousness) shines through the mind and this is what sustains life. The flow of consciousness in most people is from within moving outward. This causes them to be externalized and distracted and lose energy. Where the mind goes, energy flows. Have you ever noticed that you can "feel" someone looking at you? This is because there is a subtle energy being transmitted through their vision (which is an extension of the mind). Those who live in this externalized state of mind are not aware of the source of consciousness. Meditation as well as the other disciplines of yoga serve to reverse the flow of consciousness on itself so that the mind acts as a mirror which reveals the true Self.

Internalized consciousness of a yoga practitioner. ▶ ▶ ▶ 𓂀

Most people are unaware that there are deeper levels to their being just as they are unaware of the fact that physical reality is not "physical." Quantum physics experiments have proven that the physical world is not composed of matter but of energy. This supports the findings of the ancient sages who have taught for thousands of years that the reality which is experienced by the human senses is not an "Absolute" reality but a conditional one. Therefore, you must strive to rise beyond your conditioned mind and senses in order to perceive reality as it truly is.

"Learn to distinguish the real from the unreal."

Human beings are not just composed of a mind, senses and a physical body. Beyond the physical and mental there is a soul level. This is the realm of the Higher Self which all of the teachings of yoga and the various practices of meditation are directed toward discovering. This "hidden" aspect of ourselves which is beyond the thoughts is known as Amun, Osiris or Amenta in the ancient Egyptian system of spirituality and as Brahman, in Indian Vedanta philosophy.

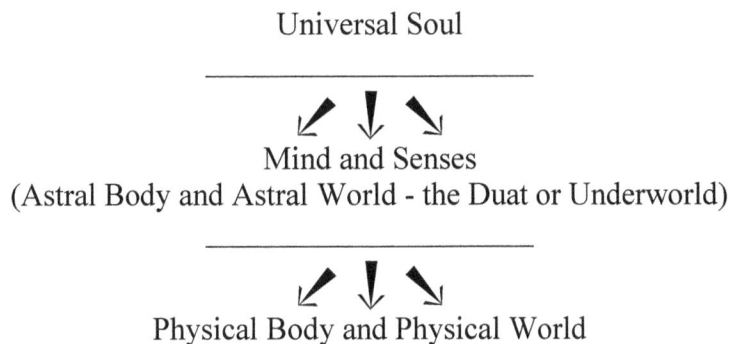

Universal Soul

↙ ↓ ↘

Mind and Senses
(Astral Body and Astral World - the Duat or Underworld)

↙ ↓ ↘

Physical Body and Physical World

When you are active and not practicing or experiencing the wisdom of yoga, you are distracted from the real you. This distraction which comes from the desires, cravings and endless motion of thoughts in the mind is the *veil* which blocks your perception of your deeper essence, Neter NETER. These distractions keep you involved with the mind, senses, and body that you have come to believe is the real you. When your body is motionless and you are thinking and feeling, you are mostly associated with your mind. At times when you are not thinking, such as in the dreamless sleep state, then you are associated with your Higher Self. However, this connection in the dreamless sleep state is veiled by ignorance because you are asleep and not aware of the experience. In order to discover this realm you must consciously turn away from the phenomenal world which is distracting you from your inner reality. The practice of yoga accomplishes this task. Meditation, when backed up by the other disciplines of yoga, is the most powerful agent of self discovery. The practice of meditation allows one to create a higher awareness which affects all aspects of one's life, but most importantly, it gives the aspirant experiential knowledge of his/his true Self.

151

What is Meditation?

Meditation may be thought of or defined as the practice of mental exercises and disciplines to enable the meditator to achieve control over the mind, specifically, to stop the vibrations of the mind due to unwanted thoughts, imaginations, etc.

Consciousness refers to the awareness of being alive and of having an identity. It is this characteristic which separates humans from the animal kingdom. Animals cannot become aware of their own existence and ponder the questions such as *Who am I?, Where am I going in life?, Where do I come from?,* etc. They cannot write books on history and create elaborate systems of social history based on ancestry, etc. Consciousness expresses itself in three modes. These are: Waking, Dream-Sleep and Dreamless-Deep-Sleep.

However, ordinary human life is only partially conscious. When you are driving or walking, you sometimes lose track of the present moment. All of a sudden you arrive at your destination without having conscious awareness of the road which you have just traveled. Your mind went into an "automatic" mode of consciousness. This automatic mode of consciousness represents a temporary withdrawal from the waking world. This state is similar to a day dream (a dreamlike musing or fantasy). This form of existence is what most people consider as "normal" everyday waking consciousness. It is what people consider to be the extent of the human capacity to experience or be conscious.

The "normal" state of human consciousness cannot be considered as "whole" or complete because if it was there would be no experience of lapses or gaps in consciousness. In other words, every instant of consciousness would be accounted for. There would be no trance-like states wherein one loses track of time or awareness of one's own activities, even as they are being performed. In the times of trance or lapse, full awareness or consciousness is not present, otherwise it would be impossible to not be aware of the passage of time while engaged in various activities. Trance here should be differentiated from the religious or mystical form of trance like state induced through meditation. As used above, it refers to the condition of being so lost in solitary thought as to be unaware of one's surroundings. It may further be characterized as a stunned or bewildered condition, a fog, stupor, befuddlement, daze, muddled state of mind. Most everyone has experienced this condition at some point or another. What most people consider to be the "awake" state of mind in which life is lived is in reality only a fraction of the total potential consciousness which a human being can experience.

The state of automatic consciousness is characterized by mental distraction, restlessness and extroversion. The automatic state of mind exists due to emotions such as desire, anger and hatred which engender desires in the mind, which in turn cause more movement, distractions, delusions and lapses or "gaps" in human consciousness. In this condition, it does not matter how many desires are fulfilled. The mind will always be distracted and agitated and will never discover peace and contentment. If the mind were under control, meaning, if you were to remain fully aware and conscious of every feeling, thought and emotion in your mind at any given time, it would be impossible for you to be swayed or deluded by your thoughts into a state of relative unconsciousness or un-awareness. Therefore, it is said that those who do not have their minds under control are not fully awake and conscious human beings.

Meditation and Yoga Philosophy are disciplines which are directed toward increasing awareness. Awareness or consciousness can only be increased when the mind is in a state of peace and harmony. Thus, the disciplines of Meditation (which are part of the Yoga) are the primary means of controlling the mind and allowing the individual to mature psychologically and spiritually.

Psychological growth is promoted because when the mind is brought under control, the intellect becomes clear and psychological complexes such as anxiety and other delusions which have an effect even in ordinary people can be cleared up. Control of the mind and the promotion of internal harmony allows the meditator to integrate their personality and to resolve the hidden issues of the present, of childhood and of past lives.

When the mind has been brought under control, the expansion in consciousness leads to the discovery that one's own individual consciousness is not the total experience of consciousness. Through the correct practice of meditation, the individual's consciousness-awareness expands to the point wherein there is a discovery that one is more than just an individual. The state of "automatic consciousness" becomes reduced in favor of the experiences of increasing levels of continuous awareness. In other words, there is a decrease in daydreaming as well as the episodes of carrying out activities and forgetting oneself in them until they are finished (driving for example). Also, there is a reduced level of loss of awareness of self during the dreaming-sleep and dreamless-sleep states. Normally, most people at a lower level of consciousness-awareness become caught in a swoon or feinting effect which occurs at the time when one "falls" asleep or when there is no awareness of dreams while in the deep sleep state (dreamless-sleep). This swooning effect causes an ordinary person to lose consciousness of their own "waking state" identity and to assume the identity of their "dream subject" and thus, to feel that the dream subject as well as the dream world are realities in themselves.

This shift in identification from the waking personality to the dream personality to the absence of either personality in the dreamless-sleep state led ancient philosophers to discover that these states are not absolute realities. Philosophically, anything that is not continuous and abiding cannot be considered as real. Only what exists and does not change in all periods of time can be considered as "real." Nothing in the world of human experience qualifies as real according to this test. Nature, the human body, everything has a beginning and an end. Therefore, they are not absolutely real. They appear to be real because of the limited mind and senses along with the belief in the mind that they are real. In other words, people believe that matter and physical objects are real even though modern physics has proven that all matter is not "physical" or "stable." It changes constantly and its constituent parts are in reality composed of "empty spaces." Think about it. When you fall asleep, you "believe" that the dream world is "real" but upon waking up you believe it was not real. At the same time, when you fall asleep, you forget the waking world, your relatives and life history, and assume an entirely new history, relatives, situations and world systems. Therefore, philosophically, the ordinary states of consciousness which a human being experiences are limited and illusory. The waking, dream and dreamless-sleep states are only transient expressions of the deeper underlying consciousness. This underlying consciousness which witnesses the other three states is what Carl Jung referred to as the "Collective Unconscious." In Indian Philosophy this "fourth" state of consciousness-awareness is known as *Turia.* It is also referred to as "God Consciousness" or "Cosmic Consciousness."

The theory of meditation is that when the mind and senses are controlled and transcended, the awareness of the transcendental state of consciousness becomes evident. From here, consciousness-awareness expands, allowing the meditator to discover the latent abilities of the unconscious mind. When this occurs, an immense feeling of joy emerges from within, the desire for happiness and fulfillment through external objects and situations dwindles and a peaceful, transcendental state of mind develops. Also, the inner resources are discovered which will allow the practitioner to meet the challenges of life (disappointments, disease, death, etc.) while maintaining a poised state of mind.

When the heights of meditative experience are reached, there is a more continuous form of awareness which develops. It is not *lost* at the time of falling asleep. At this stage there is a discovery that just as the dream state is discovered to be "unreal" upon "waking up" in the morning, the waking state is also discovered to be a kind of dream which is transcended at the time of "falling asleep." There is a form of "continuous awareness" which develops in the mind which spans all three states of consciousness and becomes a "witness" to them instead of a subject bound by them.

Further, there is a discovery that there is a boundless source from which one has originated and to which one is inexorably linked. This discovery brings immense peace and joy wherein the worldly desires vanish in the mind and there is absolute contentment in the heart. This level of experience is what the Buddhists call *Mindfulness.* However, the history of mindfulness meditation goes back to the time of ancient India and Ancient Egypt. In India, the higher level of consciousness wherein automatic consciousness is eradicated and there is continuous awareness is called *Sakshin Buddhi.* From Vedanta and Yoga Philosophy, the teaching of the "witnessing consciousness" found even greater expression and practice in Buddhist philosophy and Buddhist meditation. Buddhi or higher intellect is the source of the word *Buddha,* meaning one who has attained wakefulness at the level of their higher intellect.

The Witnessing Consciousness Teaching and Mindfulness in Ancient Egypt

In ancient Egypt, this level of awareness was called *Amun,* "the witness" or "watcher." The practice of meditation has received much publicity due to the resurgence of the interest in Eastern religions. Perhaps the earliest recorded meditation practice and instruction comes from the teaching of the "Destruction of Mankind" which is inscribed in hieroglyphic text on the walls of a chamber in the tomb of king Seti I of ancient Egypt who lived between 2000 and 1250 BCE. It describes the words of power, visualization and posture elements of meditation and the procedure for practicing the meditation. This meditation text is presented in the book *"Egyptian Proverbs: Mystical Wisdom Teachings and Meditations"* by Dr. Muata Ashby

The understanding of the "witnessing consciousness" achieved a high level of expression in the ancient Egyptian *Hymns of Amun* and in the teaching of the ancient Egyptian Trinity of Amun-Ra-Ptah. The line below from the *Hymns of Amun* explains the nature of the witnessing consciousness:

"He the One Watcher who neither slumbers nor sleeps."

The Trinity, Nebertcher: Amun-Ra-Ptah of ancient Egypt refers to the three states of consciousness and that which transcends them. Amun, the Self, is the "hidden" essence of all things. The Sun, Ra, is the radiant and dynamic outward appearance made manifest in the light of cosmic consciousness. In this aspect, Ptah represents the physical world, the solidification of the projection of consciousness (Amun) made manifest. The Triad also has a reference to the states of consciousness in the human being. The Triad refers to the subject or seer, the object or that which is seen and interaction between the two. In all human experience there is a subject-object-interaction relationship occurring all the time. This is true in the waking as well as the dream states. The seer is Amun, that which is seen is Ptah and the interacting medium or sight is represented by Ra. They are in reality projections or emanations of the transcendental underlying consciousness or Nebertcher.

Just as the subject-object-interaction consciousness of a dream is "unreal", the subject-object-interaction consciousness of the waking state is also unreal and illusory. Even though the phenomenal world experienced in the waking state appears to be abiding and solid, modern science has proven that it is not. These new findings of science confirm the ancient teachings of ancient Egyptian Yoga philosophy, Vedanta and Yoga philosophy of India, Buddhism of India and Taoism of China as well as other mystical philosophies from around the world. The study of the Trinity and the Triad of human consciousness involves an extensive study of the human mind and it is one of the most important subjects in the study of Egyptian Yoga Philosophy. Thus, a separate volume will be devoted to this study. (see the Yoga and Mystical Spirituality book series in the back section of this volume)

Meditation In Life

Meditation is not just an exercise that is to be practiced only at a certain time or at a certain place. In order for your meditative efforts to be successful, the philosophy of meditation must become an integral part of your life. This means that the meditative way of life, the yoga lifestyle, must become the focus of your life no matter what else is going on in your life. Most people who do not practice yoga cannot control the clamoring thoughts of the mind and because of this, do not experience inner peace or clarity of purpose in life. Others, beset by intensely negative thoughts, succumb to these and commit acts against their conscience and suffer the consequences of a self-defeating way of life wherein painful situations and disappointments in life are increased while happiness and contentment are decreased. The mind is weakened due to the mental energy being wasted in useless endeavors which only serve to further entangle one in complex relationships and commitments. Another source of weakening one's will to act correctly to promote situations of advancement and happiness is caused by the susceptibility to negative emotions. Negative emotions such as anger, hatred, greed, gloom, sorrow, and depression as well as excessive positive emotions such as elation serve to create mental agitation and desire which in turn cloud the intellectual capacity to make correct decisions in life.

When life seems unbearable due to the intensification of negative emotions and the obscuring of intellectual capacity, some people commit suicide in an attempt to escape or end the painful onslaught of uncontrollable thoughts. Still others prefer to ignore the messages from the deeper Self which are beckoning them to move toward introspection. Situations of stress in life are motivators whose purpose is to turn us away from the outer world because we have lost our balance. There is a place for material wealth and sensual experience (outer experiences of the senses), however, when the inner reality is ignored or when inner needs and inner development is impaired due to excess concentration on worldly goals and desires, then experiences of frustration and disappointment occur. If these situations are understood as messages from nature to pull back and find the inner balance, then personality integration and harmony can be discovered. However, if these times are faced with lack of inner strength, then they lead to suffering. Sometimes there are moments of clarity wherein the Higher Self is perceived in an intuitive flash but people usually tend to discount the occurrence as a coincidence or other curious event while others in bewilderment believe they are going mad. Others prefer to ignore the issue of spirituality altogether and simply shun any thoughts about death or the afterlife. This is a reverse-yogic movement that stunts spiritual evolution. Its root-cause is fear of the unknown and fear of letting go. The practice of yogic meditation techniques can serve to counteract any and all negative developments in the mind if the correct techniques are used and the correct understanding is adopted.

There are four main components of meditation. These are: posture, breath-life force control, sound and visualization. In the beginning stages of practice, these components may be somewhat difficult to perform with consistency and coordination but with continued effort, they become a pleasurable experience which will bring you closer to your awareness of your Self. It is difficult to control the mind in the beginning. Many aspirants loose heart because they have not obtained the results they had anticipated. They either quit prematurely or jump to different techniques without giving sufficient time for the exercises to work. They do not understand that although on occasion, profound changes will occur in a short time, for the most part it's a gradual process.

A meditative lifestyle should be developed along with one's formal meditation practices. This means acting in such a way that there is greater and greater detachment from objects and situations and greater independence and peace within. This can only occur when there is a keen understanding of one's deeper self and the nature of the world of human experience along with formal meditation practices and other activities which promote physical health (diet and exercise). Ordinarily, people "do" things in order to gain some objective or to derive some pleasure or reward. From a yogic or Buddhist perspective they are "doers of action." They act out of the unconscious and subconscious desires arising in the mind at any given time and are thus, beset with a perpetual state of unrest and agitation. The meditative way of life means that your actions are always affirmations of your higher knowledge and awareness and not based on the unconscious desires and emotions of the mind. The perfection in this discipline only comes with practice. When this art is perfected the practitioner is referred to as a "non-doer." This is because even though they may be doing many things in their life, in reality they have discovered that the true rewards of life do not depend on the outcome of an activity, its fruit or reward.

The main difference between a doer and a non-doer is that the doer is driven by desires while the non-doer is indifferent to the desires of the mind and the fruits of the actions they are performing. The non-doer acts out of wakefulness while the doer acts out of a desire filled mind. Thus, the non-doer can never be disappointed or made unhappy because of a situation in life while the doer is always engaged in a roller coaster of elation or depression, happiness or sorrow, pain or pleasure, etc., never finding an abiding peace The non-doer acts out of necessity and is primarily concerned with experiencing the moment fully while carrying out the present task to perfection, not worrying about the rewards for the task. Thus, it may be said that for the non-doer there is an immediate reward of peace and joy whereas the doer is always looking to the future or the past. Their peace and happiness does not come from expectations of the future nor do they experience sorrow due to some negative situation which occurred in the past. They have discovered a deep experience in the present which transcends both past and future. Thus, they experience a unique form of peace and happiness in an eternal present which is not affected by the various ups and downs of life. Adversity and prosperity are an integral part of human existence. The belief that life can or should only be composed of happy or positive situations is a factor of philosophical ignorance and a lack of reflection on history. A wise person realizes that life is full of adverse as well as prosperous situation. While trying to promote the prosperous situations there must be expectation of adversity as well. This wisdom leads to the understanding that the world and worldly situations cannot be relied upon as a source of happiness. There will always arise some situation which will bring any form of worldly prosperity to an end. Therefore, a wise person does not become attached to worldly objects, people or situations even while being involved with them in various situations during the normal course of a lifetime.

General society believes that actions are to be performed for the goal of attaining some objective which will yield a reward. The socialization process teaches the individual to seek to perform actions because this is the way to attain something which will cause happiness. This is the predicament of the masses of people who have not studied Yoga or Mystical Philosophies such as Buddhism, Shetaut Neter or Vedanta. The following line from the Declaration of Independence illustrates this point succinctly.

> We hold these truths to be self-evident, that all men are created equal, that they are endowed by their Creator with certain unalienable Rights, that among these are Life, Liberty and the **pursuit of Happiness**.

Yoga philosophy is not against the pursuit of happiness in the world of time and space, however, it does teach that the pursuit of happiness with a sense of attachment and dependence on objects and situations in the world of human experience will inevitably lead to disappointment and frustration and will not fulfill the deeper need of the soul. If at all they should be pursued with an attitude of detachment and dispassion. In reality, happiness does not and cannot come from objects that can be acquired or from activities that are performed. It can only come from within. Even actions that seem to be pleasurable in life cannot be considered as a source of happiness from a philosophical point of view because all activities are relative. This means that one activity is pleasurable for one person and painful for another. This leads to the realization that it is not the activity itself that holds the happiness but the individual doer who is performing the action and assigning a value to it which she or he has learned from society to assign. Therefore, if it was learned that going out to a party is supposed to be fun then that activity will be pursued as a source of happiness. Here action is performed in pursuit of the fruit of the action in the form happiness; a result is desired from the action. However, there are several negative psychological factors which arise that will not allow true happiness to manifest. The first is that the relentless pursuit of the action renders the mind restless and agitated. The second is that if the activity is not possible there will be depression in the mind. If the activity is thwarted by some outside force, meaning that something or someone prevented you from achieving the object or activity you saw as the "source of happiness" you develop anger toward it. If by chance you succeed in achieving the object or activity you become elated and this will cause greed in the mind, you will want more and more of it. When you are not able to get more at any particular time you will become depressed and disappointed. Therefore, under these conditions a constant dependence on outside activities and worldly objects develops in the mind which will not allow for peace and contentment. Even though it is illogical to pursue activities which cause pain in life people are constantly acting against their own interests as they engage in actions in an effort to gain happiness while in reality they are enhancing the probability of encountering pain later on. People often act and shortly regret what they have done. Sometimes people know even at the time of their actions that they are wrong and yet they are unable to stop themselves. This is because when the mind is controlled by desires and expectations the intellect, the light of reason, is *clouded* and *dull*. However, when the mind is controlled by the intellect, then it is not possible to be led astray due to the *fantasies* and *illusions* of the mind. When the individual is guided by their intellect, then only right actions can be performed no matter what negative ideas arise in the mind. Such a person can not be deluded into negative actions and when negative actions (actions which lead to future pain and disappointments) are not performed then unhappiness cannot exist. Thus, a person who lives according to the teachings of non-doership (without desire or expectations for the future results of their actions) lives a life of perpetual peace and happiness in the present.

Thus, true peace and inner fulfillment will never come through pursuit of actions when there is an expectation or desire for the fruits of those actions. The belief in objects or worldly activities as a source of happiness if therefore seen as a state known as *ignorance* wherein the individual is caught up in the *illusions*, *fantasies* and *fanciful notions* of the mind. However, happiness and peace can arise spontaneously when there is an attitude of detachment and dispassion toward objects and situations in life. If actions are performed with the idea of discovering peace within, based on the understanding of the philosophy outlined above, and for the sake of the betterment of society, then these actions will have the effect of purifying the heart of the individual. The desires and expectations will dwindle while the inner fulfillment and awareness of the present moment will increase. There will be greater and greater discovery of peace within; a discovery of what is truly stable and changeless within as opposed to the mind and outer world which are constantly changing and unpredictable. Along with this there is greater effectiveness and perfection in one's actions.

Actions of any type will always lead to some result. However, this result is not as predictable as people have come to believe. In reality, the only thing a human being can control is the action itself and not the fruits of the action. If there is concentration on the action without desire or expectation of the fruits of the action, then there can be peace and contentment even while the action is being performed. This is the way of the non-doer. Actions performed with expectations and desire are the way of the doer. The non-doer is free from the fruits because he/she is free from desires and expectations while the doer is dependent on the actions and is bound to the results be they positive or negative. When desires and expectation in the mind are resolved the mind becomes calm and peaceful. Under these conditions the non-doer is free from elation or depression because his/her pleasure is coming from the present action in the present moment and is not based on memories of the past of pleasurable situations which are impelling a movement to repeat those activities or on expectations for the future activities which will somehow bring happiness. The non-doer, not being bound to the memories or to the expectations is not bound by either the past nor the future and thereby discovers an eternal present. The doer is always caught up in the past or the present and thereby loses the opportunity to discover peace and true happiness. This is the condition of most people in the world. Before they realize it their entire life has gone by without their being aware of the passage of time. This is the art of true spiritual life. It leads one to detach from the world even while continuing to live in it and thereby to discover the hidden inner spiritual dimensions of the unconscious mind and what lies beyond. The doer is always bound to a form of experience which is determined by and bound to the world of time and space because only in time and space can there manifest the memories of the past and the expectations for the future. The non-doer eventually discovers a transcendental experience of expanding consciousness in the present moment.

The philosophy of meditation may seem foreign to you at first but if you reflect upon it you will discover that it holds great truth as well as great potential to assist you in discovering abiding peace and harmony in your life. When you begin to practice and discover how wonderful it is to be in control of your mind instead of being prey to the positive or negative emotions and desires you will discover an incomparable feeling which goes beyond the ordinary concept of happiness. As with other human endeavors, in order to gain success you need to study the philosophy intensively with great concentration and then practice it in your day to day life. Treat it as an experiment. The world and your life will not go away. Just ask yourself: What would happen if I was to become less attached and more in control of my mind? Follow the teachings and discover the inner resources you need to discover true happiness and to overcome the obstacles of life.

The practice of meditation requires regular and sustained practice. Failure is assured if there is no effort. Likewise, success is assured if there is sustained, regular effort. This is the key to accomplishing any goal in life and, enlightenment, is a goal like any other, albeit the highest goal. With respect to attaining the goal of enlightenment, all other goals are like dust blowing in the wind. The following instruction will serve as guidelines for meditation and is not intended to be a substitute for a competent instructor. There are many techniques of meditation. Here we will focus on basic techniques of "moving" meditations for initially calming the mind of the beginning practitioner.

Tips for Formal Meditation Practice

Begin by meditating for 5 minutes each day, gradually building up the time. The key is consistency in time and place. Nature inspires us to establish a set routine to perform our activities; the sun rises in the east and sets in the west every day, the moon's cycle is every 28 days and the seasons change approximately at the same times of the year, every year. It is better to practice for 5 minutes each day than 20 minutes one day and 0 minutes the next. Do a formal sit down meditation whenever the feeling comes to you but try to do it at least once a day, preferably between 4-6 am or 6-8 pm. Do not eat for at least 2 hours before meditation. It is even more preferable to not eat 12 hours before. For example: eat nothing (except only water or tea) after 6 p.m. until after meditation at 6 a.m. the following morning. Do not meditate within 24 hours of having sexual intercourse. Meditate alone in a quiet area, in a dimly lit room (candle light is adequate). Do light exercise (example: Chi Kung or Hatha Yoga) before meditating, then say Hekau (affirmations, prayers, mantras, etc.) for a few minutes to set up positive vibrations in the mind. Burning your favorite incense is a good way to set the mood. Keep a ritualistic procedure about the meditation time. Do things in a slow, deliberate manner, concentrating on every motion and every thought you perform.

When ready, try to focus the mind on one object, symbol or idea such as the heart or Hetep (Supreme Peace). If the mind strays, bring it back gently. Patience, self-love and self-forgiveness are the keys here. Gradually, the mind will not drift toward thoughts or objects of the world. It will move toward subtler levels of consciousness until it reaches the source of the thoughts and there commune with that source, Neter Neteru. This is the desired positive movement of the practice of meditation because it is from Neter Neteru that all inspiration, creativity and altruistic feelings of love come. Neter Neteru is the source of peace and love and is who you really are.

Rituals to Facilitate Your Meditation Practice

In the beginning the mind may be difficult to control. What is needed here is perseverance and the application of the techniques described here. Another important aid to meditation is ritualism. You should observe a set of rituals whenever you intend to practice meditation. These will gradually help to settle the mind even before you actually sit to practice the meditation. They are especially useful if you are a busy person or if you have many thoughts or worries on the mind. First take a bath. Water is the greatest cleanser of impurities. In ancient times the practitioners of yoga would bathe before entering the temples and engaging in the mystery rituals. This practice has been kept alive in the Christian practice of baptism and the prayers using the Holy Water. In the *Gospel of Peace,* water is used as an external as well as internal cleanser of the body. In modern times many Native American spiritual leaders and others use water as a means to transport negative vibrations in the body in the form of a restless mind, or other negative thoughts directed toward others or oneself out and away from the body. This may be accomplished by simply visualizing the negative feelings moving into the water as you bathe and then going down the drain and into the earth as the water is washed away. This is a very powerful means of purification because the mind controls the energies in the body. Therefore, if the mind is controlled, you will be able to control the energies of your body, your emotions, attitudes, etc. All of these must obey the command of your mind. Thus, through practice of this exercise you will gradually gain control of moods and other mental complexes. Eventually you will be able to control your mind and direct it to be calm according to your will.

Once you have bathed, put on clothing which you have specifically reserved for the practice of meditation. This will have a strong effect on your mind and will bring meditative vibrations to you because the clothing will retain some of the subtle essence of the meditation experience each time you use them. The clothing should be loose and comfortable. We recommend 100% Cotton or Silk because it is a natural material which will allow the skin to breath. Keep the clothing clean and use the same style of clothing for your meditation practice.

When you are ready, go to your special room or corner which you have set aside for meditation. Take the phone off the hook or turn off the ringer and close the door behind you, leaving instructions not to be disturbed for the period of time you have chosen. When you sit for meditation, light a candle and some incense of your choice and then choose a comfortable position maintaining the back straight either sitting on the floor in the cross-legged posture (Lotus), or sitting in a chair with feet on the floor or lying on your back on the floor in the corpse-mummy pose (without falling asleep).

Next invoke the assistance of the deity or cosmic force which removes obstacles to your success in spiritual practice. Anubis is the deity which leads souls through the narrow pathways of the Duat. Therefore, request the assistance of Anubis, who represents the discriminative intellectual ability so that you may *"distinguish the real from the unreal."*

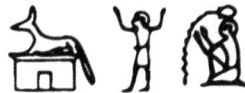

"O Apuat (Anubis), opener of the ways, the roads of the North, O Anpu, opener of the ways, the roads of the South. The messenger between heaven and hell displaying alternately a face black as night, and golden as the day. He is equally watchful by day as by night."

"May Anubis make my thighs firm so that I may stand upon them."

*"I have washed myself in the water wherein the god
Anpu washed when he performed the office of embalmer and bandager.
My lips are the lips of Anpu."*

Next invoke the presence of Isis-Maat who is the embodiment of wisdom and inner discovery of the Divine. Isis (Aset) is the mother of the universe and she herself veils her true form, as the Supreme Transcendental Self. This "veil" of ignorance is only due to ignorance. Therefore, pray for Isis to make her presence, which bestows instant revelation of her true form. This "unveiling" is a metaphor symbolizing the intuitional revelation of the Divine or Enlightenment in your mind. Isis is in your heart and only needs to be revealed. However, she can only reveal herself to the true aspirant, one who is devoted to her (the Self) and her alone. Isis says: *"I Isis, am all that has been, all that is, or shall be; and no mortal man hath ever unveiled me."* The invocatory prayer to Isis is:

"Oh benevolent Aset, who protected her brother Asar, who searched for him without wearying, who traversed the land in mourning and never rested until she had found him.

161

She who afforded him shadow with her wings and gave him air with her feathers, who rejoiced and carried her brother home.

She who revived what was faint for the weary one, who received his seed and conceived an heir, and who nourished him in solitude while no one knew where he was. . . . "

"I am the hawk (Heru) in the tabernacle, and I pierce through the veil."

Then remember your Spiritual Preceptor, the person who taught you how to meditate, thank them for their teaching and invoke their grace for success in your meditation. *"Have faith in your master's ability to lead you along the path of truth."*

"The lips of the wise are as the doors of a cabinet; no sooner are they opened, but treasures are poured out before you. Like unto trees of gold arranged in beds of silver, are wise sentences uttered in due season."

Next, utter some invocatory prayers such as the Hymns of Amun to propitiate the benevolent presence of the Supreme Being. Visualize that with each utterance you are being enfolded in Divine Grace and Enlightenment.

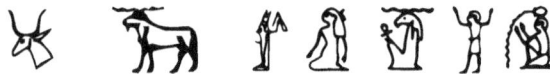

O Åmen, O Åmen, who art in heaven, turn thy face upon the dead body of the child, and make your child sound and strong in the Underworld.

O Åmen, O Åmen, O God, O God, O Åmen, I adore thy name, grant thou to me that I may understand thee; Grant thou that I may have peace in the Duat, and that I may possess all my members therein...

Hail, Åmen, let me make supplication unto thee, for I know thy name, and thy transformations are in my mouth, and thy skin is before my eyes. Come, I pray thee, and place thou thine heir and thine image, myself, in the everlasting underworld... let my whole body become like that of a neter, let me escape from the evil chamber and let me not be imprisoned therein; for I worship thy name...

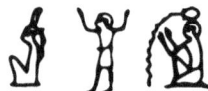

I am pure. I am pure. I am Pure.
I have washed my front parts with the waters of libations, I have cleansed my hinder parts with drugs which make wholly clean, and my inward parts have been washed in the liquor of Maat.

Now resolve within yourself that you will stay for the prescribed period of time which you have determined and then proceed with the practice as described below. Remember the following precepts: *"Have devotion of purpose"*, *"Have faith in your own ability to accept the truth"*, *"Have faith in your ability to act with wisdom."*

Simple Meditation Technique

Modern scientific research has proven that one of the most effective things anyone can do to promote mental and physical health is to sit quietly for 20 minutes twice each day. This is more effective than a change in diet, vitamins, food supplements, medicines, etc. It is not necessary to possess any special skill or training. All that is required is that one achieves a relaxed state of mind, unburdened by the duties of the day. You may sit from a few minutes up to an hour in the morning and in the late afternoon.

This simple practice, if followed each day, will promote above average physical health and spiritual evolution. One's mental and emotional health will be maintained in a healthy state as well. The most important thing to remember during this meditation time is to just relax and not try to stop the mind from pursuing a particular idea but also not trying to actively make the mind pursue a particular thought or idea. If a Hekau or Mantra (Prayer) is recited, or if a special hieroglyph is meditated upon, the mind should not be forced to hold it. Rather, one should direct the mind and when one realizes that one has been carried away with a particular thought, bring the mind gently back to the original object of meditation, in this way, it will eventually settle where it feels most comfortable and at peace.

Sometimes one will know that one has been carried away into thoughts about what one needs to do, or who needs to be called, or is something burning in the kitchen?, etc. These thoughts are worldly thoughts. Simply bring the mind back to the original object of meditation or the hekau. With more practice, the awareness of the hekau or object of meditation (candle, mandala, etc.) will dissipate as you go deeper. This is the positive, meditative movement that is desired. The goal is to relax to such a degree that the mind drifts to deeper and deeper levels of consciousness, finally reaching the source of consciousness, the source of all thought; then the mind transcends even this level of consciousness and there, communes with the Absolute Reality, Neter. This is the state of "Cosmic Consciousness", the state of enlightenment. After a while, the mental process will remain at the Soul level all the time. This is the Enlightened Sage Level.

WORDS OF POWER IN MEDITATION: Khu-Hekau, Mantra Repetition:

The word *"mantra"* in Indian Yoga signifies any sound which steadies the mind. Its roots are: "man" which means "mind" and "tra" which means "steady." In Ancient Egyptian terminology, "hekau" or word formulas are recited with meaning and feeling to achieve the desired end.

Hekau-mantra recitation, (called *Japa* in India), is especially useful in changing the mental state. The sounds coupled with ideas or meditations based on a profound understanding of the meaning can have the effect of calming the mind by directing its energy toward sublime thoughts rather than toward degrading, pain filled ones. This allows the vibrations of the mind to be changed. There are three types of recitations that can be used with the words of power: 1- Mental, 2- Recitation employing a soft humming sound and 3- loud or audible reciting. The main purpose of reciting the words of power is somewhat different than prayer. Prayer involves you as a subject, "talking" to God, while words of power - hekau - mantras, are used to carry your consciousness to divine levels by changing the vibrations in your mind and allowing it to transcend the awareness of the senses, body and ordinary thought processes.

The recitation of words of power has been explored to such a degree that it constitutes an important form of yoga practice. Two of the most comprehensive books written on this subject by Sri Swami Sivananda were *Japa Yoga* and *Sadhana.* Swami Sivananda told his pupils to repeat their mantras as many as 50,000 per day. If this level of practice is maintained, it is possible to achieve specific changes in a short time. Otherwise, changes in your level of mental awareness, self-control, mental peace and spiritual realization occur according to your level of practice. You should not rush nor suppress your spiritual development, rather allow it to gradually grow into a fire which engulfs the mind as your spiritual aspiration grows in a natural way.

Hekau-mantras can be directed toward worldly attainments or toward spiritual attainment in the form of enlightenment. There are words of power for gaining wealth or control over others. We will present Egyptian, Indian and Christian words of power which are directed to self-control and mental peace leading to spiritual realization of the Higher Self. You may choose from the list according to your level of understanding and practice. If you were initiated into a particular hekau or mantra by an authentic spiritual preceptor, we recommend that you use that one as your main meditative sound formula. You may use others for singing according to your inclination in your leisure or idle time. Also you may use shortened versions for chanting or singing when not engaged in formal practice. For example, if you choose "Om Amun Ra Ptah", you may also use "Om Amun."

Reciting words of power is like making a well. If a well is made deep enough, it yields water. If the words of power are used long enough and with consistency, they yield spiritual vibrations which reach deep into the unconscious mind to cut through the distracting thoughts and then reveal the deeper you. If they are not used with consistency, they are like shallow puddles which get filled easily by rain, not having had a chance to go deeply enough to reveal what lies within. Don't forget that your movement in yoga should be balanced and integrated. Therefore, continue your practice of the other major disciplines we have described along with your practice of reciting the hekau-mantras. Mental recitation is considered to be the most powerful. However, in the beginning you may need to start with recitation aloud until you are able to control the mind's wandering. If it wanders, simply return to the words of power (hekau-mantras). Eventually the words of power will develop their own staying power. You will even hear them when you are not consciously reciting. They will begin to replace the negative thought patterns of the mind and lead the mind toward serenity and from here to spiritual realization. When this occurs you should allow yourself to feel the sweetness of reciting the divine names.

As discussed earlier, HEKAU may be used to achieve control over the mind and to develop the latent forces that are within you. Hekau or mantras are mystic formulas which an aspirant uses in a process of self-alchemy. The chosen words of power may be in the form of a letter, word or a combination of words which hold a specific mystical meaning to lead the mind to deeper levels of concentration and to deeper levels of understanding of the teaching behind the words. You may choose one for yourself or you my use one that you were initiated into by a spiritual preceptor. Also, you may have a special hekau for meditation and you may still use other hekau, prayers, hymns or songs of praise according to your devotional feeling. Once you choose a hekau, the practice involves its repetition with meaning and feeling to the point of becoming one with it. You will experience that the words of power drop from your mind and there are no thoughts but just awareness. This is the soul level where you begin to transcend thoughts and body identification. You may begin practicing it out loud (verbally) and later practice in silence (mentally). At some point your level of concentration will deepen. You may use a rosary or "mala" (beads on a string) to keep track of your recitation. At that point your mind will disengage from all external exercises and take flight into the unknown, uncharted waters of the subconscious, the unconscious, and beyond. Simply remain as a detached witness and allow yourself to grow in peace. Listed below are several hekau taken from ancient Egyptian texts. They may be used in English or in ancient Kemetic according to your choice.

If you feel a certain affinity toward a particular energy expressed through a particular deity, use that inclination to your advantage by aligning yourself with that energy and then directing it toward the divine within your heart. Never forget that while you are working with a particular deity in the beginning stages, your objective is to delve into the deeper mystical implications of the symbolic form and characteristics of the deity. These always refer to the transcendental Self which is beyond all deities. According to your level of advancement you may construct your own Hekau according to your own feeling and understanding. As a rule, in meditations such as those being discussed now, the shorter the size of the hekau the more effective it will be since you will be able repeat it more often. However, the shorter the hekau, the more concentration it requires so as not to get lost in thoughts. You may wish to begin with a longer hekau and shorten it as your concentration builds. Words of power have no power in and of themselves. It is the user who gives them power through understanding and feeling.

When practicing the devout ritual identification form of meditation, the recitation of hymns, the wearing of costumes and elaborate amulets and other artifacts may be used. Ritual identification with the divine may be practiced by studying and repeatedly reading the various hymns to the divine such as those which have been provided in this volume, while gradually absorbing and becoming one with the teachings as they relate to you. When a creation hymn is being studied, you should reflect upon it as your true Self being the Creator, as your true Self being the hero(heroine), and that you (your true essence) are the one being spoken about in all the teachings. It is all about you. "You" are the Creator. "You" are the sustainer of the universe. "You" are the only one who can achieve transcendence through enlightenment according to your own will. When you feel, think and act this way, you are using the highest form of worship and meditation toward the divine by constantly bringing the mind back to the idea that all is the Self and that you essentially are that Self. This form of practice is higher than any ritual or any other kind of offering. Here you are concentrating on the idea that your limited personality is only an expression of the divine. You are laying down your ego on the offering mat.

In *Sadhana*, Swami Sivananda gives the following outline for the frequency of possible recitations. We have included two types of words of power: short, containing one or two syllables, medium length, containing two to three and average, containing six to eight. They are presented as guidelines for practice of hekau-mantra repetition practice.

	Number per minute			Number per hour		
	Low	Med	High	Low	Med	High
1. OM	140	250	400	8400	15000	24000
2. Hari Om	120	200	300	7200	12000	18000
3. Om Amun Ra Ptah	80	120	140	4800	7200	9000
4. Om Namo Narayanaya	60	80	120	3600	4800	7200

Generally, when the words of power are used over a sustained period of time, the benefits or *Siddhis* (psychic powers) arise. The most important psychic powers you can attain to facilitate your spiritual program are peace, serenity of mind, and concentration of the mental vibrations. Concentration opens the door to transcendental awareness and spiritual realization. Various estimates are given as to when you may expect to feel results; these vary from 500,000 repetitions to 1,200,000 or more. The number should not be your focus. Sustained practice, understanding the teachings about the Self and practicing of the virtues and self-control in an integral, balanced fashion are the most important factors determining your eventual success.

While *Om* is most commonly known as a *Sanskrit* mantra (word of power from India), it also appears in the ancient Egyptian texts and is closely related to the Kemetic *Amun* in sound and Amen of Christianity. More importantly, it has the same meaning as Amun and is therefore completely compatible with the energy pattern of the entire group. According to the Egyptian Leyden papyrus, the name of the "Hidden God", referring to Amun, may be pronounced as *Om,* or *Am*.

Om is a powerful sound; it represents the primordial sound of creation. Thus it appears in ancient Egypt as Om, in modern day India as Om, and in Christianity as Amen, being derived from Amun. Om may also be used for engendering mental calm prior to beginning recitation of a longer set of words of power or it may be used alone as described above. One Indian Tantric scripture (*Tattva Prakash*) states that Om or AUM can be used to achieve the mental state free of physical identification and can bring union with *Brahman* (the Absolute transcendental Supreme Being - God) if it is repeated 300,000 times. In this sense, mantras such as Om, Soham, Sivoham, Aham Brahmasmi are called *Moksha Mantras* or mantras which lead to union with the

Absolute Self. Their shortness promotes greater concentration and force toward the primordial level of consciousness.

There is one more important divine name which is common to both Indian as well as ancient Egyptian mystical philosophy. The sanskrit mantra **Hari* Om** is composed of Om preceded by the word Hari. In Hinduism, *Hari* means: "He who is Tawny." The definition of tawny is: "A light golden brown." This is a reference to the dark colored skin of Vishnu and Krishna. Vishnu is usually depicted with a deep blue and Krishna is depicted with a deep blue or black hue symbolizing infinity and transcendence. Hari is one of Krishna's or Vishnu's many divine names. It also means "hail" as in "hail to the great one" or it may be used as "The Great One." In the ancient Egyptian magical texts used to promote spiritual development (words of power or HEKA - mantras) the word Haari also appears as one of the divine names. Thus, the hekau-mantra Hari Om was also known and used in ancient Egypt and constitutes a most powerful formula for mystical spiritual practice. *(the spelling may be Hari or Hare)

Simply choose a hekau which you feel comfortable with and sit quietly to recite it continuously for a set amount of time. Allow it to gradually become part of your free time when you are not concentrating on anything specific or when you are being distracted by worldly thoughts. This will serve to counteract the worldly or subconscious vibrations that may emerge from the your own unconscious mind. When you feel anger or other negative qualities, recite the hekau and visualize its energy and the deity associated with it destroying the negativity within you.

For example, you may choose **Amun-Ra-Ptah.** When you repeat this hekau, you are automatically including the entire system of all gods and goddesses. Amun-Ra-Ptah is known as **Nebertcher,** the "All-encompassing Divinity." You may begin by uttering it aloud. When you become more advanced in controlling your mind, you may begin to use shorter words. For example simply utter: *Amun, Amun, Amun...* always striving to get to the source of the sound. Eventually you will utter these silently and this practice will carry your consciousness to the source of the sound itself where the very mental instruction to utter is given. Hekau-mantras are also related to the spiritual energy centers of the subtle spiritual body (Uraeus-Kundalini).

The following ancient Egyptian selections come from the ***"Book of Coming Forth by Day"*** and other ancient Egyptian scriptures:

Nuk pu NETER
I am the Supreme Divinity.

Nuk pu Ast
I am ISIS

nuk neter aa kheper tchesef
I am the great God, self created,

Ba ar pet sat ar ta.
Soul is of heaven, body belongs to the earth.

Nuk uab-k uab ka-k uab ba-k uab sekhem.
My mind has pure thoughts, so my soul and life forces are pure.

Nuk ast au neheh ertai-nef tetta.
Behold I am the heir of eternity, everlastingness has been given to me.

Sekhem - a em mu ma aua Set.
I have gained power in the water as I conquered Set (greed, lust, ignorance).

Rex - a em Ab - a sekhem - a em hati - a.
I know my heart, I have gained power over my heart.

Un - na uat neb am pet am ta.
The power is within me to open all doors in heaven and earth.

amma su en pa neter sauu - k su emment en
pa neter au tuanu ma qeti pa haru
Give thyself to GOD; keep thou thyself daily for God; and let tomorrow be as today.

Haari Om
The Divine Self, Om

Nebertcher
All encompassing existence (The Absolute)

Pa Neter
All encompassing existence (The Original One, Supreme Being)

Amun-Ra-Ptah
The Holy Trinity

Om Asar-Aset-Heru
The Holy Trinity

The following ancient Egyptian selections come from the ***"Pyramid Texts of Unas"*** (you may substitute your name where *Unas* appears):

Unas pa neb sabut
Unas is the lord (mistress) of wisdom
au aart - f em apt -f
His Uraei are on his brow

Unas pa aper-a er aab khu - f
Unas is provided with power over his spirits

au Unas kha em ur pu
Unas rises (to heaven) like a mighty one

Unas pu neb hetep
Unas is the lord of the offering

Unas pa am heka - sen
Unas has eaten the words of power of the gods

Unas aam khu - sen
Unas has eaten the spirits of the gods

Hesi - Chant, sing repeatedly, praises
Selected Smai Tawi - Kemetic Chants For Sema Institute Divine Singing and Worship

Smai Tawi (Egyptian Yoga) Daily Chants

1
Om Amun Ra Ptah
(The One Divine Self manifesting and the Trinity of Witnessing Consciousness, Mind and The Physical Universe)

2
Om Asar Aset Heru
The One Divine Self manifesting and the Trinity of the Divine Father, Mother and Child

3
Om Maati Maakheru
The One Divine Self manifesting as the dual goddesses of truth of above and below (Heaven and Earth) Assist me in attaining spiritual enlightenment.

4
Dua Ra Dua Ra Dua Ra Khepera
Adorations to Ra, Adorations to Ra in the form of the Creator

5
Dua   Ra   Cheft Uben F em aket abdet ent Pet
Adorations to Ra   when rises he in horizon eastern of   heaven
Anetej hra-k iti m Khepera, Khepera qemam   neteru
Homage to Ra, coming forth as Khepera ,   Khepera, Creator of the gods and goddesses
Cha – k uben –k pesd Mut – k Cha ti m   suten neteru
Rising thee, shinning   thee,   lighting up thy mother.   Rising as Lord, king of the gods and goddesses

6
Dua Asar Unefer Neteraah (Adorations to Asar- Pure Existence, Exalted Divinity)
Dua Asar Her Abdu (Adorations to Asar- Innermost essence of Abdu City of God)
Dua Asar Neb Djeta (Adorations to Asar- Lord of Forever)
Dua Asar Suten Heh! (Adorations to Asar- King of Eternity)

7
Net Net Dua Net Goddess Net, Goddess Net, Adorations to Goddess Net
Sefek Cheras Senhu – S Remove your vail so that I may see your true form (creation Unveiled- to see the Divine Self, i.e. spiritual enlightenment)

8
Dua Hetheru Neteritaah
Adorations to Hetheru the Great Goddess.

9

Maat Maat Ankhu Maat
Goddess Maat, Goddess Maat the source of life is Maat.

10
amma su en pa neter
sauu - k su emment enpa neter
au tuanu ma qeti pa haru
Give thyself to GOD;
keep thou thyself daily for God;
and let tomorrow be as today.

11
si neter iri mettu wadj
may God make the vascular system flourish
(An invocation of Health)

Hekau - Words of Power - Chanting Guide

The Hekau		Number of recitations per minute				Number or recitations per hour	
	Low	Med	High		Low	Med	High
Om	140	250	400		8400	15000	24000
Om Asar Aset Heru	80	120	140		4800	7200	9000
amma su en pa neter sauu - k su emment en pa neter au duanu ma qedi pa haru	6	8	10		360	480	600
Hymns of Amun					2	4	6
Chap. 125 of the Book of Coming Forth By Day					1	2	3

Prayers

Prayers are a special and potent way to charge your practice and the entire day with powerful spiritual vibrations. Prayers will be especially beneficial when the meaning is well understood. Pray with faith that you will be led to true understanding and peace.

This volume contains hekau-mantra-prayers that may be used for morning and evening prayer time as you begin and end your formal daily practices. You may consult the book *Egyptian Proverbs: TemTTchaas* for other prayers and invocatory proverbs which can be read as part of your prayer time. These serve the purpose of invoking the presence of the Divine Self to assist in directing you on your spiritual path. They bring auspiciousness to your life and uplift your mind for higher spiritual attainment.

All spiritually uplifting quotations from the ancient Egyptian texts are to be considered as words of power. Therefore, you may choose from a variety of texts according to your inner-personal feeling. Try to let your mind flow freely as it gravitates toward particular teachings and let it flow to new ones as it matures and increases in intuitional understanding. Also, as you read the teachings and study the explanations, try to allow your heart to melt into the glory and majesty of which they speak. During your time of practice, inwardly let your feelings flow toward the divine. This is very important. You must begin to understand that the teachings are talking about the Divine Self who is closer to you than anything on earth. Allow yourself to let your entire being flow in love and devotion toward the Divine. As you grow in knowledge and practice, you will discover the sweetness of divine love and cosmic union with the divine which is beyond all human experiences.

MEDITATION ON PEACE

In ancient Egyptian teachings, the word-symbol denoting supreme and transcendental peace is Hetep. What does it mean when yoga philosophy states that there is no true peace or happiness in the world of human experience?

Peace is a feeling of freedom and expansion. There are no worries when there is true peace. Also, true peace is not dependent on something that you need to do in order to have it. Usually people equate peace and happiness with things that must be done (vacation, movie, party) in order to achieve these feelings, but if you examine this mentality with the light of yoga wisdom, you will discover that this way of thinking is based on ignorance.

Supreme Peace, Hetep, is much like the peace which is experienced in the dreamless sleep state. In dreamless sleep there are no thoughts, just infinite awareness. However, because this form of experience occurs when you are asleep, your mind is veiled by ignorance and therefore, there is no transcendental awareness such as described above. The experience of Hetep transcends the most pleasurable dreams and events of the waking state. Advanced yogis can reach this level of consciousness through the practice of yoga. When they are able to abide in this state of awareness perpetually and spontaneously (without any effort), then they are considered to be fully enlightened. This state of supreme peace and transcendence of body consciousness and desires is called bliss and thus, God is known as "Bliss Absolute" and "Infinite Awareness" beyond thoughts and beyond duality. There is no more separation between you and me, the distant star, the blade of grass; there is Absolute oneness of identity with the Supreme within and Hetep.
Thus meditate:

Remain seated or lying in a comfortable, quiet place. Reflect on the meaning of *htp (HETEP-Supreme Peace)* to sublimate your physical nature, to transform the ego-personality into the instrument of your Ba (individual soul) and to melt your individual soul into the Universal Soul of GOD, the *NETER NETERU,* to become "ONE" with GOD.

If the mind strays, gently bring it back to this central idea. When it strays, remind it that any ideas it may have, any notions to the contrary, are illusions because you now know that ALL the objects of the world, including your body, are really manifestations of GOD. You are a part of them and they of you. Therefore, there is no need to crave or desire them. You are them and ALL that is because your deep inner Self, your true Self, is ONE with GOD. Allow yourself to be filled with *htp* from this awareness. Try to maintain this sense of peace at all times, not just at meditation time.

Gradually, the mind will be less and less agitated and distracted and you will experience increasing levels of peace leading to enlightenment.

Allow your ego to *htp*, to be sublimated and transformed. Submit your ego-will to the will of the Neters. *Do MAAT, Live MAAT, Speak MAAT, Be MAAT.*

MAAT is the way of the Neters; to be in harmony with the Neters is to achieve harmony, health and peace.

Practice these meditations or any others you feel work best for you and they will increase your awareness to such a degree that you will consciously realize that your Higher Self is and was always there awaiting discovery. You will leave your ignorant notions of yourself behind; you will be transformed into a oneness with GOD by leaving behind the misconceived notion (illusion) that you are a mortal personality.

Slowness Meditation Method

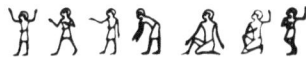

The Slowness Meditation Exercise is one of the easiest forms of practice to control the mind. As we discussed earlier, the ordinary human mind is in a constant state of motion. This motion originates from the desires which constantly compel the mind to think about ideas and how to acquire the objects it wants. These techniques are similar to the Chi Kung, Indian Yoga and Buddhist mindfulness visualizations which are designed to help you develop an awareness of the automatic consciousness so that you may gain control of your mindless tendencies. Since speed and constant movement are the main components of mindlessness or the automatic conscious state, the Slowness exercise is designed to gradually assist you in slowing yourself down at a physical, mental and finally the spiritual level. It makes use of three major components. These are 1-slowness, 2-silence, and 3- steadfastness.

Slowing the mind and body to allows concentration and meditation during any task at any time.

Silencing the body to hear the voice of NETER (GOD), the inner Self.

Steadfastness is keeping the idea ever present in the mind that you are a immortal and eternal being, made and given life by your Father-Mother CREATOR to experience the joy of living by remembering who you are, thereby becoming a God(ess) yourself.

"As You Believe So Shall You Become."

After a while, these ideas and practices will stay with you, even during your non-meditation time. You will become more conscious during work, play and other activities. Whenever possible, attempt a formal sit down meditation. The slowness exercise along with an integrated program of a vegetarian diet, reduced television or movie watching and reduced talking (eventually keeping silence for a minimum of 1 hour a day) will help calm down the restlessness which leads to the constant seeking of "fun" outside of one's self. Keeping the Highest Teaching or the Steadfast idea in one's mind at all times is also a form of meditation. You will gradually break down the illusion of what the world appears to be and gradually see it for what it is: your - Self.

Slowness- Stage One
Find a quiet room or area and with total silence proceed as follows:

The object is to train the mind to be one pointed and relaxed and to SLOW IT DOWN so as to be able to concentrate on one thing at a time.

The main activity on which one will concentrate is movement, but it MUST be slow... so slow as to be almost still.

While moving a particular limb or body part, concentrate on every movement. Every time you move a limb (i.e. arm, leg, etc.), THINK:

"Now I am moving my arm*."

*(you may move any body part, i.e. leg, arm, etc.)

Witness every movement and feel every time you take a step. Every time a limb moves concentrate on it. If something in the room catches your attention, look at it and think:

"Now I am looking at that."

You may walk in a circle, across the room, back and forth or stand in one spot and move a limb up and down. Use any movement you choose as long as it is quiet and "SLOW."

Practice this exercise for five minutes at a time gradually building up to as long a time as is comfortable. You may need to practice this stage for several days or weeks until you become aware of every movement with increasing serenity of mind. Practice daily, even if its just five minutes a day.

Slowness-Stage Two

After some time of practicing Stage One, you will feel a new consciousness above your regular "automatic" "every day" consciousness. You will begin to feel you are living more in the moment, being more conscious of what is going on every second. This process is sometimes referred to as "Mindfulness" or "The Witness." This is the Amun consciousness which is the underlying essence of your soul. You will become more aware of your every action.

Witness: You will gradually feel you are a spectator, watching yourself perform as if in a grand theatrical show or movie.

Now carry on the slow movements as in Stage One and adjust the mental attitude as follows:

The object in Stage One was to help your Ba (soul-spirit) catch up with the mind and to slow the mind down. Now we will attempt to get ahead of the mind by controlling and directing the action.

Instead of noticing you are moving, now you will direct the movements by:

1- Starting from motionless state.
2- Decide what movement, direction and limb to move.
3- Then **BEFORE** you allow any movement, say mentally: "Now I'm going to move my arm up", "Now I'm going to touch the light switch", "Now I'm going to lift my right leg to step forward", etc.

Slowness- Stage Three

Here, the emphasis will be on motion as before but unlike the previous stages, the motion will be "mental."

Sit in a chair or on the floor in any comfortable pose or lay flat on your back. Regardless of the position you choose, the most important thing is keeping the back straight so that all energy centers can flow freely.

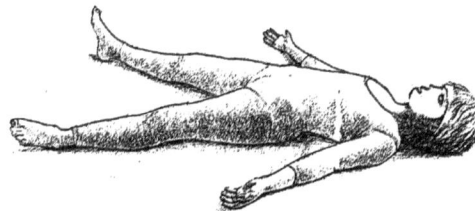

Remain completely motionless during this exercise. Now visualize yourself getting up, walking and moving as before, very slowly and deliberately. See the movement in your mind before it occurs and then send the command to your subtle body. See it moving about slowly according to your direction while you remain motionless in your meditative position. Do not allow any movement to escape your attention. Take notice of every single motion that is performed, no matter how slight.

Slowness-Stage Four

Remain motionless as in stage three. Visualize yourself traveling to far off lands, planets and universes. Imagine yourself communing with nature from the deepest recesses of the ocean to the farthest reaches of outer space - keeping motionless all throughout the exercise. Remain motionless for up to an hour and develop an awareness of yourself apart from the body. See yourself as being outside of the body and look on it as the "doer" of things in the world of time and space while "you" are the bystander who is watching the activities in the drama of the life of your body.

Meditate thus: "I am not that body, I am the spirit, immortal, eternal am I, the body dies but I live on for all eternity." "The body is not me!"

As you progress in this exercise, you will transcend the level of mental visualization. Your subtle astral body will actually leave your physical body and experience the disembodied state.

At this Astral level of existence wherein the body is transcended, there is only awareness of the mind and senses.

Slowness-Stage Five

Now remain absolutely motionless. Do not move your physical or astral body. You will begin to see that even the astral body is not the real you. You will begin to experience an awareness of being and existing devoid of your astral body. See your thoughts as they move across the firmament of your mind coming out of eternity and going back to eternity from whence they arose. Do not attempt to hold onto them. Simply observe them. This is absolute motionlessness. The real you is the motionless witness to all of the thoughts of the mind and the actions of the body. This absolute witnessing consciousness is known as Amun or Osiris and it is the support of all mental activity and all physical reality.

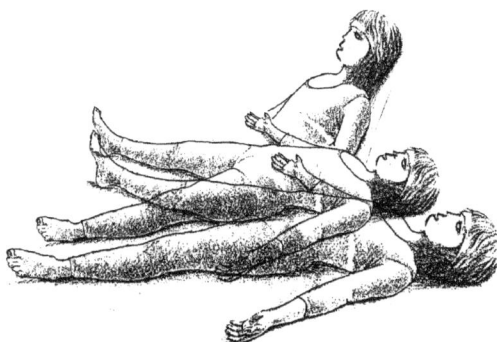

As you progress further, you will experience all pervasiveness, a oneness with all things. There will not be any place or thing wherein you are not. There will be an experience of pure consciousness. This pure consciousness is the soul and as you abide in your soul consciousness, your awareness expands until you discover that you are one with universal consciousness, God. This is the highest stage of experience wherein you strip yourself of all physical or mental actions. These actions are known as karma and when you do not identify with your pure, detached Self, you fall into identification with your thoughts and actions. This identification with your thoughts and actions which results from forgetfulness of your true Self is known as "ignorance." Therefore, true knowledge means detaching from the part of yourself that is involved in actions (thoughts, sense perceptions and physical movement) and discovering the silent, witnessing consciousness, and then consciously abiding in this knowledge regardless of the thoughts and actions you may find yourself performing in your daily life. This stage of spiritual practice is known as performing action while not performing action. This is Enlightenment. You are now steadfast or established in your essential nature, the Divine Self!

There are ancient Egyptian hieroglyphs which portray the different parts of the human being such as the soul, the shadow, the Ka, etc. separating from the body of the initiate. This is an advanced portrayal of the concept of mystical self-discovery. The process of actually experiencing the different aspects of your being and realizing that you are not just a physical body and finite, mortal personality, is what opens the door to your discovering the true Self within you. In this manner, "out of body" experiences and experiences which transcend consciousness of even the astral body, lead to the discovery of existence without your mind and senses. When this level of experience is reached, you have attained true and absolute knowledge. In contrast, knowledge which was gained through the study of the teachings and the various other practices was indirect and incomplete. This is the highest goal of meditation, to assist you to go deeper within your own being and to help you discover that part of yourself which you are not aware of.

> "I am steadfast, child of the steadfast One, conceived and born in the
> region of steadfastness. "
>
> From the Egyptian Book of Coming Forth By Day

May you discover the bliss of Silence, Slowness and Steadfastness!

*For more on the Slowness Meditation Technique see the book **"The Slowness Meditation"** and the video **"The Slowness Meditation Video"** by Dr. Muata Ashby.

THE INTEGRATED MEDITATION

As stated in the beginning of this section, there are four main components of meditation: posture, breath-life force control, sound and visualization. The previous meditation exercises have touched upon these areas but here we will use them all in an integrated fashion to achieve maximum concentration.

Before you begin, practice some light physical exercises (yoga, tai chi, etc.) for several minutes. This will serve to free up any energy blockages and wake up the mind by stimulating the circulation of the vital forces within the body.

Now choose a comfortable posture. If you consistently practice meditation, you will gradually be able to stay in one position for longer periods of time. If you practice regularly, you will discover that your body will develop a daily rhythm which will be conducive to your meditation time.

Next practice alternate nostril breathing so as to balance the positive and negative charges within the body and open up the central channel of vital energy as we discussed in the last section. Choose a particular visualization exercise or hekau. This will serve the purpose of helping to occupy the attention of the mind and prevent it from straying. It will also help you to develop sensitivity and control over the vital energy so that eventually you will be able to direct it according to your will.

A meditation on the energy centers will be used here (Kundalini Uraeus Serpent Power Tape) or you may use the format presented in the audio tape (Morning Worship and Meditation). Inhale and visualize the energy flowing up from the first energy center, through the second, and then through the third, fourth, fifth and sixth up to the seventh, the highest energy center and then as you exhale, visualize the energy flowing back through the centers from the highest to the first center at the base of the spine.* As you visualize the energy flowing from center to center, you are controlling the Life Force energy and the direction of the mind at the same time. Now we will add sound to the meditation. You may choose a hekau of your choice, one you feel especially drawn to and one that you understand the deeper meaning of, to some degree, or the one suggested by your spiritual preceptor. Repeat it with meaning and feeling as you breath, visualize and remain steady in your pose. You can link your breath and hekau repetition by reciting the first part of your hekau upon inhalation as the energy is moving up and the second part upon exhalation as the energy is moving back down. *(For more specific instructions listen to the audio tapes.)

In the beginning it may seem as though not much is happening, but within a short time, you will begin to notice changes within yourself. Your level of relaxation will improve immediately and your awareness of yourself will increase gradually. Eventually, you will begin to perceive various new sensations and psychic expansion. You will hear your heart beat. A feeling of peacefulness will develop. When you succeed in transcending your body consciousness you will be going beyond the exercises. You will not feel your arms or legs. This is an initial stage of transcendence. Your inner vision will open and you will perceive reality beyond the mind and body. At this point, do not worry about the components of the meditation. Simply relax and remain a witness to all you perceive. Do not try to run away from or to anything you notice.

Gradually allow yourself to go deeper and deeper until you become one with the source of all thoughts. This is the real you. Continue practicing this "communion" exercise with the divine until you are fully established in this level of being at all times. This is the state of Enlightenment.

Recommended Reading:

*Book- *The Glorious Light Meditation* by Dr. Muata Ashby
*Book– *Meditation The Ancient Egyptian Path to Enlightenment* by Dr. Muata Ashby

*Egyptian Yoga Meditation Video - **Experience the health of concentration and deep relaxation.**

*available through Cruzian Mystic Books

Ancient Egyptian Proverbs of The Meditation Path

"When an idea exclusively occupies the mind, it is transformed into an actual physical state."

"Reason of Divinity may not be known except by a concentration of the senses like onto it."

"Stand in a place uncovered to the sky, facing west to the sinking sun, and make your solemn worship, and the same way as he rises to the east in the morning. Now, make thy body still."

"IF THOU WILT ATTENTIVELY DWELL (MEDITATE) AND OBSERVE WITH THY HEART'S EYES, THOU'LT FIND THE PATH THAT LEADS ABOVE; NAY, THAT IMAGE SHALL BECOME THY GUIDE ITSELF, BECAUSE THE DIVINE SIGHT HATH THIS PECULIAR CHARM, IT HOLDETH FAST AND DRAWETH UNTO IT THOSE WHO SUCCEED IN OPENING THEIR EYES, JUST AS, THEY SAY, THE MAGNET THE IRON."

**Basic Instructions for the Glorious Light Meditation System-
Given in the Tomb of Seti I.
(c. 1350 B.C.E.)**

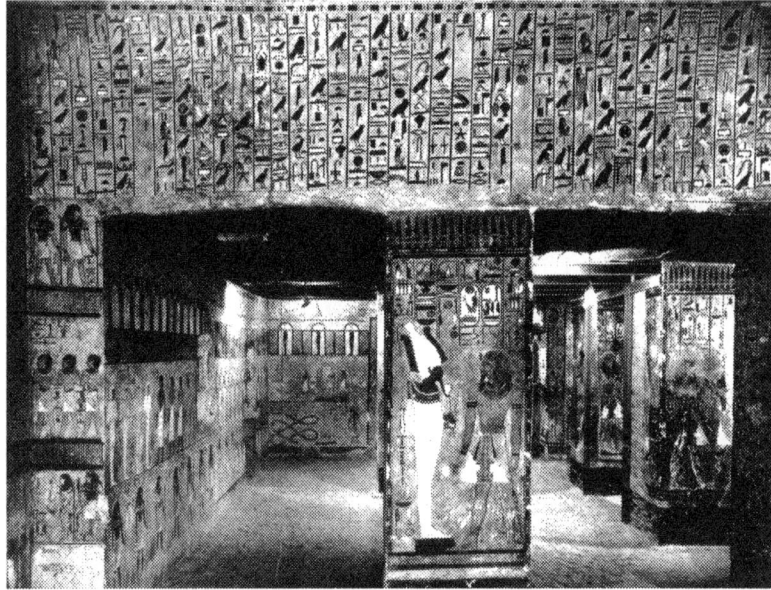

INSTRUCTIONS:

1) **To Be Practiced by Clergy and Lay Alike**
2) **Listen to the Mystical Teaching** in the Myth of Hetheru and Djehuti
3) **Be purified physically by proper hygiene**-with Nile Flood Water (leanest); wear proper clothing.
4) **Be purified by Maat** (righteousness, truth, Non-violence, non-stealing, non-killing, etc.)
5) **Sevenfold Cleansing for three days**- Serpent Power – transcend the three forms of mental expression
6) **Posture and Focus of Attention** - Make the body still, concentrating on yourself
7) **Words of power-chant**
   Nuk Hekau (I am the word itself)
   Nuk Ra Akhu (I am Ra's Glorious Shinning Spirit – Divine Light)
   Nuk Ba Ra (I am the soul of Ra)
   Nuk Hekau (I am the God who creates through sound)
8) **Visualization**- see yourself in the center of the Sundisk (circle of Ra), see yourself as Ra (Mystic Union)

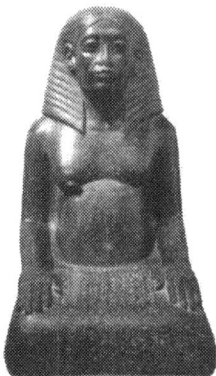

Sage Amenhotep: Kemetic Meditation Posture-Sitting With Hands on Thighs

It is well known and commonly accepted that meditation has been practiced in India from ancient times. Here we will concentrate on the evidence supporting the existence of the philosophy of meditation in Ancient Egypt.

The Paths of Meditation Practiced in Ancient Egypt	Basic Instructions for the Glorious Light Meditation System- Given in the Tomb of Seti I.

System of Meditation: **Glorious Light System**
Location where it was practiced in ancient times: **Temple of Seti I, City of Waset (Thebes)** [25]
 	
System of Meditation: **Wisdom System**
Location where it was practiced in ancient times: **Temple of Aset – Philae Island, Aswan**
 	
System of Meditation: **Serpent Power System**
Location where it was practiced in ancient times: **IN ALL TEMPLES- GENERAL DISCIPLINE**
 	
System of Meditation: **Devotional Meditation**
Location where it was practiced in ancient times: **IN ALL TEMPLES- GENERAL DISCIPLINE**
	Formal meditation in Yoga consists of four basic elements: Posture, Sound (chant-words of power), Visualization, Rhythmic Breathing (calm, steady breath). The instructions, translated from the original hieroglyphic text contain the basic elements for formal meditation.
	
	(1)-Posture and Focus of Attention
	   iuf iri-f ahau maq b-phr nty hau iu
	body do make stand, within the Sundisk (circle of Ra)
	
	This means that the aspirant should remain established as if in the center of a circle with a dot in the middle.
	
	(2)- Words of power-chant[26]
	
	(3)- Visualization
	   Iuf mi Ra heru mestu-f n-shry chet
	"My body is like Ra's on the day of his birth
	
	(Unite – become one with Ra

---

[25] For More details see the book *The Glorious Light Meditation System of Ancient Egypt* by Dr. Muata Ashby.
[26] The term "Words of Power" relates to chants and or recitations given for meditation practice. They were used in a similar way to the Hindu "Mantras."

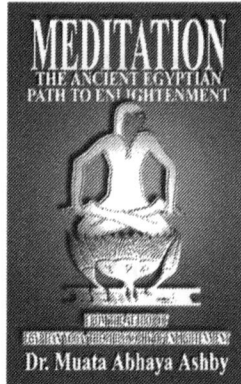

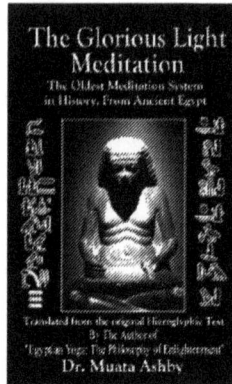

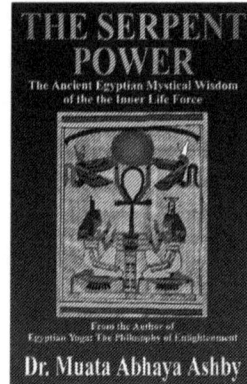

For more teachings on the path of Meditation Yoga see the books *Meditation The Ancient Egyptian Path to Enlightenment,* and *The Glorious Light Meditation* and *The Serpent Power* and by Dr. Muata Ashby

CHAPTER IIIIIII

Introduction to The Yoga of Devotion

GENERAL DISCIPLINE
In all Temples

Scripture: Prt M Hru and Temple Inscriptions.

Steps in the practice of Devotion Yoga:

1- **MYTH:** Listening to the myths and divine glories of the various forms of the divinity (god or goddess) (in this case Asar)

2- **RITUAL**: Effacement of the ego through cultivation of love for the Divine (in this case Asar)
- Hekau (words of Power) Chanting
- Praises, Hymns, Songs to the Divine

3- **MYSTICISM**: Mystical union with the Divine – "I Am Asar"

God is termed **Merri**, "Beloved One"

Love and Be Loved
"That person is beloved by the Lord." PMH, Ch 4

Offering Oneself to God-Surrender to God- Become One with God

Yoga of Devotion to the Divine

Yoga of Devotion is the process of directing the mental energies (passion and love) to the Divine. It is a process whereby one uses one of the strongest emotions, love, to overpower mental afflictions and negative thoughts leading to union with the divine object of contemplation, one's Higher Self. In much the same manner that one rises above his/her problems and ailments when he/she falls "in love" with another person, so too when one directs feelings of love to the Higher Self, one is able to transcend problems and adversities in life. In addition, since human love is only a glimpse of cosmic love, imagine how much more powerful devotion to God can be in transcending the human condition. Devotion to God, also known as "Divine Love" is an effective way to produce mental health because it easily turns the mind

185

towards the transcendental rather than towards the petty concerns of the ego. To practice Yoga of Devotion, throughout your day, feel that you are serving God when you are serving others, since all people are essentially the Self. In this way your mind does not become distracted by their personalities. When snowflakes fall, you do not become so distracted with their individual shapes that you fail to identify them as snow. Likewise, as intuitional vision of your all encompassing nature dawns in your heart, you will be able to look beyond all the different sizes, shapes, sexes and colors of people and recognize your Higher Self as the basis for their existence.

> 43. Thou art Temu, who didst create beings endowed with reason; thou makest the color of the skin of one race to be different from that of another, but, however many may be the varieties of mankind, it is thou that makest them all to live.
>
> Ancient Egyptian Hymn of Amun

> "Souls, Horus, son, are of the self-same nature, since they came from the same place where the Creator modeled them; nor male nor female are they. Sex is a thing of bodies not of Souls."
>
> —Ancient Egyptian Proverb from
> *The teachings of Isis to Horus*

When the mind is continuously directed toward the majesty and glory of God, the Neter (its Higher Self), the mind becomes imbued with that same glory and majesty. Thus devotion opens the way to the practice of the other disciplines of yoga (Yoga of Action, Yoga of Wisdom, Meditation) and these in turn lead to the experience of deeper devotion.

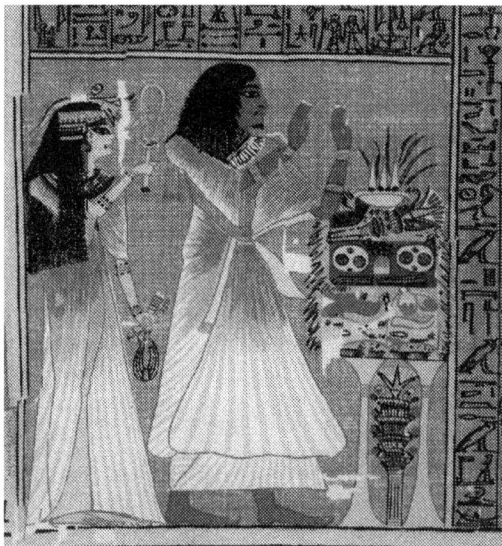

Ushet (devotion) Scene from the Papyrus of Ani- Ani in the Dua Pose- Upraised arms with palms facing out towards the Divine Image. His wife plays the sistrum to the Divinity (Asar).

Ancient Egyptian Proverbs of The Devotion Path

"If you seek GOD, you seek for the Beautiful. One is the Path that leads unto GOD - Devotion joined with Wisdom."

"O behold with thine eye God's plans. Devote thyself to adore God's name. It is God who giveth Souls to millions of forms, and God magnifyeth whosoever magnifieth God."

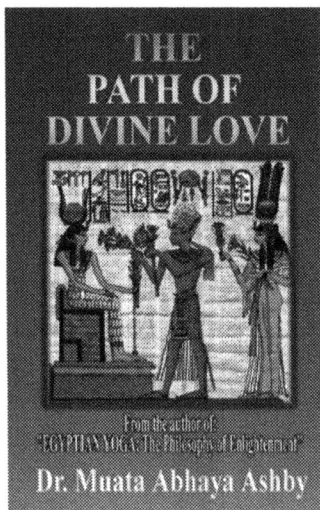

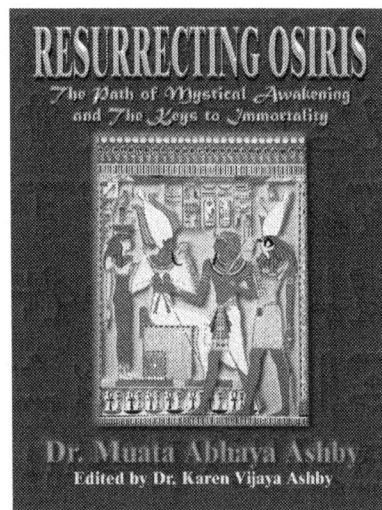

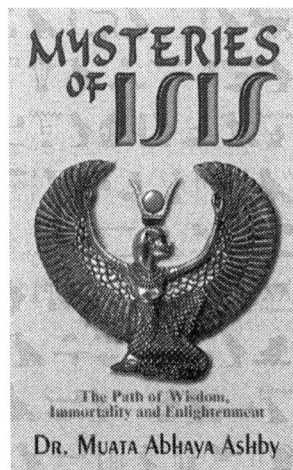

For more teachings on the path of Devotion Yoga see the book *The Path of Devotion* and *Resurrecting Osiris* and *Mysteries of Isis* by Dr. Muata Ashby

CHAPTER ||||||||

Introduction to The Yoga of Tantra

Tantric influence, however, is not limited to India alone, and there is evidence that the precepts of tantrism traveled to various parts of the world, especially Nepal, Tibet, China, Japan and parts of South-East Asia; its influence has also been evident in Mediterranean cultures such as those of Egypt and Crete.

-Ajit Mookerjee (Indian Scholar-Author)

Tantra Yoga is purported to be the oldest system of Yoga. Tantra Yoga is a system of Yoga which seeks to promote the re-union between the individual and the Absolute Reality, *"NETER"* (GOD), through the worship of nature. Since nature is an expression of GOD, it gives clues as to the underlying reality that sustains it and the way to achieve wisdom. The most obvious and important teaching that nature holds is the idea that creation is made up of pairs of opposites: Up-down, here-there, you-me, us-them, hot-cold, male-female, Ying-Yang, etc. The interaction, of these two complementary opposites, we call life and movement.

Insight (wisdom) into the true nature of reality gives us a clue as to the way to realize the oneness of creation within ourselves. By re-uniting the male and female principles in our own bodies and minds, we may reach the oneness that underlies our apparent manifestation as a man or woman. The union of the male and female principles may be effected by two individuals who worship GOD through GOD's manifestation in each other or by an individual who seeks union with GOD through uniting with his or her male or female spiritual half. All men and women have both female and male principles within themselves.

In the Egyptian philosophical system, all Neters or God principles emanate from the one GOD. When these principles are created, they are depicted as having a ***male and female*** principle. All objects and life forms appear in creation as either male or female, but underlying this apparent duality, there is a unity which is rooted in the pure consciousness of oneness, the consciousness of GOD, which underlies and supports all things. To realize this oneness consciously deep inside is the supreme goal.

In Tantrism, sexual symbolism is used frequently because these are the most powerful images denoting the opposites of Creation and the urge to unify and become whole, for sexuality is the urge for unity and self-discovery albeit limited to physical intercourse by most people. If this force is understood, harnessed and sublimated it will lead to unity of the highest order, that is unity with the Divine Self.

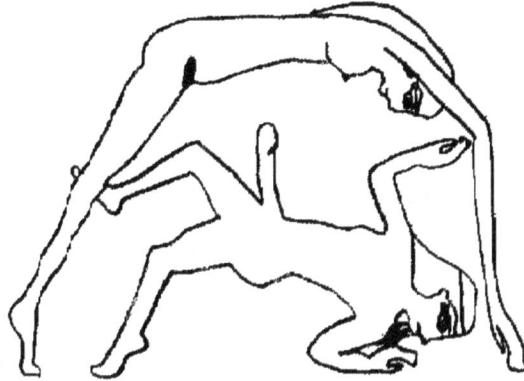

Figure 1: Above- the Kemetic God Geb and the Kemetic Goddess Nut separate after the sexual union that gave birth to the gods and goddesses and Creation. Below: three depictions of the god Asar in tantric union with Aset.

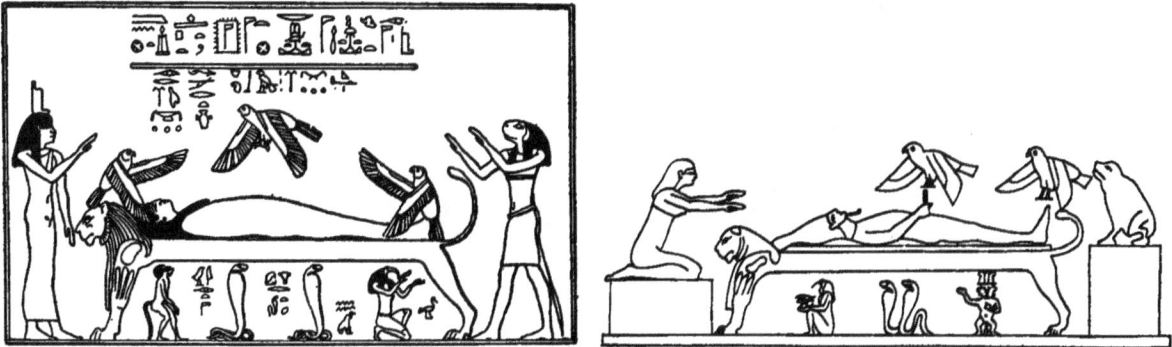

Figure 2: Above-The virgin birth of Horus (The resurrection of Osiris - higher, Heru consciousness). Isis in the winged form hovers over the reconstructed penis of dead Osiris. Note: Osiris uses right hand.

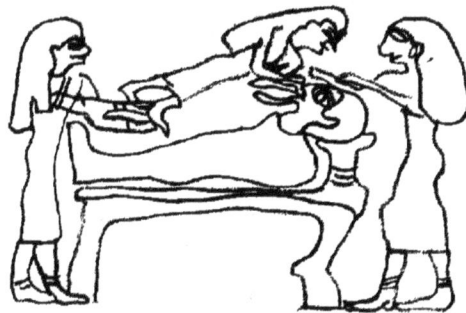

From: *Sexual Life in Ancient Egypt* by Lise Manniche

Figure 3: Drawing found in an Ancient Egyptian Building of The Conception of Heru

Isis (representing the physical body-creation) and the dead body of Osiris (representing the spirit, that essence which vivifies matter) are shown in symbolic immaculate union (compare to the "Kali Position" on the following page) begetting Horus, symbolizing to the immaculate conception which takes place at the birth of the spiritual life in every human: the birth of the soul (Ba) in a human is the birth of Horus.

-From a Stele at the British Museum 1372. 13th Dyn.

189

Tantric Iconography from Ancient Egypt

At right: **Sekhm**
She is the union
vulture, lioness,
human female
with wings,
two plumes (Isis
and Nephthys ar
phallus.

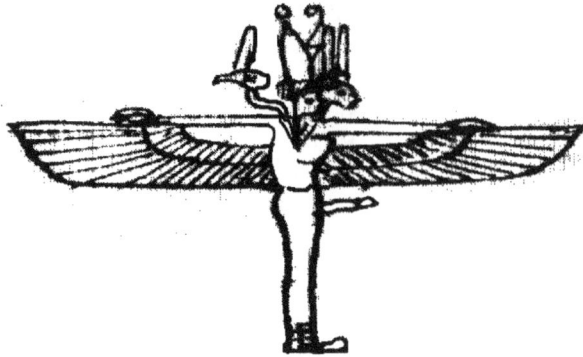

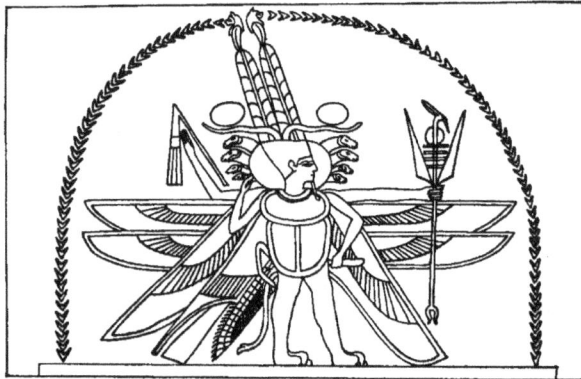

The All
Encompass
ing
Divinity.

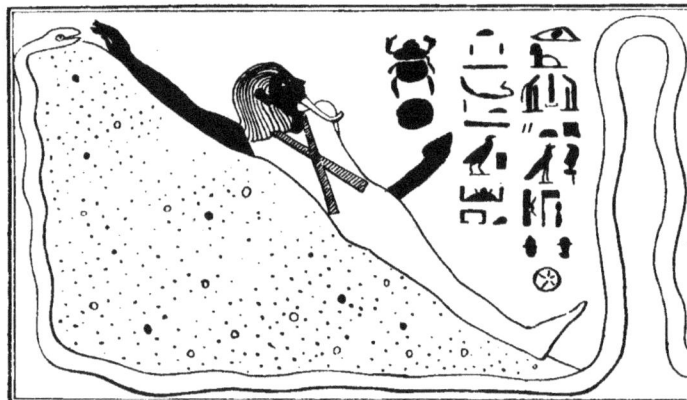

Above: Osiris as the creator who engenders Life Force energy into
creation through the Mehen Serpent (Power) of the Primeval Waters.

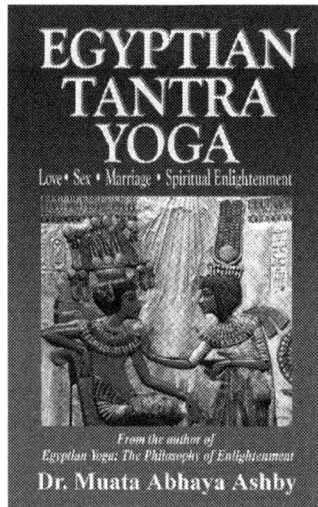

For more teachings on the path of Tantra Yoga see the book *Egyptian Tanta Yoga* by Dr. Muata Ashby

CHAPTER ∩ (10)
Introduction to The Yoga of Serpent Power

"Develop the life giving fire; few know how to use it and fewer how to master it."

"Master the fire of the back."

Ancient Egyptian Proverbs

There are five major types of Yoga under which all other forms may be classified. These are, Yoga of Wisdom, Yoga of Action, Yoga of Devotion, Yoga of Meditation, and Yoga of Sublimation of the Sexual energy and Internal Life Force. All of these yogas should be practiced in an integral fashion for optimum results in the personal spiritual discipline of the aspirant even though one may be emphasized over the others.

This Chapter will introduce the concept of the Life Force energy and its relation to human consciousness and the process of psycho-spiritual evolution. In all of the different Yogas there is a common thread which binds and unites them all. This thread is human consciousness. Human consciousness evolves over a period of many lifetimes through the process of reincarnation and transmigration of the soul, gradually rising to the higher levels of consciousness until it finally reaches awareness of the highest wisdom of its true Self.

It is important to understand that as a spiritual aspirant your goal is to raise your level of spiritual consciousness. To this end you are to use a blend of the different yogas. Each form of yoga serves to create a process by which you can raise the Life Force energy which you are trying to develop. If you are practicing Yoga of Wisdom, your consciousness will be raised through your study and understanding of the teachings. If you are practicing Yoga of Action, by your performance of actions in a selfless manner which will lead you to attain mental peace. This mental peace will allow the energy of your soul to flow in an unobstructed manner, thereby you moving towards its destined goal: the higher Self. If you are practicing Yoga of Devotion, your consciousness will be raised through directing your mind towards the Divine by attuning your emotions and feelings toward expressing love for and surrender to the Divine Self. If you are practicing Yoga of Meditation, your consciousness will be raised by calming the waves which disturb the ocean of your consciousness. When this occurs you will experience the transcendental nature of your deeper Self. If you are practicing Yoga of Sublimation of the Sexual Energy and Internal Life Force you will use the energies of the body by controlling and harnessing them. Once controlled, these constitute a formidable force to destroy the ignorance and other human faults which obstruct the soul from full expression in an individual. This last form of yoga underlies all the other forms. When the other forms are properly practiced, the internal Life Force is automatically balanced and raised. Therefore, regardless of which form of yoga you choose to concentrate on you need to have a full understanding of the Life Force energy and the process of its evolution.

Summary of Kemetic Serpent Power Yoga

Phase 1: Cleansing the Physical, and Astral Bodies
    Kemetic Yoga Postures
    Vegetarianism
    Maat-Righteous living
    Cleansing gross mental impurities through philosophy (Wisdom Teachings)

Phase 2: <u>Cultivation of the Serpent Power-Cleansing the Causal Body-</u>
    Mystical Serpent Power Psychology
    Cultivation of the Energy Centers of Psycho-spiritual Consciousness

Phase 3: <u>Special Meditations on the Highest Spheres of Psycho-spiritual Consciousness</u>
    Meditations on raising the Life Force energies to the higher Energy Centers of Psycho-spiritual Consciousness so that it may carry awareness and individual consciousness to meet and join with Cosmic Consciousness.

Note: If this form of spiritual discipline (Serpent Power Yoga) is not practiced in the format outlined above under the direction of an authentic spiritual preceptor, there may be imbalances that may lead to physical and/or mental damage to the practitioner. Phase 1 works with energy centers 1-3. Phase 2 works with centers 4-5 and phase 3 works with centers 6-7 and beyond.

The Ancient History of The Serpent Power

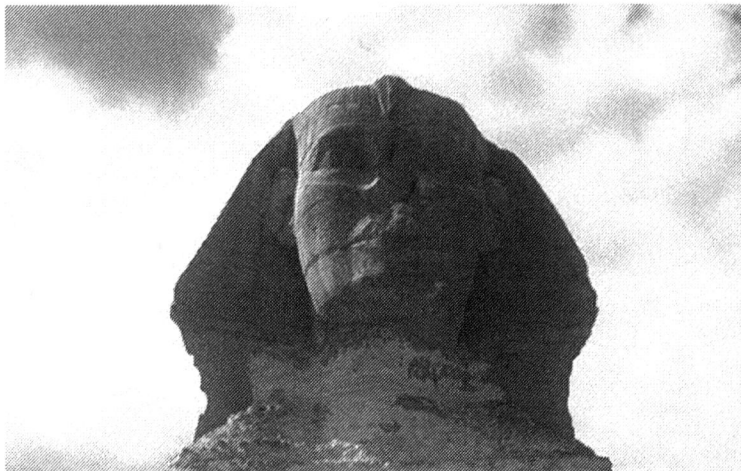

The Serpent Power Philosophy in Ancient Egypt

The Great Sphinx of Ancient Egypt. The oldest monument in the world, now dated at 10,000 B.C.E.

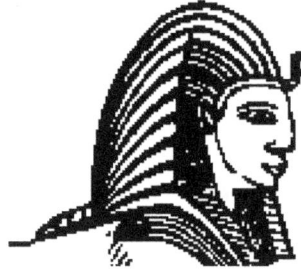

The Pharaonic headdress establishes a Serpent Power tradition in Egypt of at least 10,000 years.

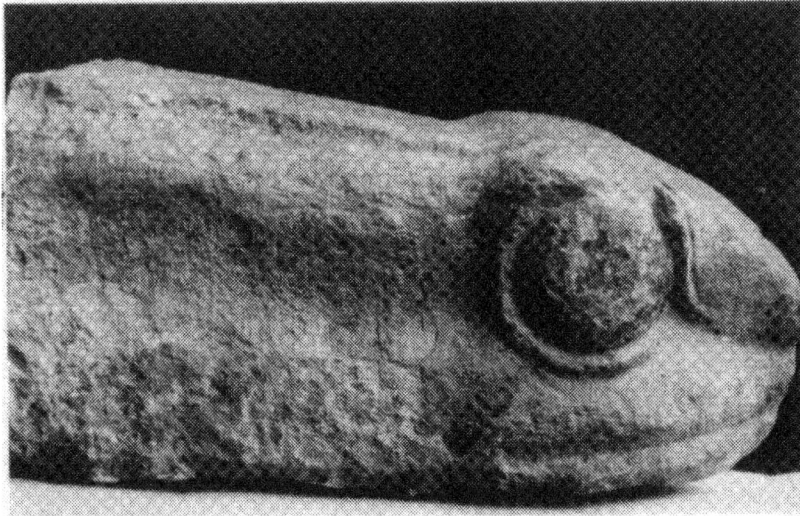

THE SPHINX SERPENT, ORIGINALLY ON THE FOREHEAD OF THE GREAT SPHINX, NOW AT THE BRITISH MUSEUM.

The ancient history of the Serpent Power begins with Ancient Egypt. The evidence for this come from the Ancient Egyptian Sphinx which has now been dated to 10,000 B.C.E. or older. Next the iconography of Indus Valley reliefs depict the practice of the serpent power technology. Next it appears in China and the rest of the world.

The Bible contains some vague references to *"seven demons"* that were *"cast out of"* Mary Magdalene, *"Jacobs Ladder," the seven seals* that are to be opened, and the *"Tree of Life."*

The Ancient Egyptian *Greenfield Papyrus* and the Egyptian *Book of Coming Forth By Day* of Kenna, which are both treatises of the Osirian Resurrection religion of Ancient Egypt, contain important teachings in reference to what is today known as Kundalini Yoga in India. We explored both of these in the book *Egyptian Yoga: The Philosophy of Enlightenment* and here we will discuss some more advanced theory related to the Serpent Power and the first level of Serpent Power Yoga meditation. There is an audio tape meditation series which follows along with this section. If you are interested in the audio workshop and meditation music contact the publisher or book distributor.

The subject of life force energy and the sublimation of sexual energy into spiritual energy existed many thousands of years in Egypt prior to its development in modern India under the name *Kundalini Yoga*. It later appears in many parts of the world but it did not find extensive documentation until the Sages of India composed the voluminous scriptures in relation to Kundalini Yoga.

As in the Indian Chakra System, the Egyptian Seven Powers are related to the seven energy centers of the subtle body. They are not visible to the ordinary eye. They are located in the same space as the physical spinal column though not in the same plane as the physical body. They are linked to the awakening of one's spiritual powers and consciousness. As one progresses on the spiritual path of evolution, while either purposely employing a yogic spiritual discipline (study and application of spiritual and philosophic scriptures, reflection and meditation) or learning through the process of trial and error, these centers will automatically open, allowing one to experience increasing communion with the Higher Self: GOD. The process of raising one's spiritual power may be aided by specific exercises such as concentration, proper breathing, meditation on the meanings of the spiritual symbols and surrendering to the will of the Higher Self (GOD). These techniques allow one to transform one's waking personality so that one may discover their innermost Self: GOD. This should be done under the guidance of a qualified teacher (spiritual master, guru, etc.).

The energy centers of the subtle body are likened to a tree which the aspirant climbs through personality integration, which leads him/her to intuitional realization of the transcendental self. In the process of creation, the creative energy manifests in the form of six planes of consciousness. This is the realm of phenomenal reality including physical, astral and mental existence. Most people function on the level of the first three energy-consciousness levels. The goal of this Yoga (Serpent Power) is to unite the six phenomenal consciousness centers with the seventh or transcendental realm of consciousness, the Absolute. This Absolute is what various religions refer to by different names such as the Kingdom of Heaven, Osiris, Krishna, Brahman, the Tao, God, Higher Self, Goddess, Christ, Buddha, etc.

Kundalini energy, known as Prana, chi, and Ra-Sekhem, flows throughout thousands of *Nadis* or energy channels. If any of the energy channels are blocked or over-sensitized, a dis-balance can arise, causing illness in the mind and physical body. There are three most important channels through which the Serpent Power flows. In India these are known as: *Sushumna, Ida and Pingala* -These are represented by the Egyptian Caduceus of Djehuti which is composed of a staff which has two serpents wrapped around it. During the ceremonies connected to the mysteries of the Uraeus serpent Goddess *Uatchet* (Udjat), the priest addresses the initiate:

The original Kamitan text relating the movement of the Serpent Power:

> *Uadjit comes to you in the form of the Serpent Goddess to anoint you on your head. She is the mistress of fire. She is also the double goddess Uadjit and Nekhebit. The rise up to your head through the left side and through the west right side also and shine there on the top of your head. Not with words (in silence, stillness) they rise to the top of your head encompassing all time, as they do for their father Ra. They speak to you from within and illumine those becoming venerable Blessed Spirits. It is they who give souls perfection, as they work their way, up to the brow, to their dwelling place on the brow, which is their throne. They firmly establish themselves on your brow as they do on Ra's brow. Not leaving, taking away the enlightenment, they stay there for you forever.*

The passage above provides an exact idea about the true nature of Isis and Nephthys. Nephthys is associated with the life which comes forth from her death in Isis. They are complementary goddess principles which operate to manifest life-death-life or the cycle of birth-death-rebirth known as reincarnation. Another important teaching presented here is that Isis and Nephthys are identified as the "the two exceedingly great uraei." They are the two forces of the Serpent Power. The Serpent Power refers to the Life Force energy which manifests in the physical human body in the form of two opposites. In Ancient Egyptian mythology and yoga these two opposites are known as "Uadjit (Uatchit, Udjat, Uatchet) and Nekhebet" or "Isis and Nephthys" or "The Two Ladies." Uadjit is the solar serpent while Nekhebet symbolizes the lunar serpent. In India they are known as "Ida and Pingala." The opposites refer to the solar pole and the lunar pole or the active and passive nature of the energies. In reality the energy is the same. It originates from the same source but it manifests as opposite due to the polarization it assumes. Thus, it may be seen as male and female. The Serpent Power energy resides at the base of the spine and when aroused through spiritual evolution (practice of yoga) it courses through the energy centers of the subtle body, finally reaching the crown of the head and re-unites into its original oneness; the poles dissolve, leaving oneness of consciousness or enlightenment.

The preceding scripture from the Ancient Egyptian embalming ceremonies is echoed in the *Book of Coming Forth By Day*. The state of enlightenment is further described in Chapters 83 and 85 where the initiate realizes that the seven Uraeus deities or bodies (immortal parts of the spirit) have been reconstituted:

"The seven Uraeuses are my body... my image is now eternal."

These seven Uraeuses, *Iarut,* are also described as the *"seven souls of Ra"* and *"the seven arms of the balance (Maat)"* (referring to the Energy Centers). Thus, we are to understand that the seven primordial powers (Uraeuses) are our true essence. Further, the same seven are GOD. Thus, GOD'S soul and our souls are identical. It is this same soul which will judge us in the balance. Therefore, we came into existence of our own free will, and we are the supreme masters (judges) of our own destiny. We may put together our divine form by attaining a purified heart or live in ignorance, ruled by passion and mortality. In Chapter 30, the initiate affirms that his / her vertebrae, back, and neck bones are firm.

Note: Arat originates as a power of the Sun God, Ra. She is often described as being the embodiment of Ra himself. As such she is the fire spitting serpent who "scorches evil." Thus, she represents the light of reason and the dynamic force of nature. In Hindu mysticism *Arati* means "light."

In the *Book of the Dead* (Chap. xvii. 30), the initiate identifies with Amsu-Min and says:

> *"I am the god Amsu (or, Min) in his coming forth; may his two plumes be set upon my head for me."* In answer to the question, *"Who then is this?"* the text goes on to say, *"Amsu is Horus, **the avenger of his father**, and his coming, forth is his birth. The plumes upon his head are Isis and Nephthys when they go forth to set themselves there, even as his protectors, and they provide that which his head lacketh, or (as others say), they are **the two exceedingly great uraei** which are upon the head of their father Tem, or (as others say), his two eyes are the two plumes which are upon his head."*

In the *Book of Coming Forth by Day*, Goddess Uatchet (Uadjit) is the destroyer of the evil forces which try to defeat the initiate. In the Osirian resurrection story she assists Isis when she is fleeing from Set. Arat was also known as "Apuat" or "Opener of Lands." The Serpents Uatchet and Nekhebet are equal to the *Ida and Pingala* respectively of Indian Kundalini Yoga. The central staff of Djehuti (caduceus) represents the Sushumna, the central astral channel. Ida is associated with lunar energy and it is cooling, coalescing, passive. Uatchet (Pingala) is associated with solar energy and it is dynamic and heating. They are both related to the left (lunar) and right (solar) nostrils. If you take notice of your breathing habits you will see that you are usually breathing out of either the left or the right nostril and rarely out of them both at the same time. This is because at particular times one form of Life Force energy may be dominant. The interaction of these two forces (solar and lunar) cause movements in the Life Force energy that is available to each living being and support their practical existence in the physical realm. This interaction is what causes the appearance of matter in the various forms of nature. However, all forms are in reality one essential essence. This is the secret of the Serpent Power. If the opposing forces were to be harmonized there would be no separation or differences between the objects of nature. In other worlds the underlying unity would emerge. This is the task of Serpent Power Yoga, to discover the underlying unity behind the multiplicity of Creation.

Thought is also intimately related to the movements in the Life Force energy, therefore, in an unenlightened personality, if there is much movement (agitation) in the mind, there will be much mental distraction and unrest. This will in turn agitate the Life Force Energy and obstruct its flow, resulting in inability to see the subtle realities beyond physical existence and also this process will engender both mental and physical tension, anxiety and disease. The object of Serpent Power Yoga is to harmonize the two opposites. When this is accomplished, there is free flow of the Serpent Power Life Force energy which may then be directed towards the *brow* and *the crown of the head* where the serpents rise up and there anoint the practitioner bestowing enlightenment, contentment, peace and bliss. This process is known as, Christhood (Christ means *anointed one*) in Christianity and the anointing of *Amrita,* the mystic nectar, in Indian Kundalini Yoga and by other names in other systems.

The two opposing forces in the Serpent Power Life Force energy of a human being are balanced by practicing the various disciplines of yoga in an integral fashion. Increasing wisdom, reflection, practice of virtues, purification of the diet, exercise and specific serpent power breathing exercises all serve to balance and harmonize the Life Force energy, enabling it to dissolve the opposites and then they rise through the central subtle channel up the spine and into the head where they eventually become established, providing a continuous shower of bliss to the practitioner.

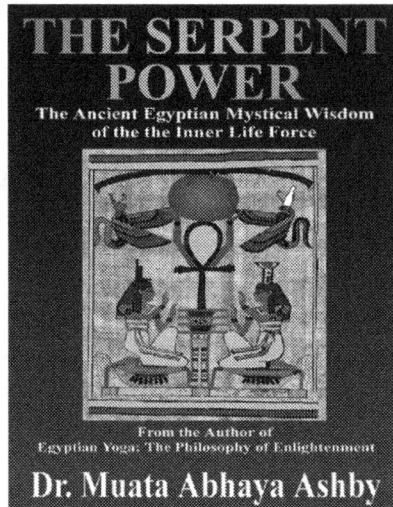

For more teachings on the path of Serpent Power Yoga see the book *The Serpent Power* by Dr. Muata Ashby

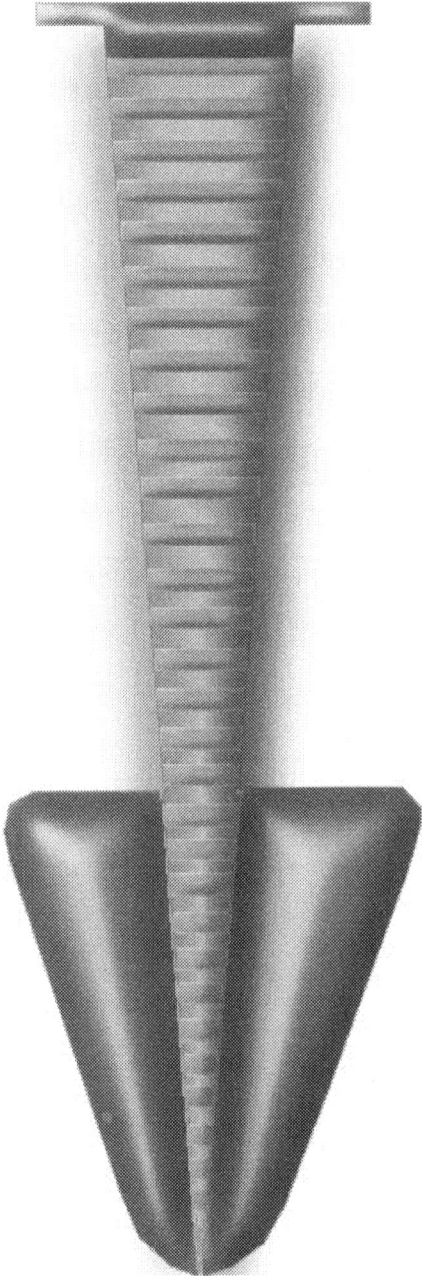

CHAPTER ∩I
Introduction to The Path Of Mystical Religion

Religion and Yoga Paths to the Same Destination

BELOW: THE PATHS TO SPIRITUAL EVOLUTION

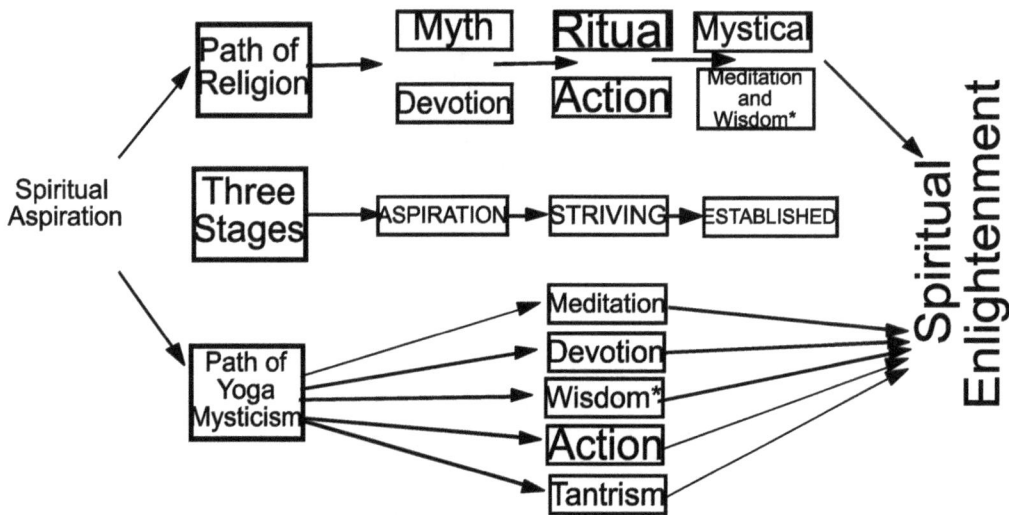

The Religious Path To spiritual realization

"When therefore, though hearest the myths of the Egyptians concerning the Gods - wanderings and dismemberings and many such passions, think none of these things spoken as they really are in state and action. For they do not call Hermes "Dog" as a proper name, but they associate the watching and waking from sleep of the animal who by Knowing and not Knowing determines friend from foe with the most Logos[49] like of the Gods."

–Plutarch (c. 46-120 AD)

Do not make the mistake to believe that the path of religion and its attendant myths are just for the ignorant masses. They also contain a higher mystical message for those who understand how to read myths and understand their higher spiritual importance and the application of their teaching in the world.

As stated earlier, religion has three stages, Myth. Ritual and Mystical. Myth is a form of language that conveys the basic tenets of the spiritual teaching and also it is a conveyor of the culture that is related to the people who practice the religion. Therefore, in order to understand

Kemitic religion, it is necessary to understand the language of Kemitic culture. The language of Kemitic religion is the story of the neteru. The word "neteru" is commonly translated as "gods and goddesses," however, word actually means "cosmic forces" or "cosmic nature of things." Understanding the neteru gives us insight into understanding ourselves since these are in effect manifestations of our own deeper divine being. The language of the myth is the activities, relationships and stories related to the neteru. When we study these it becomes clear what the origin of Creation is and what the nature of human existence is as well. This supreme knowledge leads to Spiritual Enlightenment, the great goal of religion is therefore, also the same goal as the mystic practices of yoga. Thus, understanding the origins, nature, story and interrelationships of the neteru as well as then practicing the rituals related to the worship of the neteru leads us into a mystical awareness of life and that is called *Nehast*, or Spiritual Resurrection.

The provenance, actions, relationships and impetus of each neteru reveals the mystical high secret wisdom of the Kemitic Mysteries. Therefore, understanding these is one of the major tasks of a spiritual aspirant who chooses the religious path as their main avenue to spiritual realization.

Religion and Yoga

How are the disciplines of yoga and the mysteries related to religion? The word *religion* comes from the Latin "Relegare" which means "to link back." This implies, to link the individual human soul back to its original source, the Universal soul. AS just discussed, the word *Yoga* is an Indian term meaning to "Yoke" or "Join," implying, to join individual consciousness to universal consciousness. While it is true that yogic practices may be found in religion, strictly speaking, yoga is neither a religion or a philosophy. It should be thought of more as a way of life or discipline for promoting greater fullness and experience of life. It was developed at the dawn of history by those who wanted more out of life. Yoga is the practice of mental, physical and spiritual disciplines which lead to self-control and self-discovery by purifying the mind and body so as to discover the deeper spiritual essence which lies within every human being and object in the universe. In essence, the goal of yoga practice is to unite or *yoke* one's individual consciousness with universal or cosmic consciousness. Yoga is not an escape from life but a more profound way to understand life so as to succeed in life. Therefore, Ancient Egyptian religious practice, especially in terms of the rituals and other practices of the Ancient Egyptian temple system known as *Shetaut Neter* (the way of the hidden Supreme Being), may be termed as a yoga system: *Egyptian Yoga*. In this sense, religion, in its purest form, is a yoga system, as it seeks to reunite people with their true and original source.

Religion encompasses three levels, *myth, ritual* and *mystical philosophy*. Many students of Ancient Egyptian religion have focused on the religious stories of Ancient Egypt as mythical fables or superstitious rantings from a long lost civilization. In the *Egyptian Yoga Book Series* we successfully show how the teachings of mystical spirituality were carefully woven throughout Ancient Egyptian Mythology.

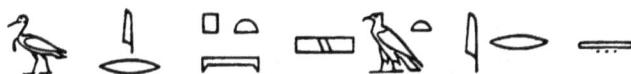

Ba ir pet Shat ir ta
"Soul is to heaven, body is to the earth"
From the Prt m Hru of the *Pyramid Texts* (3,200-2,575 B.C.E.)

Ancient Egyptian Religion centers around the understanding that every human being has an immortal soul and a mortal body. Further, it holds that creation and the human soul have the same origin. How can this momentous teaching be proven and its reality experienced? This is the task of Mystical Spirituality (religion in its three phases and / or the practice of Yoga disciplines).

The disciplines of Yoga fall under five major categories. These are: *Yoga of Wisdom, Yoga of Devotional Love, Yoga of Meditation, Tantric Yoga* and *Yoga of Selfless-Righteous Action.* Within these categories there are subsidiary forms which are part of the main disciplines.

So the practice of any discipline that leads to oneness with the Supreme Consciousness can be called Yoga. If you study, rationalize and reflect upon the teachings, you are practicing *Yoga of Wisdom.* If you meditate upon the teachings and your Higher Self, you are practicing *Yoga of Meditation.* If you practice rituals which identify you with your spiritual nature, you are practicing *Yoga of Ritual Identification* (which is part of the Yoga of Wisdom and the Yoga of Devotional Love of the Divine). If you develop your physical nature and psychic energy centers, you are practicing *Serpent Power* (*Kundalini or Uraeus*) *Yoga* (which is part of Tantric Yoga). If you practice living according to the teachings of ethical behavior and selflessness, you are practicing *Yoga of Action* (Maat) in daily life. If you practice turning your attention towards the Divine by developing love for the Divine, then it is called *Devotional Yoga* or *Yoga of Divine Love.* The practitioner of yoga is called a yogin (male practitioner) or yogini (female practitioner), and one who has attained the culmination of yoga (union with the Divine) is called a yogi. In this manner, yoga has been developed into many disciplines which may be used in an integral fashion to achieve the same goal: Enlightenment. Therefore, the aspirant should learn about all of the paths of yoga and choose those elements to concentrate on which best suit his/her personality and practice them all in an integral, balanced way.

Enlightenment is the term used to describe the highest level of spiritual awakening. It means attaining such a level of spiritual awareness that one discovers the underlying unity of the entire universe as well as the fact that the source of all creation is the same source from which the innermost Self within every human heart arises. It is a state of ecstasy and bliss which transcends all concepts and descriptions and which does not diminish and is not affected by the passage of time or physical conditions. It is in the state of Enlightenment that the absolute proof of the teachings of mystical spirituality are to be found and not in books, doctrines or dogmas. This is because intellectual knowledge is only the beginning of the road which leads to true knowledge. There are two forms of knowledge, intellectual (theoretical) and absolute (experiential). The teachings of Yoga and the advanced stages of religion can lead a person to experience the truth about the transcendental, immortal and eternal nature of the Soul and the existence of God. This is what differentiates Yoga from intellectual philosophies and debates, cults or religious dogma. In Yoga there is no exhortation to believe in anything other than what you can prove through your own experience. In order to do this, all that is necessary is to follow the disciplines which have been scientifically outlined since many thousands of years ago.

All forms of spiritual practice are directed toward the goal of assisting every individual to discover the true essence of the universe both externally, in physical creation, and internally, within the human heart, as the very root of human consciousness. Thus, many terms are used to describe the attainment of the goal of spiritual knowledge and the eradication of spiritual ignorance. Some of these terms are: *Enlightenment, Resurrection, Salvation, The Kingdom of Heaven, Moksha or Liberation, Buddha Consciousness, One With The Tao, Self-realization,*

Know Thyself, etc. Also, many names have been used to describe that transcendental essence: *God, Allah, Asar, Aset, Krishna, Buddha, The Higher Self, Supreme Being* and many others.

The Tree Stages of Religion

While on the surface it seems that there are many differences between the philosophies, upon closer reflection there is only one major division, that of belief or non-belief. Among the believers there are differences of opinion as to how to believe. This is the source of all the trouble between religions. This is because ordinary religion is deistic, based on traditions and customs which are themselves based on culture. Since culture varies from place to place and from one time in history to another, there will always be some variation in spiritual traditions. These differences will occur not only between cultures, but even within the same culture. An example of this is Christianity with its myriad of denominations.

Therefore, those who cling to the idea that religion has to be related to a particular culture and its specific practices or rituals will always have some difference with someone else's conception. In the three stages of religion, Myth, Ritual and Mysticism, culture belongs to the myth stage of religious practice, the most elementary level.

Myth → Ritual → Mysticism

An important theme, which will be developed throughout this volume, is the complete practice of religion, that is, in its three aspects, *mythology, ritual* and *metaphysical* or the *mystical experience* (mysticism - mystical philosophy). At the first level a human being learns the stories and traditions of the religion. At the second level rituals are learned and practiced. At the third level a spiritual aspirant is led to actually go beyond myths and rituals and to attain the ultimate goal of religion. This is an important principle, because many religions present different aspects of philosophy at different levels, and an uninformed onlooker may label it as primitive or idolatrous, etc., without understanding what is going on. For example, Hinduism and Ancient Egyptian Religion present polytheism and duality at the first two levels of religious practice. However, at the third level, mysticism, the practitioner is made to understand that all of the gods and goddesses being worshipped do not exist in fact, but are in reality aspects of the single, transcendental Supreme Self. This is evident in the Prt M Hru.

In the area of Yoga Philosophy and the category of Monism, there are little, if any, differences. This is because these disciplines belong to the third level of religion wherein mysticism reaches its height. The goal of all mysticism is to transcend the phenomenal world and all mental concepts. Ordinary religion is a part of the world and the mental concepts of people, and must too be ultimately transcended.

.THE RELATIONSHIP BETWEEN RELIGION AND YOGA

STEPS IN THE PRACTICE OF RELIGION

1 MYTHOLOGY	2 RITUAL	3 MYSTICISM
⬇	⬇	⬇
Learning the story of the god or goddess	*Ceremonies related to the myth*	*Meditation*
Devotion to the Deity: learning how to care for and love the Divine.	Right Living in accordance with the principles set forth by the deity in the myth.	Esoteric Wisdom about life and the spirit. Spiritual transcendence (Enlightenment)

TEXTS TO STUDY THE PATH OF RELIGION

A spiritual aspirant who feels a tendency towards approaching spiritual studies with a religious focus should concentrate on the following texts.

The Ausarian Religion and the Ausarian Trinity:
>   BOOK: *Resurrecting Asar*
>   BOOK*: Mysticism of Ushet Rekhat: Worship of the Divine Mother*

The Teachings of Anunian Theology and the Anunian Trinity:
>   BOOK*: Anunian Theology*

The Teachings of Memphite Theology:
>   BOOK*: Memphite Theology*

The Teachings of Theban Theology and the Universal Trinity
>   BOOK*: EGYPTIAN YOGA VOL. 2: The Supreme Wisdom of Enlightenment-The Mystical Wisdom of Ancient Egyptian Theban Theology*

The books above are not exclusive of each other. They each relate to one another in order to show that while you may concentrate on a particular path, you may also integrate elements of others. Also, all of the Ancient Egyptian theological systems are related. They are a coherent expression of wisdom related to the Divine as it expresses in Creation. Thus, all the volumes introduce elements from the other paths and facilitate the practice of universal religion and yoga spirituality. It is important to understand that the religious path, when practiced in its three stages, leads to the same spiritual enlightenment which is possible through Yoga Mysticism. However, if religion and yoga are practiced at the lower levels only they will not yield spiritual enlightenment but dogmas and intellectualism.

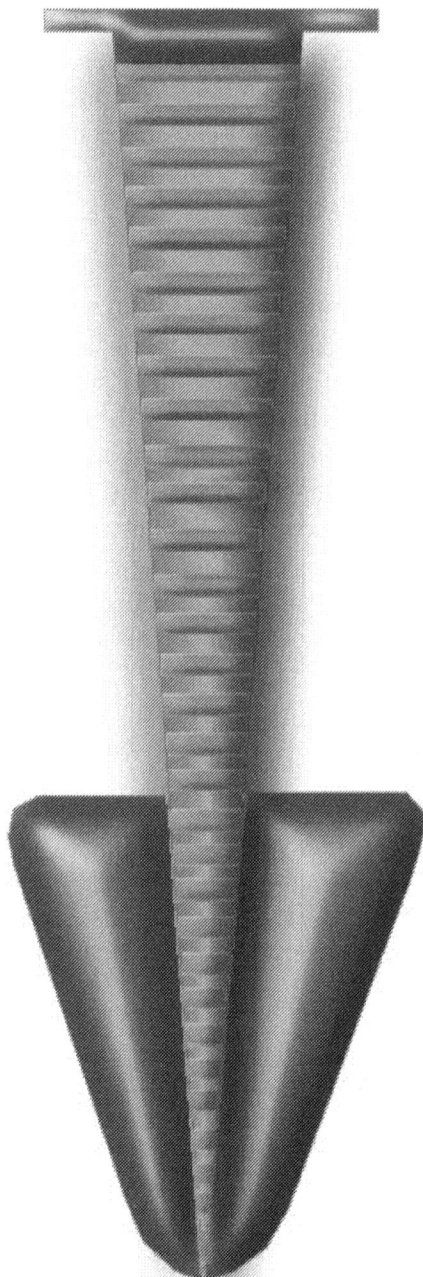

CHAPTER ∩ II

How To Get Started On the Kemetic (Ancient Egyptian) Spiritual Path

WHAT IS THE NEXT STEP?

"The lips of the wise are as the doors of a cabinet; no sooner are they opened, but treasures are poured out before you. Like unto trees of gold arranged in beds of silver, are wise sentences uttered in due season."

-Ancient Egyptian Proverb

If after reading through the first portion of this volume you feel that the Kemitic Mystery Teaching is a path you want to explore then what is your next step? The next step if you choose to practice the mysteries is to learn more about the wisdom teachings and also the initiatic (yogic) disciplines to be practiced. You must become a pure vessel for the teaching so that you may be able to understand it. Otherwise the teaching will not have any effect. If you are in a dull condition even if Heru came to speak with you in a mystical vision it would do no good. You must first practice Maat. This is the first step on the road to purity of body, mind and soul. This is the path of virtue. Then you will be ready to fathom the glorious depths of the vast spiritual teaching and you will have the capacity to behold the magnanimity of the Divine which is all around as well as within you! As you purify and refine your spiritual search you will meet a preceptor who will show you the depths of the teaching and thereby also allow you do discover the depths of your own nature.

"When the student is ready, the master will appear."

-Ancient Egyptian Proverb

The Practice of Maat dictates that you should next practice the disciplines of Kemitic Yoga. So What is Kemitic Yoga? The following section provides you a basic introduction. You should go to the books in the Egyptian Yoga Book Series in the order prescribed in the *"Egyptian Mysteries Course"* presented in the final section of this manual.

The Paths of Yoga

The Egyptian Yoga Book Series is written in such a way as to provide for the needs of various personality types. As stated earlier there are four major personality types among human beings. When those aspects are harmonized and when the person grows by developing each of those aspects it is said that they are practicing Integral Yoga. Therefore, the Egyptian Yoga Book Series has been put together in such a fashion as to offer every individual a specific discipline as well as an integrated method to practice all forms of yoga while at the same time advancing through the three stages of religion. The Ausarian Resurrection, the Teachings of Memphite Theology and the Teachings of Theban Theology are the heart of Ancient Egyptian Religion and Yoga. It is from these teachings that the various path to spiritual realization emerge.

The Paths of Yoga may be seen as the four sides of a pyramid. They all lead to the same point at the apex. The eye symbolizes the attainment of Self-knowledge, Spiritual Enlightenment. So if you are interested in a religious yogic experience, understanding the mystical symbolism of the characters in Ancient Egyptian mythology and the Devotional path of Yoga the books *Resurrecting Osiris, Egyptian Yoga Vol. 2 The Supreme Wisdom of Enlightenment-Path of Amun, Mysticism of Ushet Rekhat: Worship of the Divine Mother* and *The Path of Divine Love* will be your emphasis in the study and practice of the teachings. If you are interested in an intellectual experience of enlightening the mind by eradicating ignorance through reason and reflection, and to leading yourself to greater and greater subtlety and spiritual enlightenment and the Wisdom path of Yoga, the books *Egyptian Yoga Vol. 1 The Philosophy of Enlightenment, The Philosophy of Enlightenment, The Hidden Properties of Matter, Mysteries of Isis,* will be your emphasis in the study and practice of the teachings.

If you are interested in the path of righteous action and the selfless-service path of Yoga, the books *The Wisdom of Maati, Egyptian Yoga Vol 2. The Supreme Wisdom of Enlightenment* and *Egyptian Proverbs* will be your emphasis in the study and practice of the teachings. Also the book *Healing the Criminal Heart: Introduction to Maat Philosophy, Yoga and Spiritual Redemption Through the Path of Virtue* is good for anyone who would like to gain insight into the nature of sin (egoism) and how the practice of Maat Philosophy can lead anyone to a complete transformation, forgiveness and spiritual realization, regardless of their past.

If you are interested in the path of meditation and the Yoga of Meditation, the books *Meditation: The Ancient Egyptian Path to Enlightenment, Initiation Into Egyptian Yoga: The Secrets of Sheti, The Egyptian Yoga Exercise Workout Book* and *The Blooming Lotus of Divine Love* will be your emphasis in the study and practice of the teachings.

If you are interested in the path of Tantrism which involves discovering and developing the inner Life Force energies in order to direct them towards psychic powers and expansion in consciousness leading to union with the Divine and the Yoga of The Serpent Power and the Yoga of Tantra, the books *The Serpent Power: The Ancient Egyptian Wisdom of the Inner Life Force, Egyptian Tantra Yoga: The Art of Sex Sublimation and Universal Consciousness* and *The Egyptian Yoga Exercise Workout Book* will be your emphasis in the study and practice of the teachings.

For more on the path of Mystical Religion see the books *Resurrecting Osiris* and *Egyptian Yoga Volume 2,* and *Memphite Theology.*

Integral Path: blending the disciplines to meet the needs of your personality

The personality of every human being is somewhat different from every other. However the Sages have identified four basic factors which are common to all human personalities. These factors are: Emotion, Reason, Action and Will. This means that in order for a human being to evolve, all aspects of the personality must progress in an integral fashion. Therefore, four major forms of Yoga disciplines have evolved and each is specifically designed to promote a positive movement in one of the areas of personality. The Yoga of Devotional Love enhances and harnesses the emotional aspect in a human personality and directs it towards the Higher Self. The Yoga of Wisdom enhances and harnesses the reasoning aspect in a human personality and directs it towards the Higher Self. The Yoga of Action enhances and harnesses the movement and behavior aspect in a human personality and directs it towards the Higher Self. The Yoga of Meditation enhances and harnesses the willing aspect in a human personality and directs it towards the Higher Self.

Contentment Understanding Peace   Fulfillment
↑   ↑   ↑   ↑
Emotion   Reason   Action   Will.
↑   ↑   ↑   ↑
Devotion Wisdom   Service Meditation

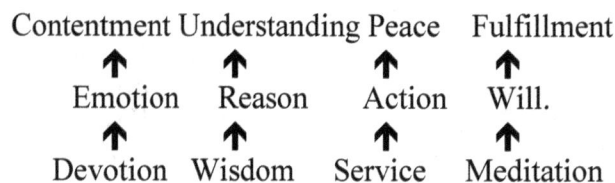

Thus, Yoga is a discipline of spiritual living which transforms every aspect of personality in an integral fashion, leaving no aspect of a human being behind. This is important because an unbalanced movement will lead to frustration, more ignorance, more distraction and more illusions leading away from the Higher Self. For example, if a person develops the reasoning aspect of personality he or she may come to believe that they have discovered the Higher Self, however when it comes to dealing with some problem of life, such as the death of a loved one, they cannot control their emotions, or if they are tempted to do something unrighteous, such as smoking, they cannot control their actions and have no will power to resist. The vision of Integral Yoga is a lofty goal which every human being can achieve with the proper guidance, self-effort and repeated practice. There is a very simple philosophy behind Integral Yoga. During the course of the day you may find yourself doing various activities. Sometimes you will be quiet, at other times you will be busy at work, at other times you might be interacting with people, etc. Integral Yoga gives you the opportunity to practice yoga at all times. When you have quiet time you can practice meditation, when at work you can practice righteous action and selfless service, when you have leisure time you can study and reflect on the teachings and when you feel the sentiment of love for a person or object you like you can practice remembering the Divine Self who made it possible for you to experience the company of those personalities or the opportunity to acquire those objects. From a higher perspective you can practice reflecting on how the people and objects in creation are expressions of the Divine and this movement will lead you to a spontaneous and perpetual state of ecstasy, peace and bliss which are the hallmarks of spiritual enlightenment. The purpose of Integral Yoga is therefore to promote integration of the whole personality of a human being which will lead to complete spiritual enlightenment. Thus Integral Yoga should be understood as the most effective method to practice mystical spirituality.

The important point to remember is that all aspects of yoga can and should be used in an integral fashion to generate an efficient and harmonized spiritual movement in the practitioner. Therefore, while there may be an area of special emphasis, other elements are bound to become part of the yoga program as needed. For example, while a yogin may place emphasis on the Yoga of Wisdom, they may also practice Devotional Yoga and Meditation Yoga along with the wisdom studies. Further, it must be understood that as you practice one path of yoga, others will also develop automatically. For example, as you practice the Yoga of Wisdom your faith will increase or as you practice the Yoga of Devotion your wisdom will increase. If this movement does not occur your wisdom alone will by dry intellectualism or your faith alone will be blind faith. So when we speak of wisdom here we are referring to wisdom gained through experience or intuitional wisdom and not intellectual wisdom which is speculative. If you do not practice the teachings through the Yoga of Action, your wisdom and faith will be shallow because you have not experienced the truth of the teachings and allowed yourself the opportunity to test your knowledge and faith. If you do not have introspection and faith, your wisdom and actions you will externalized, agitated and distracted. Your spiritual realization will be insubstantial, weak and lacking stability. You will not be able to meet the challenges of life nor will you be able to discover true spiritual realization in this lifetime or even after death. Therefore, the integral path of yoga, with proper guidance, is the most secure method to achieve genuine spiritual enlightenment. See chart of spiritual paths (below).

Integral (Wholistic) Yoga

The Process of Personality Integration

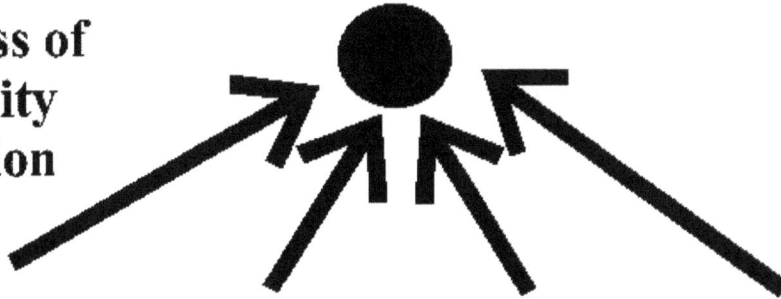

Love Contentment	Understanding	Peace	Fulfillment
↑	↑	↑	↑
Emotion	**Reason**	**Action**	**Will**
↑	↑	↑	↑
Yoga of Devotional Love	Yoga of Wisdom	Yoga of **Righteousness Virtue**	Yoga of Meditation
Control of feeling. Directed towards the Divine	Understanding the Divine, Mystical Psychology	Self-control Selfless service. Purity of Heart.	Study of Mind and development of inner powers.

The Paths of Yoga

PURPOSE OF THE INTEGRAL YOGIC DISCIPLINES

To Enlighten the Intellect	To Enlighten the Emotions	To Enlighten the Body	To Enlighten the Unconscious Mind
⬇	⬇	⬇	⬇
Yoga of Wisdom	Yoga of Devotional Love	Yoga of Right Action	Yoga of Formal Meditation

Study and Reflection

Listening should be followed by reflection upon the teachings. However, sometimes questions arise. At this time the aspirant should articulate the question and ask. Asking questions is the duty of an aspirant because it opens the door to understanding. However, once a question has been answered the answer should be reflected upon and assimilated. Sometimes an agitated mind is already thinking of the next question or a follow-up without taking care to understand the answer to the first question. This will lead to confusion. Reflection is an art and it is best carried out in silence, not only of the mouth but of the mind as well. So an aspirant should learn to ask questions and then to reflect upon them and living in accordance with the new understanding. In this manner the mind will be transformed.

"Seek to perform your duties to your highest ability, this way your actions will be blameless."
Ancient Egyptian Proverbs

There is one critical factor that every aspirant needs to understand. That is, how to balance the day to day reality with the teaching that is being learned. In the teaching you will learn how to transcend the world but this does not mean that the world is to be left behind. If you have responsibilities to maintain yourself or your family, like a job or like taking care of your children, spouse, etc. you must fulfill those responsibilities. You have gotten yourself into them by your past ignorance and you must get out of them by fulfilling your responsibility (Wisdom and righteous action). This means that if before you began studying the teaching and learning how to simplify your life and that you don't need a spouse to make yourself happy this does not mean that you go out and get a divorce. You need to fulfill your part of the relationship and understand the deeper meaning of relationships (See *Egyptian Tantra Yoga*). If you discover that you don't need a new expensive car you cannot just stop the payments. These actions would be against Maat. You must see the relationship to its conclusion even as you grow in enlightenment. You must make the car payments until you sell it and get out of dept properly. Leave nothing undone every day so that your mind may have peace everyday to study and practice the teachings and so that at the time of your death you will not be held back (reincarnation) due to unfinished business. The day to day activities have been created for your benefit. The people that you meet and the responsibilities you need to fulfill daily are the means by which the Divine Self is allowing you to work out the mystery of life by putting the teaching into action. Therefore, do not reject this gift of time, life, and activity. There should not be a contradiction between your inner life and your outer life. This contradiction is eradicated by the study of the teachings with the proper guidance. Therefore, attend as many classes as possible and listen to the tapes as often as possible. Use it wisely and you will see how your inner life and your activities in the world will work hand and hand to lead you to enlightenment. (See *The Wisdom of Maati*)

> "The nature of the body is to take delight and pleasure in complexity;
> the way of truth is that of simplicity."
>
> Ancient Egyptian Proverbs

The key to success in allowing the inner gifts of the soul and the knowledge that leads to self-discovery to unfold is simplicity. Simplicity relates not only to the teachings but to one's practical life. How many possessions do you have and how many do you really need? How many car payments, stereos, or jewelry do you have? How much concern do you have about the body? What pleasures are you running after? What are you trying to accomplish in life and why? Are you trying to get rich, famous, to be voted the sexiest person alive? All of this is perishable and fleeting. It will not bring true happiness. You must examine this question carefully. Is it for me or for the good of humanity? You only need what is necessary to fulfill your life's work. All else will be provided when needed, it will come of its own accord. The more possessions you have the more worries and concerns you have for keeping them and protecting them. Is this truly living? Worries cause mental agitation, agitation prevents peace of mind and without peace of mind there will be limited understanding of the teachings and limited ability to practice concentration and meditation. Worries and anxieties come from lack of understanding what is truly meaningful in life and ignorantly running after empty pleasures and distractions. Simplify your life! The goal of discovering the Self surpasses all worldly pleasures and all mental pleasures. Therefore, gradually make this the focus of your life and you will see how so many troubles fade and those adversities you would have led yourself into in the future are not gone forever.

> "Consume pure foods and pure thoughts with pure hands, adore celestial beings, become associated with wise ones: sages, saints and prophets; make offerings to GOD."
>
> **—From The Ancient Egyptian**
> **Stele of Djehuti-Nefer**

THE THREE MAJOR ASPECTS OF THE INITIATIC LIFESTYLE: LISTENING-REFLECTION-MEDITATION

Listening to the Teachings

"The lips of Wisdom are closed, Except to the ears of Understanding."
"Give that you may receive."

Ancient Egyptian Proverbs

Two important qualities which aspirants in a spiritual studies group need to develop are listening and speaking. In order to grow in spiritual sensitivity you must first develop the faculty of listening. Listening implies concentration on what is being listened to and one cannot concentrate if one's own ego wants to be heard. The ego of the prideful, self-important person always knows best and is not patient to hear even what the ignorant may have to say. If you want to be understood you must strive to understand others. If you want to receive compassion extend it to others. If you want harmony give harmony. Whatever you want to see eradicated from the world (violence, hatred, etc.) eradicate it from yourself and you will discover it has left the world as well. If you want to be listened to first listen to others. Listening is a special art which leads to understanding. This is why listening is the first step in the practice of the Yoga of Wisdom.

Listening to the teachings involves attending classes wherein the wisdom teachings and philosophy are imparted. The temple will include classes on mythology, meditation and wisdom of life based on the Ancient Egyptian scriptures. Also, classes will be given by advanced students in the areas of life skills, coping and lifestyles which promote the spiritual evolution of an individual.

It is important to understand that while the presence of a Spiritual Preceptor is the best form of spiritual instruction, other means of acquiring the teaching should not be overlooked. Modern technology has allowed many forms of media to be employed for the purpose of spiritual education. In ancient times it was the book. Today it is possible to use audio recordings. This is an improvement because the inflections, emphasis and other particulars can be imparted as the teaching is being given. Therefore, a spiritual aspirant should listen to the teachings over and over again and as sensitivity and the power to listen improve the same teachings will reveal more and more wisdom. There are three modes of teaching which a Spiritual Preceptor uses. The first is teaching be the actions. A preceptor shows how to act by example. Next a teacher uses speech. When the higher energy centers are unfolded in a Sage the faculty of speech blossoms. This means the power to use words un-obstructedly in speaking in order to make the teaching understood. The third method of teaching used by a Sage is subtle spiritual influence. There is a subtle spiritual influence which can occur between an aspirant and a spiritual preceptor if the aspirant allows him or her self to come under the direction of the Sage. This process occurs when a spiritual aspirant purifies him/herself by cleansing the negative thoughts and feelings from the heart and when they allow themselves to develop faith in the teacher and eradicate ignorance about the teaching. Therefore, devotion and service to the teacher and to the teaching are very important.

Service to the Teacher and the Temple

In Yogic tradition, spanning thousands of years, the highest form of service is **Service to the Mission of Spiritual Preceptor.** The task of bringing enlightenment to the world is the greatest form of selfless service and charity because it alleviates and ultimately eradicates the source of all pain and sorrow, not only of this life but of those to come in the future. Therefore, a **Spiritual Preceptor** is seen as the most compassionate being on earth. Thus, the act of following in the footsteps of an authentic spiritual personality, by your actions, words and deeds, is seen as the most laudable form of spiritual practice which an aspirant can practice. The aspirant can help the message to get out by **promoting the teachings, demonstrating them to others through programs, teaching others, helping to produce the books of the preceptor, helping with clerical tasks, etc.** of the preceptor.

- Students may assist by **transcribing the audio and video lectures** so that they may be published.
- Students may assist by **taking and filling in orders** for books and tapes.
- Students may assist by **working at presentations, lectures and workshops to schedule locations, setting up the areas**, etc.
- Students may assist by **contacting local universities and interested groups**, meeting with interested groups in order to present the teachings to them. There is a specific lecture prepared for college groups entitled *The Ancient Egyptian Origins of Philosophy and World Mythology*. It presents the origins of Greek mythology (with proof), world religions (including African Religions) and Yoga Philosophy in Ancient Egypt.
- Students may assist by **holding seminars and workshops** on the practice of *Thef Neteru* Egyptian Yoga Exercise. The exercises are an essential part of the practice since it promoted health of mind and body, which are necessary for the proper study and understanding of the teachings. They will easily draw attention to the group from those who are interested in studying the philosophy as well.
- Students may assist by **making donations to the Sema Institute**. All monies, services and property received is tax deductible and will be used for counseling, the production of books, seminars and the creation of a Yoga Center.
- Students may assist by **conducting fundraising events**. All monies, services and property received is tax deductible and will be used for the production of books, seminars and the creation of a Yoga Center.
- Students of Dr. Ashby who are attending universities or colleges may assist by creating special student affiliate groups based on the Ancient Egyptian Tradition of *Sheti* which gave rise to Greek Philosophy and the modern day Fraternities and Sororities. The Campus organization will be called *Sheti Per-Ankh* or **House of Spiritual Knowledge and Selfless Service**. Male members of the group are called Hetu (male servants of the house). Females are called Hetit (female servants of the house). All interested in this work should contact the Sema Institute for the **Sheti College Student Manual.**

INITIATION INTO SHETAUT NETER & SMAI TAWI LEVEL 1

Daily Practice (For more details see the book *Initiation Into Egyptian Yoga.*

1- Physical exercise (1 hour - Use Egyptian Yoga Exercise Video level 1) 1 hour
2- Meditation (15 minutes to 30 minutes - Use the meditation tapes)
3- Study of the philosophy (1 hour to 1 ½ hour - Follow along with the ongoing weekly class recordings from the Miami center.
4- For Reflection and Spiritual Journal writing or Study Group discussion: Answer the following questions among yourselves, allowing everyone to speak:

BEGINNING YOUR COURSE OF STUDY

Class sequence: Order the class tapes and books in the following order. The Kemitic Mystery System has been laid out in several series of lectures. These are to be approached by initiates in the following sequence unless otherwise approved by the teacher.

1. First- Book- *Initiation Into Egyptian Yoga* and begin with the Initiation lecture tape series.
2. Next- When finished with the Initiation series continue by studying *The Ausarian Resurrection* series.
3. Next: When finished with the Ausarian Resurrection series continue by studying *The Wisdom of Maati* series.
4. Next: When finished with *The Wisdom of Maati* series continue by studying the *Initiation Level 2* series.
5. Next: When finished with the *Initiation Level 2* series continue by studying *Book of the Dead* series.
6. Next: When finished with the *Book of the Dead* series contact the teacher for further instructions.

Questions for tapes and books

A- What was the message you got from this days lecture?
B- What insight have you gained into your understanding of spirituality?
C- How has this teaching affected you today?
D- How have previous lessons affected your life?
E- Describe how this lesson or any previous lesson has changed your life from your previous ways into living more in harmony with yourself, nature, humanity or God.
F- How has this or any other lesson from the Yoga series given you deeper insight into the previous religion you may have practiced?

*The student may read other books and tapes in the series as time allows but the main sequence of study should be followed as outlined above.

1- Set an official beginning and ending time for the program. It may run for a longer time but this way there will be structure and everyone can plan accordingly. The meetings should include certain specific elements and you may add your own elements as you progress. These essential elements will provide a well rounded program which includes the basic Yogic disciplines necessary to progress spiritually.
Study Group Rituals - Light candle and incense (Sandalwood first time or in a new location).

A- Opening Prayers and invocations (Yoga of Devotion)*

B- Chanting (Yoga of Devotion)†
C- Exercise Workout (Yoga of Physical Culture in preparation for the practice of Listening Reflection, Concentration and Meditation) Use the Exercise Video level one or the if you are already know the postures use the audio tape 90 minute exercise session or the 45 minute audio session.
D- Readings (Listening and Reflection- Yoga of Wisdom)**
E- Discussion period (about the readings-Yoga of Wisdom)
F- Open discussion - applying the teaching in day to day life. (Yoga of Wisdom)
G- Concentration and Meditation period (Yoga of Meditation)***
H- Closing prayers*

*see Egyptian Yoga Prayer Book or you may use the Morning Worship tape (Ushet I)
**see Yoga and Mystical Spirituality Book, Video and Audio Series by Dr. Muata Ashby.
*** see *Initiation Into Egyptian Yoga* and *Meditation The Ancient Egyptian Path to Enlightenment.*
† see Egyptian Yoga Prayer Book or you may use the Ushet Chanting Series Tapes II, III or IIII.

CHOOSING A SPIRITUAL PATH

2- Choose a format of study. You may choose the **Religious Path** or the **Yogic Path** or the **Integral Path**.

The religious path entails study of the particular myth, practice of its related rituals and entry into their metaphysical (mystical) teachings. You may study the teachings by examining the myths and discovering their mystical content. If you feel a strong affinity for the images of the divine and the glories related about them in the myths you should choose the religious path as your main but not exclusive path. Study and become well versed in the myth and its mystical implications by reading the related books, listening to the related tapes and practicing the related rituals when prescribed.

The yogic path means studying the mystical philosophy by practicing all yogic paths but concentrating on one that resonates strongly with your spiritual aspiration and your personality **(Yoga of Wisdom, Yoga of Right Action, Yoga of Devotional Love, Yoga of Meditation)**. If you feel a strong affinity for one or more of the yogic disciplines you should choose the that discipline as your main but not exclusive path. Study and become well versed in the discipline(s) you have chosen by reading the related books, listening to the related tapes and practicing the disciplines daily and regularly at the prescribed hour.

The **Integral Path** combines the two (Religion and Yoga) or you can focus on one book at a time. This is the most consuming form of practice and it it is practiced artistically it can be most effective since it leaves no aspect of the personality untouched. The integral practice means affecting the parts of the mind that yearn for a religious experience as well as that part which is scientific. This path is taken by advanced practitioners and those whishing to become advanced by adding the disciplines to fill every waking your, that is while at work practicing righteousness, while at home studying, meditating or practicing devotional rituals, etc.

3- You may contact the teacher by phone with any questions. Also anyone may feel free to contact the teacher directly for spiritual counseling.

4- The Book *Initiation Into Egyptian Yoga* should be your textbook for daily spiritual practice. It has several questions which should be answered first before beginning. It contains detailed instructions on how to set up one's own personal daily spiritual practices. The group can help to reinforce and support the individual. This is the main benefit of a study group.

5- Another important element of the spiritual practice is **community work**. your daily spiritual practices and group meetings can be seen as your formal spiritual practice. You also need to engage in spiritual practices in the outside world because this will give you the opportunity to test the validity of the teachings and to hone your spiritual skills. You will encounter **temptations** of all kinds. You may be tempted with ignorance by worldly people, drugs, sense pleasures, etc. your task is to become more spiritually strong by taking recourse to your inner Self (Djeddu). You will be able to practice understanding and self-control when you are provoked by the world. You cannot expect to progress in spiritual life if you just study the teachings, discuss them and philosophize about them. They need to be practiced in your daily life, with your family, at work, at recreation, in times of prosperity and in times of adversity. They need to go deep into your heart. So a serious spiritual aspirant must also practice them by serving humanity. This falls under the discipline of **Yoga of Action (Maat)**. As you practice the teaching what you learned intellectually is experienced and this experience purifies the heart. Purity of heart means growing in selflessness, inner peace, contentment, wisdom, etc. *Maak-heru,* a **"purified heart"** will become more sensitive to the subtler meaning of the teachings, mental peace and thus a human being can promote their movement towards sublimation of the ego. When the ego is sublimated a person can achieve meditation and spiritual enlightenment in a short time. **You should not** go into the world until you are ready however. Study and do the practices of daily spiritual life until you feel ready to expand your practice. Otherwise you will be risking frustration and failure if you move too fast. If there are any questions seek spiritual counseling first. (See the books *The Wisdom of Maati* and *Healing The Criminal Heart*)

This duty of **Selfless Service** can be carried out in several ways. A spiritual aspirant can participate in worthwhile community projects, volunteering, etc. Also, in Yogic tradition the highest form of service is **Service to the Mission of Spiritual Preceptor**. The task of bringing enlightenment to the world is the greatest form of selfless service and charity because it alleviates and eradicates the source of all pain and sorrow, not only of this life but of those to come in the future. Therefore, a Spiritual Preceptor is seen as the most compassionate being on earth. The act of following in the footsteps of an authentic spiritual personality is seen as the most laudable form of spiritual practice which an aspirant can practice. The aspirant can help the message to get out by promoting the teachings, demonstrating them to others through programs, teaching others, helping to produce the books of the preceptor. In advanced stages, when the aspirant becomes proficient he or she can begin to produce their own literature and educational materials, hold classes, etc. Even if they have not reached enlightenment, the act of teaching allows an aspirant to become motivated and proficient in the teachings. **Selfless Service to humanity** is a form of Action but it is also a form of advanced love (Yoga of Devotional Love) because it expands a person's concern to the entire world and this expands their consciousness. This point is clearly made in the Book of Coming Forth By Day Chapter 33[50] (see the book *The Egyptian Book of the Dead: Mysticism of the Prt m Hru*) and should be studied carefully. As you give wisdom you are given more wisdom by the Divine. Therefore, do not hoard anything and do not hold on to anything. Share your knowledge freely. This will allow you to grow spiritually in great strides as long as you remain free of selfishness, pride and egoism. An aspirant should always remain humble and consider him or herself as a student. This attitude will prevent egoism and this will allow their heart to purify and expand. Always feel that you have been blessed by God to have come into contact with your teacher and allow yourself to be a vessel for the teaching to touch others. Open your heart to the joy which the teachings are bringing to you, the unburdening of the mind with the pressures of life and the discoveries of long awaited answers to the most important questions of life. Share this joy with others but without attachment. Spiritual life is an internal awakening and an internal feeling. Do not expect others to agree with you, or praise you. Look only to the approval from your teacher and from the Divine. In this manner you are serving the Divine within yourself and eradicating the egoism and ignorance which is keeping you in bondage to the lower self. See the book *Initiation Into Egyptian Yoga.*

The Etiquette of Initiates and Priests and Priestesses in the Temple

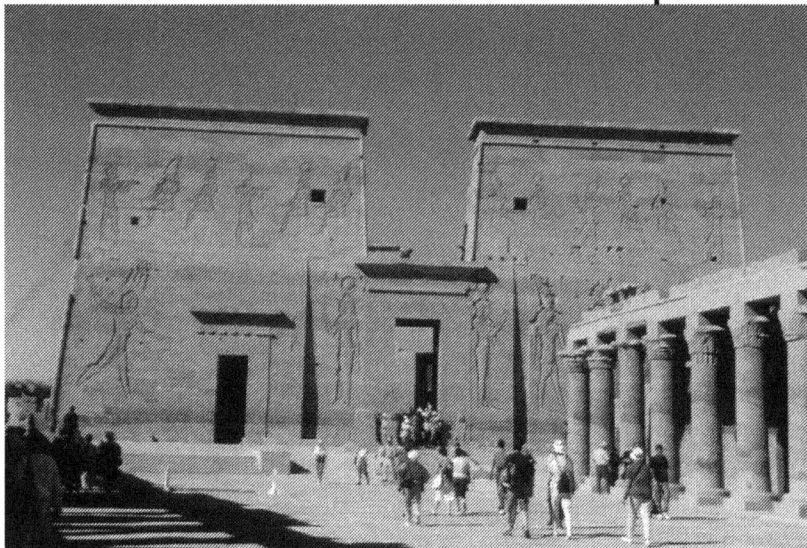

Comportment and Demeanor As an Initiate in the Spiritual Hall

In this essay, the topic will be how to conduct yourself as in initiate in the presence of the initiatic company, which is your Sheti group or in the presence of the spiritual preceptor. First of all, in ancient times when coming to a spiritual hall you would wash yourself before coming into the temple itself. This practice of the Ancient Egyptians is what later developed into the baptism ritual for the Christians. So you want to be cleansed, you must be cleansed physically, you must be cleansed in your mouth, in your speech, and you must cleansed in your mind. That means that you do not utter harsh words to anyone but if you utter harsh words to anyone you must resolve that issue before coming to the temple otherwise, your mind will be agitated and you will not draw the grace that the temple has to offer. You do not come in to the temple harboring thoughts of anger, hatred, greed, lust, jealousy, envy, and so forth. Therefore, you do not have sex before coming into the temple either. This is very disruptive to the experience of elevated spiritual vibrations. You do not eat meat before coming to the temple; it has its own worldly vibrations. You do not come to the temple with worldly possessions, you leave them at the door or put them over your coat or put them in your locker if you need one. You do not carry cell phones or pagers (beepers) you should not distract yourself or others. If you are the kind of person who does business 24 hours a day it simply means that you should be elsewhere doing that business.

Attending the class is very important to your spiritual instruction. You should attend any function prescribed by the teacher. The class is to be conducted in the manner that it has been prescribed and there should not be any deviations from that other than what has been allowed by the preceptor. It is set up that way, so that it would lead you in a proper way to develop your spiritual studies. Any deviations or adjustment are to be approved only by the preceptor and the reason for that is because you want to be managed in a proper way, you want to make sure that you are not going astray. It is the responsibility of the preceptor to shepherd you towards the correct practice and movement towards the Divine. What would happen if a train dwells? There are other students that study Egyptian Yoga Series in countries that do not have preceptorship at all, and it is great that they are making that effort. But it would be much better to also have authentic preceptorship. If this is done in a proper way it is guaranteed that you will succeed in your spiritual life.

Greeting the Spiritual Preceptor and The Term Seba

How do you greet and respect the Spiritual Preceptor. How should you approach a spiritual preceptor? When you come into the hall, when you are clean and with the right clothing, you've been allowed in to the courtyard of the temple. The first thing that you do is to prostrate yourself before the divine image and greet the priest or priestess. Prostration is being on your heels, but this time with your toes curled in, your hands in front of you resting on your elbows. Your forehead on the ground your face kissing the ground. Even if the Shrine is closed you will prostrate yourself in front of the Shrine and then take your seat. The Spiritual preceptor is known as 'Seba' in Kamitan spirituality. Sehu another term, which means spiritual counselor. Seba means preceptor, so that you can understand it, this term is similar to the Indian term 'guru'. The preceptor is greeted in the basic manner of this tradition, 'hotep' or 'hetep' whichever pronunciation you would like. The preferred manner of obeisance toward the spiritual preceptor is with both arms raised with hands facing outwards towards the preceptor and that is called the 'dua' posture. Dua means adoration and you have heard that word plenty of times in the chants: Dua Hetheru Netritaah, Dua Ra, Dua Ra Khepera, etc. And for greeting each other a simple hetep and a bow will do. This is the basic etiquette of the Sheti group.

For more insight into the term, Seba means star, it means an illuminating force, a shining object. Therefore the reason why preceptors are called Seba is because they illumine. Now , what do they illumine? They illumine the 'sebat' seba with the 't' at the end of it. In Kemetic literature, those of you who have began studying the writings, when you add a 't' to a word it makes if female. What all this means is that all of you as students are females, whether you are a male or female and the preceptor is male, whether the preceptor is male or female. What that means is that the illuminator is shining on you just like the sun shines on the moon, just as the moon, a symbol of mind, receives illumination from the sun, the student receives illumination from the teacher. That illumination is a reception or being in a female capacity just as in the sexes in an ordinary sexual relationship, the male is emitting and the female is receiving. The female receives and with that takes and creates a fertilized egg and brings forth life. In the same way the student is to allow their mind to become pregnant with the teachings and through the teachings eventually give birth to enlightened consciousness. That is the deep philosophy behind the term 'Seba'.

Similarly in India, the term 'guru' symbolizes illuminator, one who illumines the cave of heart or shines a light on there to see what is in there. In the Kemetic Culture and deep mysticism you have an artifact, which is called 'Seba-ur', Ur means great, therefore, it is 'the great illuminator.' The great illuminator is an instrument that you see being touched to the mouth in the opening of the mouth ceremony. This artifact is a symbol of a star constellation that used to be in the North Pole, there are many details about it. In short for now, for our purpose here and for your understanding, it means stars that do not move. If you were to see time-lapse photography of the north pole, you see that there are some stars that circulate around the north pole and go under the horizon and they come up again the next day. If you look at the

North Pole, the North Pole does not go under the horizon, it stays above and further, it does not move. The North Pole does not change, just like the sun does not change, but the moon has phases. So when you are a student, you are changeable some days you have very good understanding of the teachings and you are with it and some days you are going along but your mind is locked up, or your emotions are getting the best of you, that means of you have lots of past impressions coming up, you have anger, hatred, greed, lust, jealousy, envy, etc., coming out of the unconscious mind that you need to deal with and cleanse. The teachings do not want you to feel angry or greedy and so forth. That is the mind changing and that is like the moon. When you continue to receive the teachings, receiving illumination one day you do not fluctuate anymore and is what the 'Seba-ur' means.

Sitting Postures

The next important point is your posture there are several postures that are allowed in the Kemetic culture. One is the cross-legged posture, the lotus posture or the half lotus posture, which are more difficult postures to do, granted. The other posture is sitting on a chair with your legs together and your hands on both sides of your tights that one is allowed also if you need to. Another one is sitting on the ground with your feet together as if you were sitting on a chair, with your feet together or the same posture and grasping your legs side to side and holding your legs together. These are all postures that you will see in the Kemetic culture. You do not extend your feet forward, especially toward the divinity or the Sage. You do not slough over or lay down. These kinds of postures will tend to lead you toward slumber and they will also tend to impair your reasoning capacity and your mental understanding. You have a Djed Pillar in your back and if that Djed Pillar is straight, that is, vertical with the ground it is like a tree, it goes straight up and so you too must be planted as a Djed Pillar. Another posture is sitting on your knees and your heels. These postures will all lead you to attentiveness, they will lead you to wakefulness, and these features are necessary when you attend a special lecture.

Any lecture by your spiritual preceptor is to be considered as "special" and deserves your undivided attention. Usually, you will not be expected to endure a posture for more than hour and also sometimes it is preferable not to have a back on your chair or to sit against a wall because you will be leaning and resting on the back (of the chair) and you do not want to be too comfortable because again you will falling asleep, so and so forth.

Respect for the Shrine and Conduct in the Temple

The shrine, is kept closed, expect during the time when the program is being conducted and actually the shrine is only open to initiates. The shrine will be there, but it will be closed only initiates are allowed to see the Divinity, only certain initiates are allowed to manipulate or handle the Divinity, the image of the Divinity. The reason for that is that people with impure hands, those people who are not pure as we said earlier, who have not purified the body, speech, and mind, carry worldly vibrations and they carry impressions of ignorance. The secrecy regarding the image of the Divinity is to develop awe and admiration from the masses and when initiates are finally allowed to see it they are consumed by its dazzling nature. By that time they have been schooled, and have been led to understand certain things about what they will see, certain things about the image, the headdress, the staff and other things that they are going to be seeing, ankhs, scepters, the colors, etc.

Going back to the relationship inside the Temple. You want to be silent rather than talkative, introverted rather than extroverted. You want to be dedicated, meditative, if you come to the Hall and the program has not started yet, you want to come in and sit down, prostrate, do whatever is necessary and take your seat quietly. You don't want to enter and be boisterous, rowdy or loud like 'hey, you see what I did the other day and this happen to me,' that is for people outside. Cacophony, yelling, loud mouth speech, etc. is for the outside world. You want to discover the inner world. This is not a social club or social party, this is not a place for you to come so you can have a membership card, so you can say you are an initiate and put on airs, looking down on others like 'I know these things, I am higher than you.'

You are not here so you can put on Kamitan jewelry, and clothing so that people can be looking at you and be watching you; that is egoism that is not initiation. You must be in a serious mind if you enter into initiation and I want to let know what it takes, for you to succeed. Coming to class once a week is great, that is more than 99% of what the world population does. You are already elevating yourself beyond the rest of the world, but in that top 1% how many people become enlightened? Maybe one thousandths of that one percent becomes enlightened. Are you going to be in the thousandths? This is what it takes, you want to read the books thoroughly and then you go back and read them again. There are lectures that are given on the texts, listen to those lectures again because if you listen to one lecture one time you are not going to get everything that is in it. You may have to listen to it three, four times or more. After a few months pass, you may want to go back and listen to it again. You will realize that something important that was said, you missed the first or second time around or now since you have evolved further, by the third listening, you are discovering a new nuance that applies to you in a whole new way. You should listen to the tapes until the teaching is inculpated deep in your mind and until you're conscious mind is cleansed, recall that three fold cleansing that we discussed earlier.

Again, a few other little points, the chanting, the divine singing etc. are very big parts of the Kemetic Culture as I have said before, it allows you to take the teaching, elevate it with your feeling and fly to meet the Divine with it. Devotion in your worship, Divine Love, is the essential key, but devotion without wisdom is, as I have said before, blind faith. Wisdom without devotion is dry intellectualism. After you learn to love this Divinity, if you do not know that Divinity, or how that Divinity relates to you, or what it is, how can you truly come close to the Divine? How can you love someone you do not even know? You must get to see a connection, develop a connection or feeling, and understand also. When feeling and understanding are harmonized and cultivated there is no stopping your spiritual evolution.

You need to learn he chants by heart and this should not be too difficult if you are practicing them on a daily basis. In fact, it should become automatic, so you may use the sheets to begin with, but I want you to know that you have to put the sheets down, also eventually at least for the basic chants and prayers. Otherwise they will be like crutches, and that is not the ideal. If you do that it will not allow you to relax with it and to flow with it and this is something that needs to happen in your devotional feeling. The flow is going to constantly be interrupted and your mind will be constantly drawn into the paper and you need to be able to allow your thoughts as well as your feelings to flow towards the Divine in an unobstructed manner. The same goes for the drumming, cymbal playing or sistrum playing.

Spiritual Clothing

The very clothing itself has spiritual meaning, the way the hair is done, and all of these different items carry a special mystical meaning. At the time of initiation, you should have been cleansed, and have your white or light colored clothing, upon entering the spiritual hall. You do not come to the spiritual hall with your lowly worldly clothing, you should have special clothes for the spiritual teachings. The garb is an absolute necessity, it is an augmentation, it is something that helps the practice. It is symbolic of putting on a new body, a new consciousness, a new birth, like the snake as it sheds its old skin and becomes reborn as it were into a new body and thereby has a new life in a bigger body. So too the aspirant has an expanded consciousness.

Part of the ritual of initiation is that you must be preparing yourself with the right clothing. It is taking a bath, it is making sure that you smell properly. In Kemetic philosophy, hygiene is of utmost importance for your health, not only physically but also for mental and physical health. If there is no hygiene there is going to distraction because you are going to have disease and disease will take you away from your spiritual disciplines. How are you going to come to a spiritual hall if you are on the bed, laid up with disease? In a practical sense it cannot work. Hygiene of your body, speech, and of your mind are the three main concerns for an initiate. What do you do when you go out in the street? You go out you do your business and take a shower when you come home. In the same way you should take a shower for your mouth, a shower for your mouth is uttering the Divine Chants, Divine Singing. The shower for your mind is the practice of meditation, it allows all that day activity to wash away, to be cleansed away.

Therefore just as you take a shower daily you should do your chants daily, you should do the meditation daily, and of course we have tapes that are already set up for that purpose, to help you to do your practices at home on a daily basis. You may be meeting once a week as a group, but on a daily basis as initiates you are expected to play the Morning Worship Tape and beyond that your are expected to enter into individual studies on the teachings, the philosophy. Taking your own initiative to follow up on teachings that you have received by the Spiritual Preceptor. This requires you to spend more time than just attending classes on Sunday and doing your morning worship. Like I have suggested previously, you can play lecture tapes on your way to work, in your car, or if you have a walk-man, a cassette player or any such devices.

Also, in your personal bodies you must realize that given the nature of the teachings that you are trying to learn that the body is not your ultimate abode. It is not your only existence. The perpetual worrying or running after the body, putting oils on the body and the body must have nice clothing to look good, then it must have jewelry, and it must have nice oils for the hair, special shampoo, and this and that, or tattoos, or piercing. All of this is counterproductive to the teaching and therefore, it is not enjoined in the teaching. This understanding excludes the spiritual clothing and certain other aspects. They have a spiritual symbolism that turn your mind actually towards the teaching, but not including piercing, not including use of chemicals on the body that transform the way your body naturally wants to manifest itself. Things that have a healthful nature are allowed. Things like synthetic chemicals for bleaching the skin, dying the hair, or straightening the hair; or things that will be make you unnaturally sexually alluring are all counterproductive to the teachings.

Handling the Mind and Engaging in the Disciplines

You must learn how to handle your mind, so that your mind is very open to listening to a lecture. Sometimes it just wants to relax and listen to music; sometimes you would want to hear chanting, or sometimes you do not want anything, then be quiet and meditate. You have to learn how to work with your mind. That is why the teaching has been set up, so that in anyone of those different manifestations of the mind you would be able to handle it and you can adjust the teachings to suit its desire. This is why you find that when we begin our program with the chanting, its setting up the vibrations, cleansing out the mind, and at the end of the chanting session you can be silent for few minutes, in quiet contemplation. You see that we do not go immediately into a talk on the philosophy or on some historical issues.

Doing the basic practices is fine for those who do that, but for those who want to advance in the spiritual philosophy, in the mystical philosophy, those who wants to become Sages and Saints you must do more than that. The mind cannot be enlightened just by reading or intellectualizing it won't work, it has never worked that way. All the books that are written by many others on history and philosophy will fail and it has failed. Some people believe that all they need to do is read books to become enlightened and eradicate unrighteousness and learn about self. This does not work because the books are wrong, the books are wonderful, but they need to be part of a concerted spiritual discipline. The discipline should include chanting, formal meditation, as well as meditation in the form of the postures. Initiates should practice a complete, holistic discipline that takes care of the whole personality. This is called Integral Yoga. It takes your whole personality into account. In spiritual philosophy it is recognized that you have four main aspect to your personality. One of them is your intellect; the other one is the emotions, people know about the emotions a lot; but you also have a physical constitution, people are getting more health conscious, they want to exercise; but even going beyond that, your body needs to be brought in line with your spiritual life. So just because you exercise does not mean that your body is in line with your spiritual life. You can go joggling, you can play tennis, or you can do gymnastics, but it does not necessarily mean that your body is in tune with your spiritual direction. That is why the discipline of physical postures such as Yoga from India, Tai Chi and Qi Gong from China, or Aikido from Japan were developed. These were designed to bring your body in line that is in harmony with your spiritual consciousness. The Kemetic Thef Neteru (Sema Paut) systems are postures that you can find, inscribed on the walls of the Temples of Ancient Egypt. These were initiates getting into these postures. Those of you who live in New York you have these large China Town areas. I am sure at some point you have seen many people gathering in one morning all together doing the Tai Chi. Can you imagine what was going on in the courtyards of the temples of Ancient Egypt, the exercises that were being practiced, the ritual that was engaged, the meditations that were being conducted? When you walk there you look everywhere, and everywhere you turn there is an inscription, an image or a ritual. The inscriptions on our temple hall give you a little ideal of what it needs to be. Go to any Kamitan temple and there is not one square foot that does not have any inscription. Wherever you look there is a meditation in there. If you want to be successful at this your mind has to be constantly turned toward the Divine, continuously. Not in a fanatical way, mind you, but in a way that is balanced, in a way that is insightful, in a way that you are not stressed. Meaning for instance that you emotionally may want to do something, but your intellect is not with it, your intellect is like "no I don't feel like it." You are unbalanced. It is like going to the airport and then you realize you have left your bags at home. You have to go back home and get your baggage but when you get to the airport you found out that you left your keys, so you have to go back and get your keys. By the time you come back the plane is gone. Your movement has to be ordered. It has to be balanced. You have to allow what is called the Oodja, which is the Divine fire that is in you to grow slow and steady to a blazing desire for spiritual enlightenment that your mind and hart are in agreement with. And all of this process is called Shemsu. Shemsu means that you are a follower, a devotee. This process is engaged through the sheti group. Sheti is the study and penetration of the mysteries, the discovery of the mysteries. Sheti or Shedy is that study that allows you to develop spiritual enlightenment or Maakheru (truth of speech) or Nehast (spiritual awakening, resurrection).

The Relationship Between Initiates

Now to your relationship with each other as initiates, and your relationship first of all with each other people form the outside. Your relationship with each other should be cordial, friendly, to the standpoint of the etiquette's we just described, to the standpoint of ordinary civility. Your relationship should not be sentimental with each other. Your relationship should not be friendly in a worldly sense. Familiarity breeds contempt. You want to develop a business like and detached attitude, but friendly. You do not go exchanging personal family issues; you could do that outside with other people. You are initiates brothers and sisters, you are here to learn the teachings and not to carry on a worldly relationship, in the Hall. Those who want to do that should stay outside, that is your prerogative, that is fine for then. You are here to learn the teachings, you are here not to disrupt the conduct of that process, because you are here as initiates presumably because you understand that this is the higher reality of life. What is in the world is a misconception, you are here to learn the reality even as you go out in the world, you continue to uphold, the ordinary necessities of life. You go to work, you pay your bills and all those kinds of things. Even that, you are also trying to spiritualize those activities as well. If you are doing a job that is unrighteous, activities that are not useful to people, you want to change those. If you are defrauding people in some business or if you are in sales and you selling things that are not useful to people, or just to make money then you would want to do something righteous, helpful to people. In this manner you can make your business activities part of your spiritual disciplines and be thereby closer to the teaching in day-to-day life.

The Personal Life and Relationships of an Initiate

As far as your personal life is concerned, the teachings do not require you to divorce your family or to go into some place out in the forest and be alone. What you need to do is to learn how to developed an internal detachment and dispassion and understanding about the world. However, going on retreats, spending time at the temple, away from the world so that you can immerse yourself in the teachings is enjoined by the scriptures and should be done if it is within your means. The teaching does not require or advocate fanaticism. Fanaticism is actually detriment to the true understanding of the teachings, for understanding the teachings properly. It prevents you from enlightening your whole personality, you are actually blocking the true teaching from coming into your heart, into your mind. Fanaticism makes your personality imbalanced and extremes agitate the mind and cloud the intellect. Fanaticism breeds blind faith or dry intellectualism, intellectual knowledge without feeling. That is why the teachings enjoin that there should be a balanced practice for the intellect and emotions. So you need the music, the postures, meditation and righteous action. If there is a conflict amongst each other that conflict is to be discussed amongst yourselves and the group leader, the acting officiating priest or priestess. If there is no resolution based on the teachings that you already know, that problem is to be brought to the 'Seba' for resolution. Once that answer is given, that answer is to be accepted without question and it is to follow without question. Its wisdom will be revealed to you as you go along. However, if the conduct is as prescribed by the teachings (outlined in this essay), there should be minimal occurrences that require that kind of communication. However, from time to time conflicts come out with all people even initiates and that is understood, but as initiates you must realize that you are first and foremost ready to handle conflicts not as worldly people but as people with higher ideals so you are ready to forgive and along with that forgiveness there should be understanding.

If you think that somebody did something to you, something wrong to you, somebody is egoistic and then you harbor that in you unconscious mind. You keep that in your heart and say this person did something it could be a year ago, it could be two years ago, or three years ago, the relationship with the person is constantly tainted and that person may not even know that you are harboring that ill feeling against them. You're harboring those feelings are preventing you from striving ahead concerning the teachings, that ignorance that you are holding in your mind is working to cloud your intellect. The intellect and heart need to be cleansed of all anger, hatred, greed, guilt, envy, lust, etc. as all of these are detrimental to your spiritual evolution.

Selfless Service

Your duty as initiates is to serve and we will discuss that a little bit. What is your duty as selfless servants? When you assist others, providing clothing, food, shelter, etc. you are practicing the service that is prescribed in the Pert m Heru text. When you help the preceptor to deliver the message of the spiritual teachings you are practicing the highest service to humanity. You helped to bring the message out, you helped to coordinate it and in so doing you have aligned yourselves with the living process of divine grace which God has set forth and which operates through the preceptor and touches people all over the world. Certain things may go wrong, books may not arrive where they were suppose to, things run late, etc. these things will always happen, the question is how do you deal with it. That makes you an initiate or a worldly person. That makes you an ignorant slave of the world or a master of life. If you are an initiate you understand and even expects mishaps and since you are committed to the teachings and to the work, you are not disturbed, rather you press on and you ultimately succeed. If you understand that in the end it is going to work out you will not be disturbed. Everything that happens, happens for a reason. So you see, illusions are developing in mind about the teachings such as the teachings are hard. The reason it is hard is because you make it so. Just like life is hard because you make it so, because you cant get what you desire and somehow you have learned that you deserve what you desire and when life disappoints you, you complain and you shout, you holler, you scream, you not only make your situation worse but you are also harboring new impressions of that screaming for the next time that is going to make you even doubly upset. You want to be quiet you want to move ahead, you do not want to squirm, you do not want to cry out and that is the Maatian way of action, that is Maat in action. When it is all over you are going to realize that you have gained something, you gained inner peace, you have gained understanding, you have gained power because you can say look at all these adversities I had but look how I did it anyway. What can I not do?

So that kind of service is very valuable to the preceptor and to God. It is very appreciated and you must realize that another thing happens, another benefit that you have that ordinary people do not have is that this kind of service allows you to be closer to the teacher and thereby gain greater insight into the nature of enlightened beings. You are able to asks questions and be able to discuss things in a way that ordinary people cannot. You were able to spend more time to get a feel for how the teacher is, what he/she thinks and how they look at things. Which is actually what you need to learn, how the teaching is to be applied in life. Enlightenment is a way of thinking, feeling, looking and acting in life and understanding of how the teaching applies gives insight into the enlightened state. Those people who are out there who talk about liking Egyptian Yoga or about being interested in meeting Dr. Muata Ashby, that talk does not lead them to enlightenment, it is the righteous action based on the teachings that leads one to enlightenment. When you draw yourself closer to the teaching and the teacher by making a way for lectures to be given, supporting the temple, engaging in service to the community, and the world, etc., that is why you get greater benefit and more advanced instruction, because you initiated the action and came into close association with the teacher. People who talk, who just read books and other intellectual pursuits, they do not go beyond these limited actions, they do not receive the higher benefits.

Foundational Books in the Kamitan Yoga

There are some of the books in the series that you need to have and give special consideration to like the Kemetic Diet. That is part of the foundation of your whole life, your diet, your food, you physical food, your mental food, and your soul food. Egyptian Yoga The Philosophy of Enlightenment, the Initiation Into Egyptian Yoga book and the African Origins book are like foundational books for the entire discipline. You should be generally well versed in what is contained in the Egyptian Yoga Volume 1: The Philosophy of Enlightenment. If somebody comes up to you off the street and says, "what is Egyptian Yoga?" what are you going to tell them? Would you say 'I don't know, it is something that Dr. Ashby teaches when you go to class.' You want to be proper ambassadors for the teachings, not going around proselytizing or bringing loud speakers and a soapbox, so that everybody can hear the teachings, or play a tape about Dr. Ashby on loud speakers. We do not need that. If in your travels, in your day-to-day communication with people, they ask you or say somebody comes up to you, a coworker, and ask you. Or you have seen someone in need, perhaps walking by in the hall and you have seen they are crying, you go up to them to say what is going on? and they reply 'oh I am having this trouble in my life and you seem so calm. You had this same trouble the other day and how is it that you are not upset? What are you going to tell them? I practice meditation, and I am into studies that give me insight so and so forth. It is called Kemetic Yoga. Why don't you come and join me for classes and see for yourself if you like, so and so forth.' This is what you can do as an initiate. You can do big things but also you can in a subtle and quiet way help others by your very balanced way of dealing with life and then with the right words at the right time and in the right way lead them to greater insight and a more sublime way of life.

Beginning Your Studies

Introduction to the Egyptian Yoga Book Series

Now you can study the teachings of Egyptian Yoga wisdom and Spirituality with the ***Egyptian Yoga and Mystical Spirituality Book Series***. The books take you through the Initiation process and lead you to understand the mysteries of the soul and the Divine, to attain the highest goal of life: ENLIGHTENMENT. The ***Book Series*** takes you on an in depth study of Ancient Egyptian mythology and their inner mystical meanings. Each Guide Book is prepared for the serious student of the mystical sciences and provides a study of the teachings along with exercises, assignments and projects to make the teachings understood and effective in real life. The series is ideal for study groups or individuals on the spiritual path of religion and/or Yoga mysticism.

The first ingredient in spiritual practice is the aspirant. There must be spiritual aspiration, FAITH, a burning desire to transcend limitation and discover Divinity, and a strong belief that there is something beyond ordinary human experience. Next, in order to practice the teachings effectively there should be proper guidance. This is the purpose for which the books, *Egyptian Yoga: The Philosophy of Enlightenment, Initiation Into Egyptian Yoga: The Secrets of Sheti, Meditation: The Ancient Egyptian Path to Enlightenment* and *The Egyptian Yoga Exercise Workout Book,* were written. *Egyptian Yoga: The Philosophy of Enlightenment* provides a comprehensive background to the teachings of Ancient Egypt and places them in a context of world religion, Indian Yoga and modern science, for all to understand. Sheti means Spiritual discipline or program, to go deeply into the mysteries, to study the mystery teachings and literature profoundly, to penetrate the mysteries. This volume describes the various paths for spiritual development and provides guidelines for setting up your schedule of daily spiritual practices as part of the various spiritual disciplines. It is a "How to" manual for beginning to practice the teachings from the first day and it also outlines the qualifications of a spiritual aspirant, an Initiate, the teacher disciple relationship, diet and health, introduction to meditation, prayer and chanting. This volume is the first book in the Egyptian Yoga Course Program. Together they form the foundation for an effective effort in the study and practice of Egyptian Yoga.

TIME REQUIREMENT TO SUCCED IN THE TEACHINGS

Many aspirants ask about the time required to study the mysteries and this is a very good question from the aspect of the masses. Everything is in terms of time or in terms of money profited or in pleasure gained. In the mystical field the time spent and the rewards reaped are irrelevant since Spiritual Enlightenment is not a thing that can be quantified in terms that the ego or the intellect can understand. However, for beginning aspirants it is expressed in the following way.

The time required to attain spiritual realization depends on the current level of spiritual evolution, the effort in the practice of the disciplines and the level of preceptorship. If one is currently at a very degraded state, beset with encrusted egoism, low mental vibrations (anger, hatred, greed, lust, jealousy, envy etc.) then much cleansing work needs to be done in order to progress. To the extent that those negative aspects of the personality, which are termed "fetters," exist in the personality to that extend the progress will be hampered.

However, even the most degraded personality can attain spiritual realization even in a single lifetime if they apply themselves fully to the task of spiritual enlightenment. By keeping good association and study of the teachings (Sheti) and humbling to an authentic spiritual master (Seba) and the personality is transformed in time. This time may be in the realm of weeks, months, days, years or lifetimes. Thus, the time is not important but that you should begin and turn towards the teaching is, because your desire and anxiety will also be an obstacle. Questions like how long will it take? Is this the right path? Etc. are distracting to the mind and also misguided. If you are a righteous aspirant and you have discovered an authentic teacher, then you need not worry about anything. Your salvation is assured and guaranteed. Therefore, do not ask how long but rather ask at what time is class being given and make sure to not miss even one session with the teacher, until the final goal is attained. Do not allow your ego to fool you into thinking that you know the path or that you have heard it all before or that you have achieved some great height or that you need no direct contact with a teacher or that letters and the telephone or videos are good substitutes for being in the presence of the teacher. Many an aspirant have fallen due to such notions.

How to Overcome Failure on the Spiritual Path

Question: Having heard the teaching and after some time if you have not having attained spiritual enlightenment what is there to do?

Many aspirants study the teaching for some time, even years, and find that they have not achieved the ultimate goal of which the teachings speak, that great *Nehast,* the spiritual awakening that bestows the knowledge of nature and the Divine, that wisdom that opens the doors to eternity, that teaching that bestows immortality, supreme joy, peace and God consciousness which is spoken about so much and is the objective of all spiritual aspirants worldwide. What should an aspirant do if she or he finds her/him self in this predicament? The aspirant should take recourse to

1. Repeated effort and
2. Dispassion (becoming free from delusion about the world and desire and hatred) which clouds the intellect.
3. devotion with form
   a. this secures divine grace-

Repeated effort means: at this level of practice (in the teaching for some time-even years), not just listening to the teachings and going about one's worldly business. It means diligence in the practice of the teachings and the disciplines enjoined by the teachings. There must be uncompromising meticulousness and fastidiousness and strictness in the practice. Not sporadic or irregular practice. Some aspirants practice salad-bar spirituality, picking and choosing what they want to do. Some come to some lectures, some rituals, some meditation gatherings, some meetings and then wonder why they have not succeeded, yet they have not attended to the teaching in a full way. There will be only limited success until the teaching and its disciplines are attended to fully by an aspirant. Some aspirants allow gaps of years in the practice of the teachings, falling in and out of worldly entanglements. This is not the path to the ultimate success because it is not the highest and best practice of the teachings- *Sdjm* –heeding the teaching. Even while living in the world an aspirant must find a way to handle the worldly responsibilities –this is righteous and proper-for without this there is no basis for practice of the teachings. But worldly responsibilities are not to be pursued beyond necessity.

"Neither let prosperity put out the eyes of circumspection, nor abundance cut off the hands of frugality; they that too much indulge in the superfluities of life, shall live to lament the want of its necessaries."

-Ancient Proverb of Shetaut Neter

Worldly responsibilities that are performed for the sake of promoting spiritual practice are to be considered Divine actions, -part of the spiritual disciplines as opposed to those that are performed for the sake of promoting more pursuit of worldly pleasures and worldly desires. Repeated effort also means working to become less entangled with the world and to lead a simple life-pay off mortgages, get a car for transportation and not as a status symbol, seeking the company of spiritually minded (others who study the teaching-not religious people) people as opposed to worldly minded, living within one's means, etc. Having taken care of the worldly duties-providing for ones food, shelter and health- the attention is to be turned towards the teaching exclusively, meaning that the actions are to be performed for the sake of the Divine and not for the egoistic self.

Lack of Dispassion- without dispassion the teaching will not the mind and second step of assimilation of the teaching will not occur or will occur imperfectly and the third stage will not be possible at all. There are three stages in the process of study of the teaching, Listening, Reflection and Meditation. Reflection is the second stage. When the teaching has been heard then it needs to be reflected upon deeply and this reflection process leads to assimilation of the teaching into the depth of the mind and finally there is meditation on the teaching, the single-minded and singular experience of the deeper meaning of the teaching in one's own experience.

Maturity to Succeed in the teaching does not occur until there is sufficient frustration with the pursuit of worldly desires. A person's capacity to practice dispassion emerges when they realize the futility of trying to fulfill their egoistic desires through worldly pleasures and so dispassion is a reaction to frustration but if the dispassion is based on ignorance-the lack of spiritual teaching, then it will be short-lived. That person will experience dispassion only for a short time and then be back to worldly pursuits.

"Neither let prosperity put out the eyes of circumspection, nor abundance cut off the hands of frugality; they that too much indulge in the superfluities of life, shall live to lament the want of its necessaries."

-Ancient Proverb of Shetaut Neter

Dispassion is the gradual freedom achieved when the mind becomes released from the mood swings caused by desire and hatred due to ignorance about the world and passionate desire to fulfill desires through the world of time and space. These desires are a product of a deluded mind that does not realize the futility of trying to fulfill desires through a fleeting world of human experiences. This search causes the mind to be clouded with ignorance and there can be no peace due to the constant mental swings themselves and the deluded concepts that the mind subscribes to. The movements of the mind cloud the intellect and prevent right thinking. The ignorant concepts act as impenetrable canvases or images of the world in accordance with the desires of the mind. This renders the world not as it is but as a deluded notion of reality based on the internal egoistic notions and desires. In this state of mind objects and worldly pursuits are chased after without regard for truth because the desire has blotted out the negative aspects and painted a picture of happiness in the object or pursuit. This deluded notion renders the mind incapable of assimilating the teachings in a proper way.

"God sheds light on they who shake the clouds of Error from their soul, and sight the brilliancy of Truth, mingling themselves with the All-sense of the Divine Intelligence, through love of which they win their freedom from that part over which Death rules, and has the seed of the assurance of future Deathlessness implanted in him. This, then, is how the good will differ from the bad."

-Ancient Proverb of Shetaut Neter

Divine Grace = God does not grant Nehast (Spiritual awakening-enlightenment) This is not within God's power to give. As a spark of the Divine every human being is essentially one with God and as such partakes in Divine Power. The soul, as that spark, has led itself to ignorance and so by itself must lead itself to awakening. Practicing devotion to God has the effect of turning the mind towards the Divine and this leads to purity of feeling and thinking. Essentially it is a worship of the Divinity within oneself. When the divinity within is worshipped as opposed to the world, it allows that divinity to emerge as the preeminent aspect of life and the mind AWAKENS to its presence and the true nature of the personality which is not the egoistic notion but the heretofore unknown Divine Spirit-God within. Devotional exercises bestow propitious conditions to practice and advance in spiritual attainment. God does not grant enlightenment but only opens the door. Propitious conditions includes peace of mind, encounters with spiritual preceptors, reduction of pressure of egoistic tendencies that act as obstacles to spiritual attainments. When Divine Grace dawns the aspirant gains spiritual strength and increasing desire to study and practice the teaching as well as increasing pleasure and fulfillment through the practice and increasing dispassion about the worldly objects and worldly desires. Divine Grace is propitiated through Devotion to the Divine and Right Action-righteousness.

"Seekest thou God, thou seekest for the Beautiful. One is the Path that leadeth unto It - Devotion joined with Knowledge."

-Ancient Proverb of Shetaut Neter

Devotion to God allows the depth of the teaching to be revealed. Approaching the teaching intellectually will only promote a superficial understanding and therefore a limited attainment. Intellectual study allows the teaching to be thought about but this thinking process can become circular if the depth of the teaching is not approached. Devotion-Divine Love towards God allows the depth of the teaching to be approached. In essence the teaching must be felt as well as known. Intellectual knowledge must be augmented by feeling the teaching. The feeling aspect of the soul, when tapped into, does not allow the intellectual aspect to become deluded. In fact, it will plague the intellect with insecurities, torment the intellect with doubts until the right path is pursued this is the deeper conscience of a person-whose source is their own soul. This cannot occur of the divine feeling is dulled due to delusion and worldly desire. Devotional exercises and rituals allow the intellectual teaching to be experience as well as thought.

"O behold with thine eye God's plans. Devote thyself to adore God's name. It is God who giveth Souls to millions of forms, and God magnifyeth whosoever magnifieth God."

-Ancient Proverb of Shetaut Neter

<u>Super-conscious state</u> – in order for the process of spiritual evolution to occur there must be experience of the superconscious state of mind. The mind must experience going beyond the bounds of its own constrictive concepts and desires and the world of time and space. Otherwise, the teaching and the feeling of the spiritual process will remain short of the highest attainment no matter how pious the person may be or how elevated the mind and personality may appear to be. All the disciplines lead to a meditative experience in which time and space are transcended and all-encompassing, eternal existence and unlimited expanded consciousness is discovered. First in small measure and eventually in full splendor. Even a short glimpse which is merely a preview, unlocks lifetimes of mental fetterings and sparks the true awakening if the final phase of the march towards spiritual awakening.

<u>Meditation</u> is the key to opening the mind to the experience of superconsciousness and this can only be achieved when the mind and personality has been cleansed of delusion, passion, attachment for worldly objects and desires. This purity leads to spiritual strength and spiritual strength is the key factor needed to attain entry into the superconscious state. In order to attain the highest meditative state, concentration and extended practice of mental focus is required. Without mental purity, and peace concentration is impossible and the superconscious state will elude even the cleverest intellect.

<u>Spiritual Strength</u> – In order to succeed on the spiritual path an aspirant needs spiritual strength. Spiritual strength is the strength that emerges when the mind is freed of ignorance, delusion and passion. The ignorant, deluded and passionate mind is fettered by its conscious and subtle desires and misconceptions. The conscious desires lead to worldly pursuits but this process, being unfulfilled, leaves residues of unfulfilled desire and also produces new subtle desires for other pursuits (if this desire did not work, maybe another will-etc. For Example: the deluded mind may reason thus- If a blue car did not make me happy, maybe a red one will) and these all become lodged in the unconscious level of mind. This constitutes a continued fettering of the mind in the present and in the future. These fetter the minds power because each subtle desire locks a portion of will power with itself in the unconscious level of mind. So even a person who appears to be free of desires may harbor these in the unconscious mind and thereby be weak willed. Such a person cannot resist worldly desires, nor can they sit still for meditation because thoughts constantly emerge to disturb the mind and even if thought do not seem to be emerging at some particular time there are energy disturbances throughout the body and there is illusory discomfort and the person claims they cannot succeed in meditation. So mental restlessness due to subtle desires, or energies must be resolved (cleansed and transcended by the mind) in order to succeed on the spiritual path. This is done by

    <u>a</u>-practice of devotion to god
    <u>b</u>- practice of right action
    <u>c</u>- practice of dispassion and detachment for the world
    <u>d</u>- practice of attachment to the teaching
    <u>e</u>- repeated effort in the above (a-d) until there is ultimate success

<u>Desires are of three types:</u> Heavenly (Maatian), Worldly (Un-Maatian) and mixed. Those who seek success on the spiritual path must turn away from the worldly to the mixed and then from the mixed to the Divine. When Maatian (principles of right action based on truth) actions are practiced the personality becomes purified, the mind becomes unburdened

from vises and egoistic tendencies. Then the personality is capable of understanding and experiencing the higher consciousness talked about in the teachings. Therefore, desire the for worldly attainments but be replaced with desire for spiritual attainments in the form of increasing Divine Love, increasing dispassion and increasing peace and desire to study the teachings and be in the company of those who espouse it. Thus, spiritual evolution entails turning away from worldly desire and towards desire to attaine spiritual awakening. Therefore, desire is not the problem, what is the problem is what is desired. The right desire leads to freedom and enlightenment. The wrong desire leads to ignorance, delusion, fettered bondage to the world and its accompanying virtually boundless source of human suffering, unfulfillment and sorrow.

Diligence on the Path- Mature aspirants need to grow up- arrange their priorities, conserve resources and invest in their own evolution, pay their dues (seminar fees, etc.), not leaving each other and the temple to shoulder the burdens, drop childish worldly entanglements that distract from the teaching, drop competing philosophies and infantile teachings that foment confusion so they can concentrate on what they proclaim to be following. Diligence on the spiritual path is not independent self-will. Those who want to practice salad bar spirituality or seek the advice of oracles or create their own independent classes should do so on their own. One cannot be a Shemsu in this way, by mixing teachings, following confused ideologies, following popular culture as the individual finding his or her own way. These are illusions of a decadent time that were always there but now in epidemic proportions due to the modern capacity to have a plethora of sensory bombardments, misinformations and complexities which play on the ignorant and distracted mind. Aspirants have no choice as to what the practice of the teaching needs to be in order to attain success. They do have a choice in the intensity of their level of practice and devotion to the teaching and these determine to the level or degree of success that is attained and when.

If you want to succeed be consistent with your studies. Do not attend classes sometimes, practice the postures sometimes, meditate sometimes, and then also carry on in the world as a worldly person. Do you eat sometimes, sleep sometimes? As these things are done daily so should the teaching be done as well. If you want success concentrate on this teaching and drop others. Follow the instructions carefully and meticulously and when there is faltering, pick yourself up and try again and again. Practice the teachings in this manner until the goal is attained, no matter how long it takes or where you need to go to receive it.

A qualified aspirant will not wait for the teaching but will make a way for it. He or she will not sit around hoping to find a teacher. The first task is to make yourself a qualified aspirant, purify yourself physically and mentally and be diligent in the studies under the guidance of your own conscience in the beginning, But there is a time when you must seek out a teacher. You must have the attitude that if I must travel to the other side of the world then that is what needs to be done. If you do not want to leave your family, your friends, job, etc. to pursue the teaching and enlightenment then you should not because you will not succeed even if you forced yourself, so realize that you are not yet fit for advancement in the teachings. Even college students leave home to pursue their dreams. What could be said about those who do not want to pursue the greatest goal of life because they are holding on to worldly things?

These are the keys for all who wish to excel in the teaching but they should be the special focus for all who have studied the teaching for some time and yet find themselves without success beyond a specific point. A DETERMINED ASPIRANT MUST SEE THE ENDEAVOR OF SPIRITUAL AWAKENING TO ITS END. If this is not done the aspirant will for ever wander in the wilderness of life, deluded and suffering or self-aggrandized, believing they have attained when in reality they are projecting on the world their notion of reality reflecting within their illusion of sagehood. Such personalities walk the earth without the necessary humility to realize their own degraded state and thereby deprive themselves of the illuminating association with an authentic teacher. Others, convinced they have practiced correctly do not seek out counseling and so their dispassion turns to morose and sometimes even morbid discontent with all things including the teaching.

The Spiritual Checklist

In the last issue I began a two part series on how to overcome failure on the spiritual path. This brought up certain issues that are very important for aspirants to understand. Many times as aspirants get into the teaching for some time they may get into a rut as it were. They practice as many of the teachings and disciplines as they can but as they do that sometimes they get to a point where they must drop certain disciplines in order to practice others due to lack of time. In this circumstance a certain irregularity in the practice of the disciplines develops and the quality of all the disciplines suffers. The worldly activities and relations become intermingled with the disciplines and the spiritual program becomes haphazard. The aspirant may believe they are doing so many disciplines, chanting, classes, exercises, diet, etc. but in reality they may come for class once a week, do postures once or twice a week, take vitamins three times a week, do morning worship twice a week, etc. then next week these disciplines are left our in favor of others. What results is a situation where so many things are being done but the quality of those things is degraded and they do not have the effect of purifying the mind and shielding it from worldly entanglements. In fact the disciplines when practiced in this way can have the opposite effect and lead to a degraded personality because the effort put into the practice and then frustration when the feelings of anger, hatred, greed, lust, etc. still remain leads to the idea that the teaching does not work or the aspirant may simply get caught in the worldly experiences. Then the aspirant will come back to the teacher and ask what they can do, where did they go wrong, etc. They receive encouragement and advice but then the cycle begins all over again and there is no ultimate progress. This is because at that stage what is most important is to practice the disciplines. Spiritual counseling is necessary sometimes but if the disciplines are not practiced the counseling will also not be effective. For this reason the following list has been prepared. It contains the practices and disciplines that should be taken care of so that aspirants may understand when they are actually practicing the teaching and when they are actually not. Before calling the preceptor look at this list and see if you are truly following the instructions or not. If you find that you are not then make the necessary adjustment in your spiritual practice. Then if assistance is still needed call for advice. Keep a spiritual diary along with the table below. Note over time how your personality is changing and seek to avoid the mistakes of the past. See the book Initiation into Egyptian Yoga for more details. HTP

In the table below you must be able to check off ✓each item daily, weekly, monthly and annually in order to consider yourself as practicing the teaching of Shetaut Neter and Sema Tawi. It is important to practice the daily disciplines daily because this regular practice will be most effective to transform the mind. However, if one practice is missed then double up (to make up) the next day if possible or on the weekend, etc. do not say, "the yesterday is passed and I cannot go back so let me forget about it and start today."

235

Essential Daily practices	Essential Weekly practices		Essential Monthly practices		Essential Annual practices	
	✓		✓		✓	
Nutrition: vitamins and supplements	Keep company with elevated personalities at least 1 hour per week		Give 1/10 donation		Attend annual conference	
Nutrition: vegetarian diet	Selfless service 1 hour					
No smoking	Fasting 1 day per week		Celibacy: no sex more than once per month**		Make annual observance of the Kemetic New Year	
No drugs or alcohol						
Daily worship						
8 hours sleep						
Go to bed by 12 am						
Wake up early by 8 am						
Study of spiritual scripture- Ex. reading systematically the *Pert M Hru* text						
Abstain from company with negative personalities						
Silent meditation 20 minutes twice daily						
Practice breathing rhythmically 10 minutes twice daily						
Practice physical exercises 15 minutes daily						
*Observe the 42 Precepts of Maat (especially no lying, cheating, stealing, killing, hurting others***, etc.						
No talking for 1 hour (during waking hours)						

*At the end of the day read 42 Precepts of Maat and see if any were broken practice penitence for each transgression on an equal time basis (if the transgression lasted 1 hour practice the penitence to redress that transgression for at least 1 hour). First make a vow and then practice a penance for a period of time- you must observe the full period of the vow of penitence. Example of penitence: 1 hour of silence, not watching television for one day, not going to beach for one week, not eating the ice cream, not playing the music, not meeting with friends, etc. (Choose one penitence per transgression, it must be something that your ego desires otherwise it will have no effect on your personality. The idea is to assert your will over your ego by subjecting it to the regulation of Maat and not the unconscious desires. See your penitence as an austerity, a sacrifice period to redress the transgression and purify the heart.

**If this practice has not been kept skip you planned encounter of the future. Sleep separate from your partner for a period of time. Keep in mind that for advanced practice celibacy is to be observed for a 7 year period. Monastic aspirants maintain separate sleeping quarters. The advice given above is for householder aspirants. Remember that children will add more responsibilities and duties to your life that will leave less time for the practice of the teachings so use appropriate contraception in accordance with your desired level of practice. See book *Egyptian Tantric Yoga.*

***If you hurt someone by word or deed apologize to them and practice the austerity in * above. If you hurt someone by thought simply recognize the error and practice the austerity

Epilogue

In order to become a follower of Shetaut Neter an aspirant must become a member of the Shemsu Congregation of converted devotees of Shetaut Neter

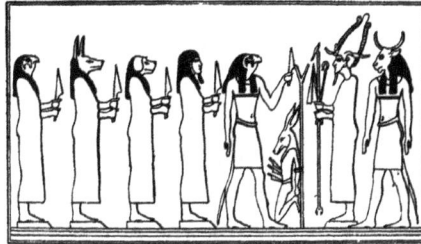

What is the Philosophy of Shems:

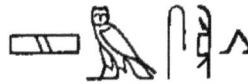

"Shems"
{to follow }

Shems means "follow." *Shemsu Shetaut Neter* are the followers of the Neterian Path. What does it mean to follow something? Why should some things be followed and others not? What should be followed in life and why? These are certainly some of the most important questions in life because if serious thought is put to them, they involve the crucial questions of life, who am I? Why am I here? What is my purpose? etc. which are or should be the most important concerns in life. This treatise suggests some answers. They are offered from the perspective of an Ancient Egyptian concept and its attendant teachings as developed by the sages of Shetaut Neter-African religion in ancient times.

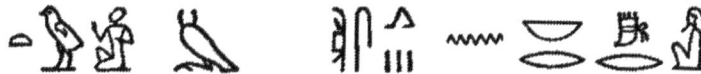

tu-a m shems n Neberdjer
I am a follower of Neberdjer

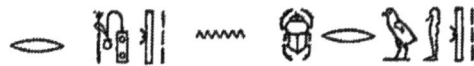

er sesh n Kheperu
in accordance with the writings of
Lord Kheperu"

The answer to the important questions of life was given by the sages of ancient times as following the spiritual path. In ancient times that path was known as *Shetaut Neter*. The "teachings" were given by the Creator, *Kheperu* in the form of outward appearances, shapes and objects of creation. *Lord Djehuti* codified those into the hieroglyphic texts and these teachings were passed on through history to succeeding generations of sages, priestess and priestesses of Neterian Religion. Why is it important for you to become a member of the Shetaut Neter tradition and what does it mean to be a follower of the Shetaut Neter spiritual teaching? If you are reading this it is because at one time or another you have come to the recognition of the important work being conducted by those who currently are following *Shetaut Neter* for the

237

betterment of humanity, but also to promote your own ⬚🦅▱👁 *Nehast* {spiritual awakening and emancipation, resurrection}. In order to reach the state of consciousness known as *Nehast* there must first be ⬚🦅⌐👁 *Nehas* {wakefulness, being awake}. Being awake implies wakefulness towards the teaching, that is, attentiveness, spending time, desire, etc. for spiritual pursuits. This means being mature enough to have grown beyond childish pursuits and interests, the worldly ideals of life. It is easy to think one is mature when one hears the Ancient Egyptian Proverb: *"Searching for one's self in the world is the pursuit of an illusion."* However, why is it that these same ones who have heard and agree continue to *shems* (pursue) worldly illusions instead of applying themselves fully to the teaching? Needing to have a job to support oneself and one's family should not be an impediment to intensive practice. However, it will become an obstacle if that job or career is the main objective in life. The teaching should be the main objective and the job should be a means to finance the intensification of the practice of the teachings. We must conclude that until the action follows the thought the thought is not being held as a reality or a priority. So there is insufficient maturity in such a person to pursue the teaching in an intensive and advanced way. Their choice action reveals their lower state of maturity and aspiration. Such people should follow at the level of practice that includes devotional practices, rituals, and the study of Maat ⚖👤ꟾꟾꟾ teachings to develop purity or heart until a higher level of aspiration develops. The focus here is to develop 👁⚖ꟾꟾꟾ *arit maat* {"offering righteous actions, living life righteously"}.

The opposite of *nehas* i 𓃭🦅👁 *Nem* {"sleep, slumber, slothfulness, immaturity"}. A person who is immature cannot adopt the teaching properly and will thus not be able to follow it rightly. What is needed is wakefulness towards higher perspectives in life and slothfulness towards what is degraded. This means an aspirant should be awake as opposed to ordinary worldly people who are asleep towards the higher perspective and wakeful towards what is base, degraded and illusory in life. Once there is wakefulness, spiritual sensitivity, spiritual aspiration, respect for the sages and reverence towards the spiritual teaching and the Divine there should be ⬚🦅👁 *Snehas* {"Wakefulness, watchfulness, alertness, vigilance"}. There are many who follow spiritual teachings of all traditions who at times appear to have grown and at others seem to have fallen back to their old habits and degraded passions and desires *aba* ꟾꟾ🐆. In order to truly follow an ideal one must be steady on the path and watchful so that negative behaviors and patterns do not draw one back into earlier, lower states of consciousness.

The work of following a spiritual teaching requires the follower's financial support but also their psychic support as well as their physical support. When a person becomes a member they are taking an important step in sustaining the dissemination of the ▱ꟾꟾꟾ *shetit*, "teachings" of 🦅 *Shetaut Neter*- "Ancient Egyptian-African Religion" for themselves and for the world. As the membership grows and the pooling of resources increases, it will be possible to affect more lives and create more powerful programs to better facilitate the practice of the

238

teachings. It is important to take the step of membership because this shows to oneself, the world and to others of like mind that there are others who believe, feel and aspire as they do and this develops *udja* [hieroglyphs] spiritual strength and in a mysterious way allows every individual member to have a subtle means of support that urges them on to success on the spiritual path wherever they may be. So *shems* is the means to have [hieroglyphs] *knumt-nefer* –"good association, divine association, joining others, together." This is a special association, unlike the worldly kinds of groups that have worldly goals and objective or religious goals and objectives. *Shems* is the coming together of followers of the Divine for the purpose of promoting righteousness and order in society and also spiritual awakening and enlightenment for those who are ready to tread the path to [hieroglyphs] *rech-m-ab* –"self-knowledge, higher consciousness" and [hieroglyphs] *an-menit* –"immortality."

Anyone can join the Shemsu if they are sincerely desiring to follow this path. Becoming part of the Shemsu means you will gain support from others who are trying to overcome immaturity but you also must put forth effort to act, think and speak with maturity and integrity. So those who want to put forth effort towards self-improvement and worthiness to progress in the teachings, should take the oath of Shetaut Neter. The oath is a pledge to apply yourself to the teaching of Shetaut Neter to your best capacity in order for its teaching to be revealed. Those who take the oath are considered as official followers of the Shetaut Neter Religion so it is a rite of conversion to Shetaut Neter. Becoming a follower is the first serious step on the path. The next is initiation. In order to take the oath it must be performed in the presence of a qualified priest or priestess of Shetaut Neter.

The Oath of the Followers of Shetaut Neter

In order to become a follower, an aspirant, of Shetaut Neter a person must:

Resolve to have faith in the Neterian path as laid out by Lord Heru.
Resolve to listen to the teaching of Shemsu and study Shetaut Neter philosophy.
Resolve to practice the threefold worship daily.
Resolve to observe the 42 precepts of Maat in your day-to-day life to your best ability.
Take the oath of Shems- pledge your faith to the Neterian Path and the teachings of Lord Heru-outlined below.
  After making the offering of incense, water libation, food, over an image or icon of Lord Heru, repeat the oath 7 times (From the PertmHeru text, Chap 1 verse 7).

nua   amtu –   k   Heru

I am one of those who support and believe in Heru, your son who redeemed your name after Set murdered you. (Repeat Seven Times)

NOTE: THOSE WHO DO NOT HAVE ACCESS TO A PRIEST OR PRIESTESS MAY PERFORM THIS CEREMONY THEMSELVES AND AFTERWARDS CONSIDER THEMSELVES NETERIAN FOLLOWERS.

Types of Aspirants:

There are basically 5 types of aspirants and of course there are gradations within these criteria. Sometimes aspirants develop advanced qualities of a higher designation but may still possess lower qualities. The lower qualities that are deemed as **_critical_** to the spiritual discipline are to be considered obstacles to advanced initiation. The Critical deficiencies are those that are deemed unworkable for higher spiritual practice and are listed in the designations for *Distracted* and *Wayward aspirants*- listed below. As for the imperfection of the qualities listed in the higher aspirant designations (Monastic, Well-trained, In-training) those are deemed workable.

There are three levels of Temple teaching and these correlate to the different areas of the temple. The outer region: Open Court, relates to neophyte teachings. The Hypostyle Hall relates to advancing philosophical and mystical teachings. The Inner Shrine relates to advanced ritual performance and experience of the Divine. The first level relates to Shemsu Initiation. The second level relates to Asar Initiation. The third level relates to Hem Initiation. Those who are admitted to Asar and Unut are being admitted to Level 2 temple teachings -Hypostyle Hall- metaphysics and advanced philosophy which requires maturity and seriousness.

Level 1 Open Court Temple Introductory teachings-	Level 2 Hypostyle Hall Metaphysics and Advanced philosophy	Level 3 Inner Shrine -mysticism

The Shems level or –Open Court Temple- level teachings are for introduction to the teachings, intro to Maat, Intro to Worship and Intro to Meditation. This level is dedicated to cleaning the gross impurities of the personality (controlling emotions and desires) and to instill ethics, devotion, and developing will power for the road ahead. The Shedy disciplines are the key to success at this level.

Those who excel in the Open Court may be admitted to the Covered Court of the temple when the Hem may notice advancement and maturity.

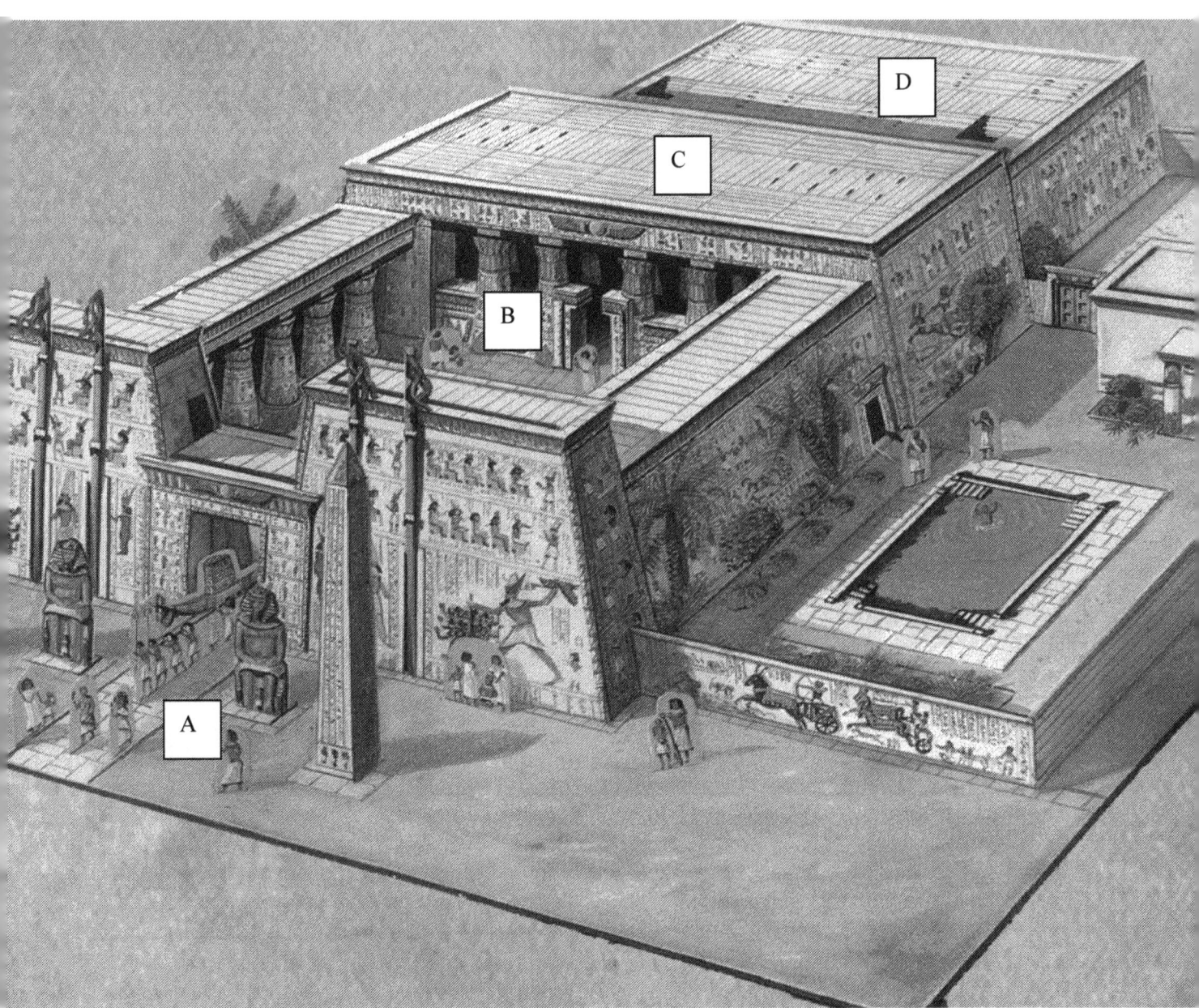

The Neterian Temple

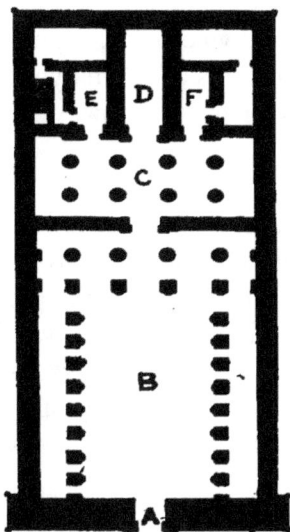

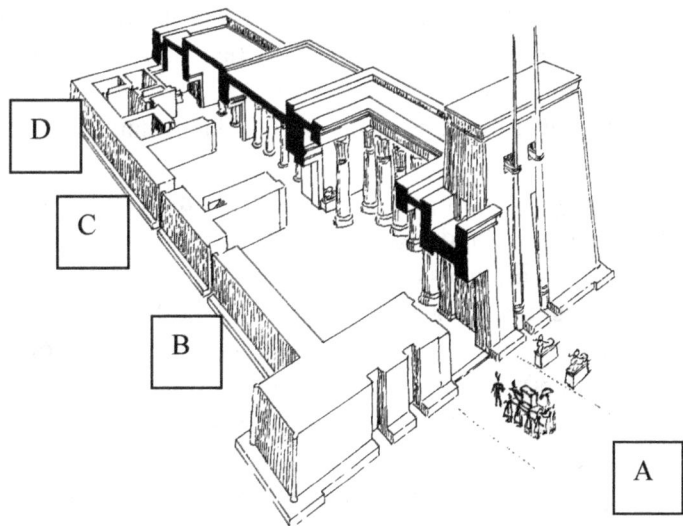

After making the proper propitiation at the entrance of the temple and having shown sufficient devotion and respect over a period of time an aspirant may be allowed to enter the Temple through the pylons (A), but will only be allowed to enter the outer court area: the Peristyle Hall. The typical Neterian Temple has three sections: (B) Peristyle Court, (C) Hypostyle Hall, and D) Holy of Holies. These represent the areas where different levels of worshippers may enter. This follows generally the nomenclature of the triads of spirituality:

- The three levels of mind: **Unconscious - Subconscious – Conscious.**
- The three levels of relative consciousness (waking, dream, sleep) constitute the ego-personality of a human being.
- Religion encompasses three levels, *myth, ritual* and *mystical philosophy.*
- The Great Trinity of creation: Amun-Ra-Ptah.

The Three sections of the Temple, B-Open Court (Peristyle Hall), C-Hypostyle Hall (covered), D-Inner Shrine (Holy of Holies), also represent the three stages of religion and the Neterian three levels of aspiration:

1- **The Mortals**
2- **The Intelligences**
3- **The Creators or Beings of Light**

The Basic Levels of Aspirants below relate to the Mortals and The Intelligences. The Creators of Light have transcended aspirant status:

Monastic: Dedicated to advanced practice, teaching and temple management and capable of independent life-without temple support. This is an extraordinary aspirant who may practice any type of sema (yoga disciplines), demonstrates the following virtues: great energy, enthusiasm, charm, heroism, scriptural knowledge, the inclination to practice, freedom from delusion, orderliness, youthfulness, moderate eating habits, control over the senses, fearlessness, purity, skillfulness, liberality, the ability to be a refuge for all people, capability, stability, thoughtfulness, patience, good manners, observance of the moral and spiritual law, the ability to keep his struggle to him/her self, kind speech, faith in the scriptures, the readiness of the divine, knowledge of the vows in his/her particular level of practice, and the active pursuit of all forms of –Sema-yoga and Shetaut Neter. Mastery over food, sex and ego-desires. Spontaneously practices celibacy, fasting and control over the mind. (Qualifies for Hem status)

Well trained –Lucid- The exceptional aspirant is someone who shows such qualities as firm understanding, aptitude for meditative absorption, self-reliance, liberal-minded-ness, bravery, vigor, faithfulness, willingness to defer authority to and respect the teacher, and delight in the practice of Semayoga and Shetaut Neter, ritual and the Shedy practices and the willingness to do whatever is desired by the teacher. Has attained proficiency in control over food, sex and ego-desires (lower energy centers); has attained proficiency in controlling emotions and desires. (An aspirant that has become proficient in these areas -qualifies for advanced Asar status or consideration for Unut status)

In training, but devoted to the Temple, assisting the Unut and learning the disciplines. The aspirant is endowed with even-minded-ness, patience, a desire for virtue, kind speech, and the tendency to practice moderation in all things and the willingness to do whatever is desired by the teacher. Displays balance in personal and spiritual life, compassion and charitable nature. Has attained basic skill in controlling emotions and desires- may not always be successful but recognizes errors when pointed out and works diligently to correct them. (An aspirant that has become proficient in these areas qualifies for Asar status)

Probationary status: *Those aspirants who have been part of the program previously (as Asar) and who may even have excelled intellectually with the teaching but have not progressed in devotion and feeling or who have left the temple of their own volition, due to distraction or contumacy issues, and who may in the future seek to rejoin will be accepted on a probationary status for 1 year. They will work with a mentor who will oversee their practice and studies with the assistance of the Asar Council. If the council deems they have the capacity to rejoin the ranks of Asar they will be readmitted with full status recognition after 1 year of consistent practice. During the 1-year probationary period the aspirants on probation may not be accepted into advanced classes (Temple Level 2).*

Distracted: Agitated-Struggling- Interested in the teachings but caught up in the world, confused with different teachings and spiritual traditions, not centered on 1. Sometimes devoted, sometimes attends classes-sometimes not, sometimes deferent-sometimes contumacious, sometimes agreeable and peaceful and at other times willful and irreverent; this is disjointed practice that will not be successful and such a person cannot be promoted. They need more time practicing the Shemsu disciplines (cleaning the gross impurities of the personality (controlling emotions and desires) and to instill ethics, devotion, and developing will power). This level of aspiration may include egoism, the desire to advance in the teachings without humility or patience, etc. (Does not qualify for Asar status)

Wayward, contumacious (Dull-weak aspirant- is unenthusiastic, foolish, fickle, timid, ill, dependent, rude, ill-mannered, and un-energetic.) This aspirant may obey commands but with an ill will, and murmuring, not only with lips but also in the heart and so is not acceptable to the Temple or to God. This level of aspiration may include egoism, the desire to advance in the teachings without humility or patience, etc. This personality may suffer from psychological disturbances that prevent them from conducting a balanced life or concentrating on the teachings. (Does not qualify for Asar status)

How to Begin Your Studies?

Where do I start? This is a very important question because you do not want to become overwhelmed with all that the teaching has to offer and also an aspirant should tread the path that he or she is qualified to pursue. Many times beginners are so amazed at what they have been missing that they throw themselves into the teaching not realizing they have entered at a level they are not yet ready for. Others pursue areas that are not suited to their needs and so their evolution is strained.

The chart below was designed to assist you in determining what level of study you are ready for and how to go about pursuing the knowledge of the teachings. Read the questions and follow the instructions to the area of study you are interested in. The references are for the SEMA INSTIUTE CATALOG or the SEMA INSTITUTE WEB PAGE where more information is contained. Serious Novices should start with ASSISTED STUDIES.

If you are working, have a family to support and want to advance in the teachings begin with ASSISTED STUDIES.

If you are not settled financially, or have family issues begin with ASSISTED STUDIES and resolve those issues before considering further advanced studies.

If you have problems with drugs begin with ASSISTED STUDIES and also start the Kemetic Diet Program

If you have been receiving ASSISTED STUDIES for a year or more and are interested in teaching the Kemetic Diet System or the Tjef Neteru System go to the Teacher Certification information

If you have been studying/practicing and/or already teaching for more that 2 years and are interested in advanced studies go to the Academic Degree information.

If you have been studying/practicing and/or already teaching for more that 2 years and are interested in advanced studies and dedicating your life to the teaching go to the Academic Degree program information.

The main areas of study are:

INDEPENDENT STUDIES - For those interested in studying and reading books on their own
 Go to Home Study information

Go to Neterian Awakening Newsletter information
Go to Book reading page - how to read the books -which book to read first, etc.
Go to the Virtual Temple and learn to practice the Daily Worship Program and Glorious Light Meditation System

ASSISTED STUDIES - For those interested in studying and reading books and receiving counseling and direct instruction - in addition to the resources for Independent Studies:
Go to Membership Program
Go to the Internet Classes
Go to the Spiritual Counseling

ACADEMIC DEGREE -For those interested in becoming advanced practitioners or teachers of Shetaut Neter Religion or Sema Tawi -Egyptian Yoga Disciplines
Go to Sema University Degree programs

Step 1: WHICH BOOK TO READ FIRST?
A- Become of Member of the Shetaut Neter Association and receive the monthly *Neterian Awakening Newsletter-Guide*
B- Begin reading the main books in the book series in the following order.

Neterian Awakening Guide	Introduction to Ancient Egyptian Religion Yoga and their influence on world religion and spirituality	What is the teaching all	Documented History and African Origins of Shetaut Neter and Sema Tawi

Step 2: How to Start the *Shedy* Disciplines of Kamitan Spirituality?

Shedy: program of studies and disciplines to penetrate the mysteries

Step 3: The Main Paths of *Shetaut Neter* (Kamitan) Mystic Religion

The Main Neterian Traditions and their Mystery Systems

Anunian Theology of the God Ra	Asarian Theology of the God Osiris	Memphite Theology The God Ptah	Mysticism of the Goddess	Mystical Journey Form Jesus to Christ (Ancient Egyptian Gnostic Christianity)

Step 4: The Four Mystic Paths of *Smai Tawi* (Egyptian Yoga)

	Wisdom	Action	Devotion	Meditation
The paths and disciplines to attain Self-Mastery	Wisdom Philosophy	Maat Philosophy	Feeling and Emotion Philosophy	Meditation Philosophy

THE KAMITAN MYSTERIES COURSE

The teachings presented in the Egyptian Yoga Book Series may be approached as a comprehensive program of study in the mystical yoga and religious sciences. In essence this is how the books have been designed and the purpose for which they were written. Those interested in such a path may observe the following program of study, working through the volumes in the order listed below, following the instructions and questions in each volume.

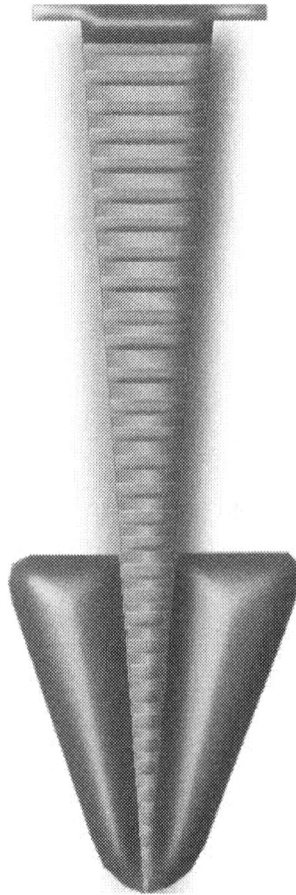

May the goddess grant you peace, joy and health and spiritual enlightenment!

Yours in the Lord
Sebai Maa

May you discover the glory of initiation and the unfoldment of spiritual living.

INDEX

Other Books From C M Books

P.O.Box 570459
Miami, Florida, 33257
(305) 378-6253 Fax: (305) 378-6253

This book is part of a series on the study and practice of Ancient Egyptian Yoga and Mystical Spirituality based on the writings of Dr. Muata Abhaya Ashby. They are also part of the Egyptian Yoga Course provided by the Sema Institute of Yoga. Below you will find a listing of the other books in this series. For more information send for the Egyptian Yoga Book-Audio-Video Catalog or the Egyptian Yoga Course Catalog.

Now you can study the teachings of Egyptian and Indian Yoga wisdom and Spirituality with the Egyptian Yoga Mystical Spirituality Series. The Egyptian Yoga Series takes you through the Initiation process and lead you to understand the mysteries of the soul and the Divine and to attain the highest goal of life: ENLIGHTENMENT. The *Egyptian Yoga Series*, takes you on an in depth study of Ancient Egyptian mythology and their inner mystical meaning. Each Book is prepared for the serious student of the mystical sciences and provides a study of the teachings along with exercises, assignments and projects to make the teachings understood and effective in real life. The Series is part of the Egyptian Yoga course but may be purchased even if you are not taking the course. The series is ideal for study groups.

Prices subject to change.

1. EGYPTIAN YOGA: THE PHILOSOPHY OF ENLIGHTENMENT An original, fully illustrated work, including hieroglyphs, detailing the meaning of the Egyptian mysteries, tantric yoga, psycho-spiritual and physical exercises. Egyptian Yoga is a guide to the practice of the highest spiritual philosophy which leads to absolute freedom from human misery and to immortality. It is well known by scholars that Egyptian philosophy is the basis of Western and Middle Eastern religious philosophies such as *Christianity, Islam, Judaism,* the *Kabala,* and Greek philosophy, but what about Indian philosophy, Yoga and Taoism? What were the original teachings? How can they be practiced today? What is the source of pain and suffering in the world and what is the solution? Discover the deepest mysteries of the mind and universe within and outside of your self. 8.5" X 11" ISBN: 1-884564-01-1 Soft $19.95

2. EGYPTIAN YOGA II: The Supreme Wisdom of Enlightenment by Dr. Muata Ashby ISBN 1-884564-39-9 $23.95 U.S. In this long awaited sequel to *Egyptian Yoga: The Philosophy of Enlightenment* you will take a fascinating and enlightening journey back in time and discover the teachings which constituted the epitome of Ancient Egyptian spiritual wisdom. What are the disciplines which lead to the fulfillment of all desires? Delve into the three states of consciousness (waking, dream and deep sleep) and the fourth state which transcends them all, Neberdjer, "The Absolute." These teachings of the city of Waset (Thebes) were the crowning achievement of the Sages of Ancient Egypt. They establish the standard mystical keys for understanding the profound mystical symbolism of the Triad of human consciousness.

3. THE KEMETIC DIET: GUIDE TO HEALTH, DIET AND FASTING Health issues have always been important to human beings since the beginning of time. The earliest records of history show that the art of healing was held in high esteem since the time of Ancient Egypt. In the early 20th century, medical doctors had almost attained the status of sainthood by the promotion of the idea that they alone were "scientists" while other healing modalities and traditional healers who did not follow the "scientific method' were nothing but superstitious, ignorant charlatans who at best would take the money of their clients and at worst kill them with the unscientific "snake oils" and "irrational theories". In the late 20th century, the failure of the modern medical establishment's ability to lead the general public to good health, promoted the move by

many in society towards "alternative medicine". Alternative medicine disciplines are those healing modalities which do not adhere to the philosophy of allopathic medicine. Allopathic medicine is what medical doctors practice by an large. It is the theory that disease is caused by agencies outside the body such as bacteria, viruses or physical means which affect the body. These can therefore be treated by medicines and therapies The natural healing method began in the absence of extensive technologies with the idea that all the answers for health may be found in nature or rather, the deviation from nature. Therefore, the health of the body can be restored by correcting the aberration and thereby restoring balance. This is the area that will be covered in this volume. Allopathic techniques have their place in the art of healing. However, we should not forget that the body is a grand achievement of the spirit and built into it is the capacity to maintain itself and heal itself. Ashby, Muata ISBN: 1-884564-49-6 $28.95

4.   INITIATION INTO EGYPTIAN YOGA Shedy: Spiritual discipline or program, to go deeply into the mysteries, to study the mystery teachings and literature profoundly, to penetrate the mysteries. You will learn about the mysteries of initiation into the teachings and practice of Yoga and how to become an Initiate of the mystical sciences. This insightful manual is the first in a series which introduces you to the goals of daily spiritual and yoga practices: Meditation, Diet, Words of Power and the ancient wisdom teachings. 8.5" X 11" ISBN 1-884564-02-X   Soft Cover $24.95 U.S.

5.   *THE AFRICAN ORIGINS OF CIVILIZATION, MYSTICAL RELIGION AND YOGA PHILOSOPHY* HARD COVER EDITION ISBN: 1-884564-50-X $80.00 U.S.   81/2" X 11"   Part 1, Part 2, Part 3 in one volume 683 Pages Hard Cover First Edition Three volumes in one. Over the past several years I have been asked to put together in one volume the most important evidences showing the correlations and common teachings between Kamitan (Ancient Egyptian) culture and religion and that of India. The questions of the history of Ancient Egypt, and the latest archeological evidences showing civilization and culture in Ancient Egypt and its spread to other countries, has intrigued many scholars as well as mystics over the years. Also, the possibility that Ancient Egyptian Priests and Priestesses migrated to Greece, India and other countries to carry on the traditions of the Ancient Egyptian Mysteries, has been speculated over the years as well. In chapter 1 of the book *Egyptian Yoga The Philosophy of Enlightenment,* 1995, I first introduced the deepest comparison between Ancient Egypt and India that had been brought forth up to that time. Now, in the year 2001 this new book, *THE AFRICAN ORIGINS OF CIVILIZATION, MYSTICAL RELIGION AND YOGA PHILOSOPHY,* more fully explores the motifs, symbols and philosophical correlations between Ancient Egyptian and Indian mysticism and clearly shows not only that Ancient Egypt and India were connected culturally but also spiritually. How does this knowledge help the spiritual aspirant? This discovery has great importance for the Yogis and mystics who follow the philosophy of Ancient Egypt and the mysticism of India. It means that India has a longer history and heritage than was previously understood. It shows that the mysteries of Ancient Egypt were essentially a yoga tradition which did not die but rather developed into the modern day systems of Yoga technology of India. It further shows that African culture developed Yoga Mysticism earlier than any other civilization in history. All of this expands our understanding of the unity of culture and the deep legacy of Yoga, which stretches into the distant past, beyond the Indus Valley civilization, the earliest known high culture in India as well as the Vedic tradition of Aryan culture. Therefore, Yoga culture and mysticism is the oldest known tradition of spiritual development and Indian mysticism is an extension of the Ancient Egyptian mysticism. By understanding the legacy which Ancient Egypt gave to India the mysticism of India is better understood and by comprehending the heritage of Indian Yoga, which is rooted in Ancient Egypt the Mysticism of Ancient Egypt is also better understood. This expanded understanding allows us to prove the underlying kinship of humanity, through the common symbols, motifs and philosophies which are not disparate and confusing teachings but in reality expressions of the same study of truth through metaphysics and mystical realization of Self. (HARD COVER)

6.   AFRICAN ORIGINS BOOK 1 PART 1 African Origins of African Civilization, Religion, Yoga Mysticism and Ethics Philosophy-Soft Cover $24.95 ISBN: 1-884564-55-0

7.   AFRICAN ORIGINS BOOK 2 PART 2 African Origins of Western Civilization, Religion and Philosophy(Soft) -Soft Cover $24.95 ISBN: 1-884564-56-9

8.   EGYPT AND INDIA (AFRICAN ORIGINS BOOK 3 PART 3) African Origins of Eastern Civilization, Religion, Yoga Mysticism and Philosophy-Soft Cover $29.95 (Soft) ISBN: 1-884564-57-7

9.   THE MYSTERIES OF ISIS: The Path of Wisdom, Immortality and Enlightenment   Through the study of ancient myth and the illumination of initiatic understanding the idea of God is expanded from the mythological comprehension to the metaphysical. Then this metaphysical understanding is related to you, the student, so as to begin understanding your true divine nature. ISBN 1-884564-24-0 $24.99

10.   EGYPTIAN PROVERBS: TEMT TCHAAS *Temt Tchaas* means: collection of ——Ancient Egyptian Proverbs How to live according to MAAT Philosophy. Beginning Meditation. All proverbs are indexed for easy searches. For the first time in one volume, ——Ancient Egyptian Proverbs, wisdom teachings and meditations, fully illustrated with hieroglyphic text and symbols. EGYPTIAN PROVERBS is a unique collection of knowledge and wisdom which you can put into practice today and transform your life. 5.5"x 8.5" $14.95 U.S   ISBN: 1-884564-00-3

11.   THE PATH OF DIVINE LOVE The Process of Mystical Transformation and The Path of Divine Love This Volume will focus on the ancient wisdom teachings and how to use them in a scientific process for self-transformation. Also, this volume will detail the process of transformation from ordinary consciousness to cosmic consciousness through the integrated practice of the teachings and the path of Devotional Love toward the Divine. 5.5"x 8.5" ISBN 1-884564-11-9 $22.99

12.   INTRODUCTION TO MAAT PHILOSOPHY: Spiritual Enlightenment Through the Path of Virtue Known as Karma Yoga in India, the teachings of MAAT for living virtuously and with orderly wisdom are explained and the student is to begin practicing the precepts of Maat in daily life so as to promote the process of purification of the heart in preparation for the judgment of the soul. This judgment will be understood not as an event that will occur at the time of death but as an event that occurs continuously, at every moment in the life of the individual. The student will learn how to become allied with the forces of the Higher Self and to thereby begin cleansing the mind (heart) of impurities so as to attain a higher vision of reality. ISBN 1-884564-20-8 $22.99

13.   MEDITATION The Ancient Egyptian Path to Enlightenment   Many people do not know about the rich history of meditation practice in Ancient Egypt. This volume outlines the theory of meditation and presents the Ancient Egyptian Hieroglyphic text which give instruction as to the nature of the mind and its three modes of expression. It also presents the texts which give instruction on the practice of meditation for spiritual Enlightenment and unity with the Divine. This volume allows the reader to begin practicing meditation by explaining, in easy to understand terms, the simplest form of meditation and working up to the most advanced form which was practiced in ancient times and which is still practiced by yogis around the world in modern times. ISBN 1-884564-27-7 $24.99

14.   THE GLORIOUS LIGHT MEDITATION TECHNIQUE OF ANCIENT EGYPT ISBN: 1-884564-15-1$14.95 (PB) New for the year 2000. This volume is based on the earliest known instruction in history given for the practice of formal meditation. Discovered by Dr. Muata Ashby, it is inscribed on the walls of the Tomb of Seti I in Thebes Egypt. This volume details the philosophy and practice of this unique system of meditation originated in Ancient Egypt and the earliest practice of meditation known in the world which occurred in the most advanced African Culture.

15.   THE SERPENT POWER: The Ancient Egyptian Mystical Wisdom of the Inner Life Force.   This Volume specifically deals with the latent life Force energy of the universe and in the human body, its control and sublimation. How to develop the Life Force energy of the subtle body. This Volume will introduce the esoteric wisdom of the science of how virtuous living acts in a subtle and mysterious way to cleanse the latent psychic energy conduits and vortices of the spiritual body. ISBN 1-884564-19-4 $22.95

16.   EGYPTIAN YOGA MEDITATION IN MOTION Thef Neteru: *The Movement of The Gods and Goddesses* Discover the physical postures and exercises practiced thousands of years ago in Ancient Egypt which are today known as Yoga exercises. This work is based on the pictures and teachings from the Creation story of Ra, The Asarian Resurrection Myth and the carvings and reliefs from various Temples in Ancient Egypt 8.5" X 11" ISBN 1-884564-10-0 Soft Cover $18.99   Exercise video $21.99

17. EGYPTIAN TANTRA YOGA: The Art of Sex Sublimation and Universal Consciousness This Volume will expand on the male and female principles within the human body and in the universe and further detail the sublimation of sexual energy into spiritual energy. The student will study the deities Min and Hathor, Asar and Aset, Geb and Nut and discover the mystical implications for a practical spiritual discipline. This Volume will also focus on the Tantric aspects of Ancient Egyptian and Indian mysticism, the purpose of sex and the mystical teachings of sexual sublimation which lead to self-knowledge and Enlightenment. 5.5"x 8.5" ISBN 1-884564-03-8 $24.95

18. ASARIAN RELIGION: RESURRECTING OSIRIS The path of Mystical Awakening and the Keys to Immortality NEW REVISED AND EXPANDED EDITION!   The Ancient Sages created stories based on human and superhuman beings whose struggles, aspirations, needs and desires ultimately lead them to discover their true Self. The myth of Aset, Asar and Heru is no exception in this area. While there is no one source where the entire story may be found, pieces of it are inscribed in various ancient Temples walls, tombs, steles and papyri. For the first time available, the complete myth of Asar, Aset and Heru has been compiled from original Ancient Egyptian, Greek and Coptic Texts. This epic myth has been richly illustrated with reliefs from the Temple of Heru at Edfu, the Temple of Aset at Philae, the Temple of Asar at Abydos, the Temple of Hathor at Denderah and various papyri, inscriptions and reliefs. Discover the myth which inspired the teachings of the *Shetaut Neter* (Egyptian Mystery System - Egyptian Yoga) and the Egyptian Book of Coming Forth By Day. Also, discover the three levels of Ancient Egyptian Religion, how to understand the mysteries of the Duat or Astral World and how to discover the abode of the Supreme in the Amenta, *The Other World*   The ancient religion of Asar, Aset and Heru, if properly understood, contains all of the elements necessary to lead the sincere aspirant to attain immortality through inner self-discovery. This volume presents the entire myth and explores the main mystical themes and rituals associated with the myth for understating human existence, creation and the way to achieve spiritual emancipation - *Resurrection.* The Asarian myth is so powerful that it influenced and is still having an effect on the major world religions. Discover the origins and mystical meaning of the Christian Trinity, the Eucharist ritual and the ancient origin of the birthday of Jesus Christ. Soft Cover ISBN: 1-884564-27-5 $24.95

19. THE EGYPTIAN BOOK OF THE DEAD MYSTICISM OF THE PERT EM HERU $26.95   ISBN# 1-884564-28-3 Size: 8½" X 11" I Know myself, I know myself, I am One With God!–From the Pert Em Heru "The Ru Pert em Heru" or "Ancient Egyptian Book of The Dead," or "Book of Coming Forth By Day" as it is more popularly known, has fascinated the world since the successful translation of Ancient Egyptian hieroglyphic scripture over 150 years ago. The astonishing writings in it reveal that the Ancient Egyptians believed in life after death and in an ultimate destiny to discover the Divine. The elegance and aesthetic beauty of the hieroglyphic text itself has inspired many see it as an art form in and of itself. But is there more to it than that? Did the Ancient Egyptian wisdom contain more than just aphorisms and hopes of eternal life beyond death? In this volume Dr. Muata Ashby, the author of over 25 books on Ancient Egyptian Yoga Philosophy has produced a new translation of the original texts which uncovers a mystical teaching underlying the sayings and rituals instituted by the Ancient Egyptian Sages and Saints. "Once the philosophy of Ancient Egypt is understood as a mystical tradition instead of as a religion or primitive mythology, it reveals its secrets which if practiced today will lead anyone to discover the glory of spiritual self-discovery. The Pert em Heru is in every way comparable to the Indian Upanishads or the Tibetan Book of the Dead." Muata Abhaya Ashby

20. ANUNIAN THEOLOGY THE MYSTERIES OF RA The Philosophy of Anu and The Mystical Teachings of The Ancient Egyptian Creation Myth Discover the mystical teachings contained in the Creation Myth and the gods and goddesses who brought creation and human beings into existence. The Creation Myth holds the key to understanding the universe and for attaining spiritual Enlightenment. ISBN: 1-884564-38-0 40 pages $14.95

21. MYSTERIES OF MIND AND MEMPHITE THEOLOGY Mysticism of Ptah, Egyptian Physics and Yoga Metaphysics and the Hidden properties of Matter   This Volume will go deeper into the philosophy of God as creation and will explore the concepts of modern science and how they correlate with ancient teachings. This Volume will lay the ground work for the understanding of the philosophy of universal consciousness

and the initiatic/yogic insight into who or what is God? ISBN 1-884564-07-0 $21.95

22.   THE GODDESS AND THE EGYPTIAN MYSTERIESTHE PATH OF THE GODDESS THE GODDESS PATH The Secret Forms of the Goddess and the Rituals of Resurrection The Supreme Being may be worshipped as father or as mother. *Ushet Rekhat* or *Mother Worship*, is the spiritual process of worshipping the Divine in the form of the Divine Goddess. It celebrates the most important forms of the Goddess including *Nathor, Maat, Aset, Arat, Amentet and Hathor* and explores their mystical meaning as well as the rising of *Sirius,* the star of Aset (Aset) and the new birth of Hor (Heru). The end of the year is a time of reckoning, reflection and engendering a new or renewed positive movement toward attaining spiritual Enlightenment. The Mother Worship devotional meditation ritual, performed on five days during the month of December and on New Year's Eve, is based on the Ushet Rekhit. During the ceremony, the cosmic forces, symbolized by Sirius - and the constellation of Orion ---, are harnessed through the understanding and devotional attitude of the participant. This propitiation draws the light of wisdom and health to all those who share in the ritual, leading to prosperity and wisdom. $14.95 ISBN 1-884564-18-6

23.   *THE MYSTICAL JOURNEY FROM JESUS TO CHRIST* $24.95   ISBN# 1-884564-05-4 size: 8½" X 11" Discover the ancient Egyptian origins of Christianity before the Catholic Church and learn the mystical teachings given by Jesus to assist all humanity in becoming Christlike. Discover the secret meaning of the Gospels that were discovered in Egypt. Also discover how and why so many Christian churches came into being. Discover that the Bible still holds the keys to mystical realization even though its original writings were changed by the church. Discover how to practice the original teachings of Christianity which leads to the Kingdom of Heaven.

24.   THE STORY OF ASAR, ASET AND HERU: An Ancient Egyptian Legend (For Children)   Now for the first time, the most ancient myth of Ancient Egypt comes alive for children. Inspired by the books *The Asarian Resurrection: The Ancient Egyptian Bible* and *The Mystical Teachings of The Asarian Resurrection, The Story of Asar, Aset and Heru* is an easy to understand and thrilling tale which inspired the children of Ancient Egypt to aspire to greatness and righteousness. If you and your child have enjoyed stories like *The Lion King* and *Star Wars you will love The Story of Asar, Aset and Heru.* Also, if you know the story of Jesus and Krishna you will discover than Ancient Egypt had a similar myth and that this myth carries important spiritual teachings for living a fruitful and fulfilling life. This book may be used along with *The Parents Guide To The Asarian Resurrection Myth: How to Teach Yourself and Your Child the Principles of Universal Mystical Religion.* The guide provides some background to the Asarian Resurrection myth and it also gives insight into the mystical teachings contained in it which you may introduce to your child. It is designed for parents who wish to grow spiritually with their children and it serves as an introduction for those who would like to study the Asarian Resurrection Myth in depth and to practice its teachings. 41 pages 8.5" X 11"   ISBN: 1-884564-31-3 $12.95

25.   THE PARENTS GUIDE TO THE AUSARIAN RESURRECTION MYTH: How to Teach Yourself and Your Child the Principles of Universal Mystical Religion.   This insightful manual brings for the timeless wisdom of the ancient through the Ancient Egyptian myth of Asar, Aset and Heru and the mystical teachings contained in it for parents who want to guide their children to understand and practice the teachings of mystical spirituality. This manual may be used with the children's storybook *The Story of Asar, Aset and Heru* by Dr. Muata Abhaya Ashby. 5.5"x 8.5"   ISBN: 1-884564-30-5 $14.95

26.   HEALING THE CRIMINAL HEART BOOK 1 Introduction to Maat Philosophy, Yoga and Spiritual Redemption Through the Path of Virtue   Who is a criminal? Is there such a thing as a criminal heart? What is the source of evil and sinfulness and is there any way to rise above it? Is there redemption for those who have committed sins, even the worst crimes?   Ancient Egyptian mystical psychology holds important answers to these questions. Over ten thousand years ago mystical psychologists, the Sages of Ancient Egypt, studied and charted the human mind and spirit and laid out a path which will lead to spiritual redemption, prosperity and Enlightenment.   This introductory volume brings forth the teachings of the Asarian Resurrection, the most important myth of Ancient Egypt, with relation to the faults of human existence: anger, hatred, greed, lust, animosity, discontent, ignorance, egoism jealousy, bitterness, and a myriad of psycho-spiritual ailments which keep a human being in a state of negativity and adversity. 5.5"x 8.5" ISBN: 1-884564-17-8 $15.95

27. THEATER & DRAMA OF THE ANCIENT EGYPTIAN MYSTERIES: Featuring the Ancient Egyptian stage play-"The Enlightenment of Hathor' Based on an Ancient Egyptian Drama, The original Theater - Mysticism of the Temple of Hetheru $14.95   By Dr. Muata Ashby

28. GUIDE TO PRINT ON DEMAND: SELF-PUBLISH FOR PROFIT, SPIRITUAL FULFILLMENT AND SERVICE TO HUMANITY Everyone asks us how we produced so many books in such a short time. Here are the secrets to writing and producing books that uplift humanity and how to get them printed for a fraction of the regular cost. Anyone can become an author even if they have limited funds. All that is necessary is the willingness to learn how the printing and book business work and the desire to follow the special instructions given here for preparing your manuscript format. Then you take your work directly to the non-traditional companies who can produce your books for less than the traditional book printer can. ISBN: 1-884564-40-2 $16.95 U. S.

29. Egyptian Mysteries: Vol. 1, Shetaut Neter ISBN: 1-884564-41-0 $19.99 What are the Mysteries? For thousands of years the spiritual tradition of Ancient Egypt, Shetaut Neter, "The Egyptian Mysteries," "The Secret Teachings," have fascinated, tantalized and amazed the world. At one time exalted and recognized as the highest culture of the world, by Africans, Europeans, Asiatics, Hindus, Buddhists and other cultures of the ancient world, in time it was shunned by the emerging orthodox world religions. Its temples desecrated, its philosophy maligned, its tradition spurned, its philosophy dormant in the mystical Medu Neter, the mysterious hieroglyphic texts which hold the secret symbolic meaning that has scarcely been discerned up to now. What are the secrets of Nehast {spiritual awakening and emancipation, resurrection}. More than just a literal translation, this volume is for awakening to the secret code Shetitu of the teaching which was not deciphered by Egyptologists, nor could be understood by ordinary spiritualists. This book is a reinstatement of the original science made available for our times, to the reincarnated followers of Ancient Egyptian culture and the prospect of spiritual freedom to break the bonds of Khemn, "ignorance," and slavery to evil forces: Såaa .

30. EGYPTIAN MYSTERIES VOL 2: Dictionary of Gods and Goddesses ISBN: 1-884564-23-2 $21.95 This book is about the mystery of neteru, the gods and goddesses of Ancient Egypt (Kamit, Kemet). Neteru means "Gods and Goddesses." But the Neterian teaching of Neteru represents more than the usual limited modern day concept of "divinities" or "spirits." The Neteru of Kamit are also metaphors, cosmic principles and vehicles for the enlightening teachings of Shetaut Neter (Ancient Egyptian-African Religion). Actually they are the elements for one of the most advanced systems of spirituality ever conceived in human history. Understanding the concept of neteru provides a firm basis for spiritual evolution and the pathway for viable culture, peace on earth and a healthy human society.   Why is it important to have gods and goddesses in our lives? In order for spiritual evolution to be possible, once a human being has accepted that there is existence after death and there is a transcendental being who exists beyond time and space knowledge, human beings need a connection to that which transcends the ordinary experience of human life in time and space and a means to understand the transcendental reality beyond the mundane reality.

31. EGYPTIAN MYSTERIES VOL. 3 The Priests and Priestesses of Ancient Egypt ISBN: 1-884564-53-4 $22.95 This volume details the path of Neterian priesthood, the joys, challenges and rewards of advanced Neterian life, the teachings that allowed the priests and priestesses to manage the most long lived civilization in human history and how that path can be adopted today; for those who want to tread the path of the Clergy of Shetaut Neter.

32. THE KING OF EGYPT: The Struggle of Good and Evil for Control of the World and The Human Soul ISBN 1-8840564-44-5 $18.95   Have you seen movies like The Lion King, Hamlet, The Odyssey, or The Little Buddha? These have been some of the most popular movies in modern times. The Sema Institute of Yoga is dedicated to researching and presenting the wisdom and culture of ancient Africa. The Script is designed to be produced as a motion picture but may be addapted for the theater as well. 160 pages bound or unbound (specify with your order) $19.95   copyright 1998 By Dr. Muata Ashby

33.   FROM EGYPT TO GREECE: The Kamitan Origins of Greek Culture and Religion ISBN: 1-884564-47-X $22.95 U.S. FROM EGYPT TO GREECE   This insightful manual is a quick reference to Ancient Egyptian mythology and philosophy and its correlation to what later became known as Greek and Rome mythology and philosophy. It outlines the basic tenets of the mythologies and shoes the ancient origins of Greek culture in Ancient Egypt. This volume also acts as a resource for Colleges students who would like to set up fraternities and sororities based on the original Ancient Egyptian principles of Sheti and Maat philosophy. ISBN: 1-884564-47-X $22.95 U.S.

34.   THE FORTY TWO PRECEPTS OF MAAT, THE PHILOSOPHY OF RIGHTEOUS ACTION AND THE ANCIENT EGYPTIAN WISDOM TEXTS ADVANCED STUDIES This manual is designed for use with the 1998 Maat Philosophy Class conducted by Dr. Muata Ashby. This is a detailed study of Maat Philosophy. It contains a compilation of the 42 laws or precepts of Maat and the corresponding principles which they represent along with the teachings of the ancient Egyptian Sages relating to each. Maat philosophy was the basis of Ancient Egyptian society and government as well as the heart of Ancient Egyptian myth and spirituality. Maat is at once a goddess, a cosmic force and a living social doctrine, which promotes social harmony and thereby paves the way for spiritual evolution in all levels of society. ISBN: 1-884564-48-8 $16.95 U.S.

Music Based on the Prt M Hru and other Kemetic Texts

Available on Compact Disc $14.99 and Audio Cassette $9.99

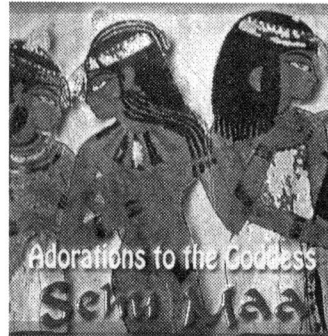

Adorations to the Goddess

Music for Worship of the Goddess

NEW Egyptian Yoga Music CD
by Sehu Maa
Ancient Egyptian Music CD
Instrumental Music played on reproductions of Ancient Egyptian Instruments– Ideal for
<u>meditation</u> and
reflection on the Divine and for the practice of spiritual programs and <u>Yoga exercise sessions.</u>

©1999 By Muata Ashby
CD $14.99 –

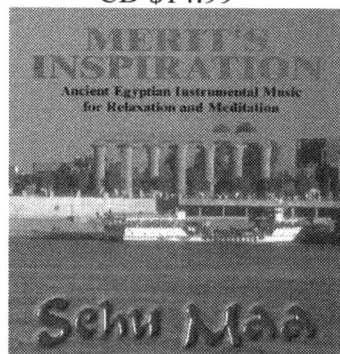

MERIT'S INSPIRATION
NEW Egyptian Yoga Music CD
by Sehu Maa
Ancient Egyptian Music CD
Instrumental Music played on
reproductions of Ancient Egyptian Instruments– Ideal for <u>meditation</u> and
reflection on the Divine and for the practice of spiritual programs and <u>Yoga exercise sessions.</u>
©1999 By
Muata Ashby
CD $14.99 –

UPC# 761527100429

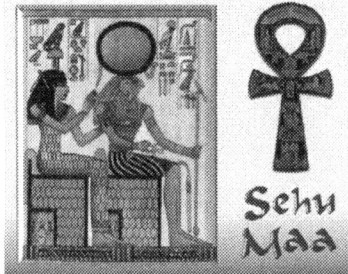

ANORATIONS TO RA AND HETHERU
NEW Egyptian Yoga Music CD
By Sehu Maa (Muata Ashby)
Based on the Words of Power of Ra and HetHeru
played on reproductions of Ancient Egyptian Instruments **Ancient Egyptian Instruments used: Voice, Clapping, Nefer Lute, Tar Drum, Sistrums, Cymbals** – The Chants, Devotions, Rhythms and Festive Songs Of the Neteru - Ideal for meditation, and devotional singing and dancing.

©1999 By Muata Ashby
CD $14.99 –
UPC# 761527100221

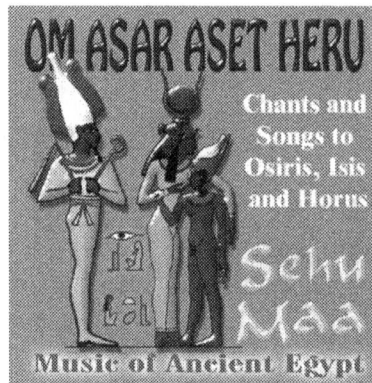

SONGS TO ASAR ASET AND HERU
NEW
Egyptian Yoga Music CD
By Sehu Maa
played on reproductions of Ancient Egyptian Instruments– The Chants, Devotions, Rhythms and Festive Songs Of the Neteru - Ideal for meditation, and devotional singing and dancing.
Based on the Words of Power of Asar (Asar), Aset (Aset) and Heru (Heru) Om Asar Aset Heru is the third in a series of musical explorations of the Kemetic (Ancient Egyptian) tradition of music. Its ideas are based on the Ancient Egyptian Religion of Asar, Aset and Heru and it is designed for listening, meditation and worship. ©1999 By Muata Ashby
CD $14.99 –
UPC# 761527100122

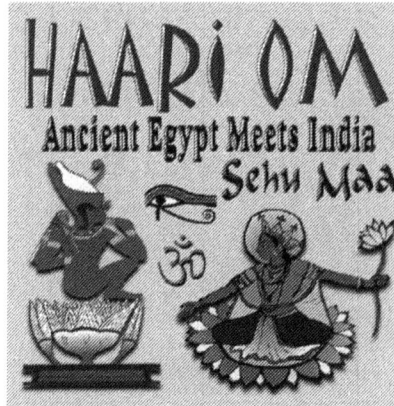

HAARI OM: ANCIENT EGYPT MEETS INDIA IN MUSIC
NEW Music CD
By Sehu Maa

The Chants, Devotions, Rhythms and
Festive Songs Of the Ancient Egypt and India, harmonized and played on reproductions of ancient instruments along with modern instruments and beats. Ideal for meditation, and devotional singing and dancing.
Haari Om is the fourth in a series of musical explorations of the Kemetic (Ancient Egyptian) and Indian traditions of music, chanting and devotional spiritual practice. Its ideas are based on the Ancient Egyptian Yoga spirituality and Indian Yoga spirituality.
©1999 By Muata Ashby
CD $14.99 –
UPC# 761527100528

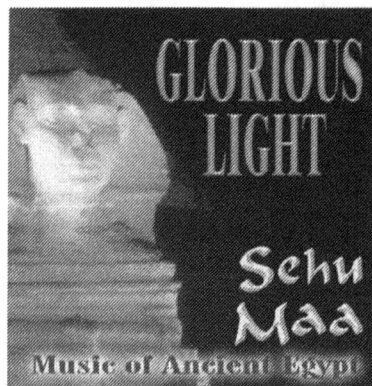

RA AKHU: THE GLORIOUS LIGHT
NEW
Egyptian Yoga Music CD
By Sehu Maa
The fifth collection of original music compositions based on the Teachings and Words of The Trinity, the God Asar and the Goddess Nebethet, the Divinity Aten, the God Heru, and the Special Meditation Hekau or Words of Power of Ra from the Ancient Egyptian Tomb of Seti I and more...
played on reproductions of Ancient Egyptian Instruments and modern instruments - Ancient Egyptian Instruments used: Voice, Clapping, Nefer Lute, Tar Drum, Sistrums, Cymbals
— The Chants, Devotions, Rhythms and Festive Songs Of the Neteru – Ideal for meditation, and devotional singing and dancing.
©1999 By Muata Ashby
CD $14.99 –
UPC# 761527100825

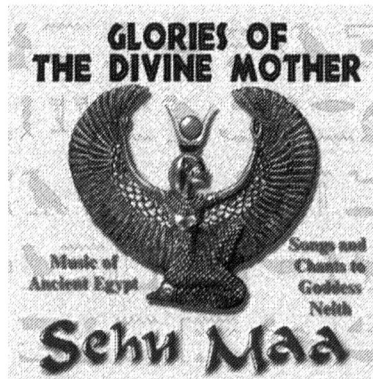

GLORIES OF THE DIVINE MOTHER
Based on the hieroglyphic text of the worship of Goddess Net.
The Glories of The Great Mother
©2000 Muata Ashby
CD $14.99 UPC# 761527101129`

Order Form

Telephone orders: Call Toll Free: 1(305) 378-6253. Have your AMEX, Optima, Visa or MasterCard ready.

Fax orders: 1-(305) 378-6253   E-MAIL ADDRESS: Semayoga@aol.com

Postal Orders: Sema Institute of Yoga, P.O. Box 570459, Miami, Fl. 33257. USA.

Please send the following books and / or tapes.

ITEM

_____Cost \$_____

_____Cost \$_____

_____Cost \$_____

_____Cost \$_____

_____Cost \$_____

Total \$_____

Name:_____

Physical Address:_____

City:_____ State:_____ Zip:_____

Sales tax: Please add 6.5% for books shipped to Florida addresses

_____Shipping: \$6.50 for first book and .50¢ for each additional

_____Shipping: Outside US \$5.00 for first book and \$3.00 for each additional

_____Payment:_____

_____Check -Include Driver License #:

_____

_____Credit card: _____ Visa, _____ MasterCard, _____ Optima, _____ AMEX.

Card number:_____

Name on card:_____ Exp. date:_____/_____